The Health Gap

Robert L. Kane, whose commitment to community medicine extends to both teaching and research in this emergent discipline, is on the faculty of the Department of Family and Community Medicine of the University of Utah College of Medicine. A graduate of the Harvard Medical School, Dr. Kane was formerly medical director of the Indian Health Service's Navajo unit at Shiprock, an assignment that led to his first book for Springer, *Federal Health Care (With Reservations!)*, written in collaboration with his wife Rosalie A. Kane. His most recent book (also published by Springer) is *The Challenges of Community Medicine*. Dr. Kane is the editor of the *Journal of Community Health*.

Josephine M. Kasteler (Ph.D., Utah) is a medical sociologist in the Division of Behavioral Science, Department of Family and Community Medicine of the College of Medicine, University of Utah. Her primary research interests are in utilization, compliance, and gerontology.

Robert M. Gray is professor of sociology at the University of Utah. Dr. Gray (Ph.D., University of Chicago) was formerly Chief, Division of Behavioral Science, in the Department of Community and Family Medicine, University of Utah College of Medicine.

THE HEALTH GAP
Medical Services and the Poor

EDITED BY

Robert L. Kane,
Josephine M. Kasteler,
Robert M. Gray

Springer Publishing Company / New York

Library of Congress Cataloging in Publication Data
Main entry under title:

The Health gap.

  Bibliography: p.
  1. Poor—Medical care—United States.   2.   Medical care—United States—Utilization.   3.   Health attitudes—United States.   4.   Community health services—United States—Citizen participation.   5.   Poor—Medical care—United States—Bibliography.   I.   Kane, Robert Lewis, 1940–   II.   Kasteler, Josephine M., 1914–
III.   Gray, Robert M.
RA418.5.P6H4   362.1'0973   75-30563
ISBN 0-8261-1860-7
ISBN 0-8261-1861-5 pbk.

Printed in U.S.A.

Contents

Preface

This book is intended to serve two purposes. First, it is an introduction for those interested in learning why the poor do not make full use of the health-care facilities and services available to them. Readings have been assembled to illustrate the multiple dimensions of this problem. Second, it provides comprehensive bibliographical information for those familiar with the subject but interested in pursuing it in greater depth.

The book was born out of frustration. We were familiar with the large number of theories and pronouncements regarding health-care utilization by the poor. Yet rarely were there specific data to corroborate these theories. In a similar vein, numerous solutions have been proposed for the dilemmas of the poor, including health-care delivery, but again data documenting the effectiveness of these solutions are scarce. We therefore started a systematic search of the literature in order to construct an annotated bibliography that would classify the reasons given for inadequate utilization of health-care services by the poor and clarify the extent to which these reasons could be documented. This search was then expanded—we sought to study not only the definition of the problems but also the proposed solutions. A bibliography of over six hundred references resulted, a distilled portion of which makes up a significant part of this volume.

We have organized, under four topic headings (Parts II-V), a series of readings intended to illustrate the type of information available, in terms of both actual data and theoretical perspectives. For some topics, certain works stood out as classics in their field. In other areas, the existence of many good articles made the choice far more difficult. While our choices are not necessarily definitive, we do feel that they typify the information available on each topic.

Part I introduces the general subject of utilization of health services and facilities by the poor. It includes illustrative data on the differences in health status between the poor and the rest of the population, as well as a discussion of the general problems of providing health care as it relates to utilization. Some of the models currently used to define health and illness behavior are also summarized.

Parts II–V contain the readings, grouped according to topic. Each group of readings is preceded by a brief introduction, which includes a list of cross-references to the annotated bibliography.

In Part VI we summarize and project future health-care delivery trends in this country and their potential impact on utilization patterns by the poor.

Part VII contains the annotated bibliography, which represents an extensive search of the literature through July 1974.

It is our hope that this book will provide both background and stimulus for further research in the area of providing more and better health care for the poor.

The Health Gap

Part I

POVERTY, ILLNESS, AND MEDICAL UTILIZATION: AN OVERVIEW

The 1960s in America represent an era of major concern for the poor. President Johnson's War on Poverty poured great sums of money through the Office of Economic Opportunity, and drew public attention to the unequal distribution of goods and services and to the plight of lower-income groups. Not that the unequal distribution was by any means new, but for the first time in the country's history the attention of the entire nation was turned toward efforts to raise the standard of living of the poor.

These efforts were apparently not in vain. In 1959, 40 million people (22 percent) were living below the poverty level. In 1972, there were 24 million, or 12 percent of the population, in the poverty group.[1] However, with today's inflationary trend this percentage should be adjusted. There are a number of ways to determine poverty level. One definition establishes a given amount of income at a particular economic state of the nation: all families falling below that line are labeled "poor." The poverty level criterion used for the figures just cited is defined by the Social Security Administration and takes into account the Department of Agriculture's economy food plan; it reflects the differing consumption needs of families based on size, composition, age, and location of residence.

One of the inequities that received special attention during the 1960s was the delivery of medical care. That disparity is with us still, although some strides have been made toward rectifying it. But whether we use the terms "persons below the poverty level," "the near poor," "lower-income groups," or any other classification of a disadvantaged population, one fact remains constant—economic deprivation is associated with poorer health, and the quantity and quality of medical care received by the poor is below the national

3

average. Poorer health may possibly be a direct consequence of less medical care. However, the reasons for the receipt of less than average medical care are many and varied. One important factor is the poor utilization of medical services by lower-income people, even when adequate services are available.

HOW THE POOR VIEW THEIR HEALTH

Health workers in underprivileged areas are quick to attest that people from these areas share similar attitudes, superstitions, and value judgments concerning their health and the health of their neighbors. Very often their beliefs about what constitutes ill health and what should be done about it set them apart from other groups with more scientifically based attitudes.[2]

Considerable diversity exists in definitions of the term "health" because such definitions are greatly influenced by culture. Disorders endemic to whole groups may be taken as a matter of course rather than defined as illness. On the other hand, being sick in some ethnic groups may not even be accompanied by clinically definable symptoms.[3] Jahoda claims that social customs and norms often determine whether particular behaviors are considered normal or sick.[4] A group of people, whether family, neighborhood, community or society, must label a condition a *disease* or *disability* before it can be considered a health problem to that group.[5] The frequency of such problems usually determines the health norm, or the status of health considered appropriate for its members. Often the more frequently a disease occurs, the more likely it will be considered normal rather than ill health. The common cold is a case in point: most sufferers will protest that they are not sick, they just have a cold. Sigerist reports on the Kuba of Sumatra who do not view serious skin diseases as symptoms of illness,[6] and Stiles makes note of diseases such as hookworm and cattle tick that are regarded as normal among tribes in North Africa even to the degree that eradication is resisted.[7] Fluoridation attempts and pollution-related problems in the United States are other examples of variance in definitions of health across subcultures.

The poor's interpretation of health is a natural consequence of their style of life. Their entire orientation is colored by the fact that they live with other poor people; they take on the perspectives of those around them and reinforce each other's beliefs and values. The way they cope with health problems is "traceable either to the material situation of poverty itself, to the social structure of poverty, or to aspects of the life outlook of poverty—the ideals, values, and beliefs to which the poor man adheres."[8]

Relationships between the social environment and definitions of illness are pointed out by Cherkasky. He maintains that one must know what sort of family the person has, where he lives, what kind of clothes he wears, what food he eats, what kind of job he has, and how he feels about all these factors if one is to understand his definition of illness. When a person declares himself ill and if in fact he is ill, these factors may be more indicative of the origin of his disease than the germ that has been isolated from his sputum.[9]

One's position in the occupational scale appears to have a great deal to do with one's perception of illness. The white-collar worker, who is usually more knowledgeable about disease symptoms and who generally can better afford to seek medical care, views the presence of symptoms as a sign of ill health. The unskilled or semi-skilled worker, on the other hand, may not recognize symptoms as readily, even when they are brought to his attention, he may view them as inconsequential and look upon "running to the doctor" as a sign of weakness. He thus fails to seek care even when necessary simply because he wishes to perceive himself as being indestructible, a perception he has acquired from the expectations of his fellow workers. In general, the blue-collar worker must be incapacitated before he acknowledges that he is ill. Koos found that less than a fourth of those in his lower-class population recognized a loss of appetite, persistent coughing, low back ache, joint and muscle pain, swelling of the hands and ankles, shortness of breath, and frequent headaches as symptoms.[10]

When health priorities are considered, social class differences are pronounced. When a household is operating with a minimum of material necessities, the family's desires are for physical improvements, i.e., a better or larger home, better household equipment, a new car. Health comes further down the list unless a crisis is threatening. When income is more than sufficient for one's basic needs, then one can insist on freedom from pain and physical discomfort and can take preventive health measures to provide for future health; only then can one think of physical examinations as routine. On the other hand, when income is uncertain and inadequate for food and rent, health is likely to be defined as the ability to keep working, and treatment is postponed until disability is threatened.[11] Among the many reasons, then, for poor utilization of health services by the poor are their definitions of health and illness.

THE HEALTH STATUS OF THE POOR

For the average person, health is defined in terms of the meanings acquired from his culture. In a statistical sense, health is defined relatively—by the number of health problems existing in one group as compared with another. By this definition, lower-income groups have an abundance of health problems. English, in examining the dimensions of poverty, explains that being poor means more than not having an adequate income with which to maintain a minimum standard of living.[12] It means living under conditions that undermine both physical and mental health. It means struggling with malnutrition, with inadequate housing, heating, and sanitary facilities, all of which are contributing factors when it comes to poor health.

Recent statistics, gathered mostly through national health surveys, evidence the comparatively poorer health status of lower-income people. Sixty percent of the children coming from families defined as poor have never seen a dentist.[13] Thirty percent of their parents have one or more chronic diseases.[14] Incidence of all forms of cancer is inversely related to income.[15] Heart disease and diabetes are more prevalent among the poor.[16] The poor have four times as many heart problems, six times as many cases of hypertension, arthritis, and rheumatism, eight times as many visual impairments, and far more psychiatric illnesses, especially schizophrenia, than the more affluent.[17]

Death rates from tuberculosis, influenza, syphilis, pneumonia, and vascular lesions of the central nervous system are twice as high among poor blacks as among middle-class whites.[18] The poor are troubled with liver and stomach problems at a rate of two to one over the more affluent.[19] There are nearly four times as many cases of emphysema in the poverty groups as among persons where annual family income is $15,000 or more.[20] And there exists twice as much disability from accidents among the poor when the two groups are compared.[21] Infant mortality rises considerably as income decreases; and the poor's risk of dying under age twenty-five is four times the national average.[22]

These figures clearly document the fact that by national standards the health status of the poor is far below that of other income groups in the United States. The question is, does illness lead to poverty, or does poverty contribute to high rates of illness? There is much to be said for the logic of the Drift Hypothesis, which states that people who are burdened with heavy expenses because of frequent or prolonged illness drift down into poverty neighborhoods. On the other hand, environmental conditions that usually accompany poverty status are incongruous with freedom from disease. A third position is that people who become ill under poverty circumstances do not have the resources for early and adequate treatment and thus remain ill for longer periods of time than would be the case were they in a higher income bracket or part of a higher social class way of life. This latter factor dramatically influences rates of disease and illness.

INEQUITIES IN THE DISTRIBUTION OF MEDICAL CARE

Although the poor have more health problems than the affluent, they do not use a larger share of the health care offered. The reverse is true. Medical care has been shown to be less available to lower-income people than to those in upper strata; the inequity is further compounded by the underutilization of available health services by the economically disadvantaged.

Achieving an equitable distribution of services in the health field has been the aim of those who believe that health care is a right, not a privilege. In the United States the expectation has been increasing that all pregnant women will receive prenatal care; that infant mortality will remain at the lowest possible level; that well-baby clinics, or their functional equivalent in private care, will be accessible to all; that all children will be immunized against communicable disease; that infectious diseases will be promptly treated; that persons involved in accidents or in need of other emergency care will have a place to go whether they can afford it or not; and that chronic disease will be diagnosed and treated early. The degree to which these expectations are met appears to follow income-level lines in a very definite pattern.

Efforts to diminish these social class differences in medical care are evident in a number of health delivery programs. Writing on the use of health services, Lefcowitz declares, "There is almost universal agreement that the poor are short-changed on medical care in both quality and quantity. The Neighborhood Health Center programs sponsored by OEO and HEW were designed primarily to redress the imbalance."[23] Whether the neighborhood health centers are making inroads in reducing the deficit remains to be seen, but efforts like this and Medicare, Medicaid, Model Cities, and Regional Medical Programs represent the beginnings of a national policy for a more equitable distribution of medical care.

The National Health Surveys have shown that there is not only a positive relationship between social class and frequency of medical services used, but also between social class and type of service used, with a greater percentage of care among upper classes going for preventive services.[24] The poor's approach to medical care is usually one of emergency care and crisis situations. Preventive care or treatment of minor illnesses are beyond the coping capacity of most poor people.

Concern for equality of care is not exclusively the province of the federal government; the theme of the 1972 meetings of the American Orthopsychiatric Association was that a national emergency exists in the delivery of health services to the poor.[25] A great many people have exerted an enormous amount of effort to meet that emergency. The poor probably have more services available to them now in their own neighborhoods, at lower cost to themselves, than ever before. Yet the problem of utilization has become a formidable one.

This book brings together some of the most informative articles on the extent to which physician's services, hospitals, clinics, and other health-care facilities and services are used by the poor, and to delineate some of the reasons why lower-income people fail to utilize available services more extensively. For the purposes of this book, utilization is defined as *the degree to which individuals use various types of medical services and facilities in seeking help for, or in preventing, health-related problems.*

REASONS FOR POOR UTILIZATION AMONG LOWER-INCOME PEOPLE

The picture is quite clear about patterns of utilization—increases in the number of services and facilities used by families are closely correlated with an increase in family income, with striking differences evident between the lower- and higher-income groups, in that the latter use these services much more extensively. In addition, family size tends to decrease with an increase in family income, making the differential even more pronounced.[26]

The literature is replete with studies showing a relationship between income and the receipt of medical care. Yet it is well recognized that it is not low income per se, but the concomitant and intervening factors associated with low income that provide the basis for explaining poor utilization. Studies are accumulating to clarify these links between low income and poor utilization. Factors associated with being poor would include:

1. cultural differences in perception of illness and treatment required;

2. social class differences in orientation toward illness;

3. psychological variations in attitudes, such as feelings of alienation, self-image, and confidence in the medical care system;

4. social factors, such as expectations of family and friends, peer pressure, and social support;

5. unequal purchasing power;

6. ability to be absent from work, either for illness or medical appointments;

7. ignorance of where to go for help;

8. failure to understand the importance of medical care;

9. differential knowledge of health and illness;

10. structural factors, such as housing, sanitary conditions, transportation facilities, and baby-sitting problems;

11. inadequate nutrition;

12. differential priorities.

There can be little doubt that illness and the cost of medical care have serious consequences for the poor. The problem is cyclical in nature; where considerable illness exists in a low-income family, it is only natural to assume that the costs involved (both direct and indirect) will help to maintain the poverty status. The availability and accessibility of medical care, and relations between the providers and consumers of care, are other factors that either facilitate or impede utilization.

There is evidence of a new migration of city people to small towns for medical care.[27] It is strongly suspected that some of the reasons are that care in the country is (1) more personal, (2) more accessible, (3) less expensive, (4) provided more promptly, and (5) easier to understand. Andrus and Fenley hold health science schools (Medicine, Nursing, Pharmacy, Health Education) accountable for many of the problems in health-care delivery, especially to rural populations.[28]

Quite in contrast to the care usually provided in large medical centers and clinics is the care received by respondents in a study conducted in the lower Rio Grande Valley. The curandera, or healer, according to Madsen, receives the patient in his home, is carefully attentive to his description of symptoms, makes a diagnosis that he explains in terms that have meaning for the patient, and recommends treatment congruent with the myths and legends of his belief system.[29] The curandera may be 10 percent healer and 90 percent bedside manner, but he meets the psychological needs of the patient in ways that are satisfying to him and his family. When one compares this mode of treatment with the cool impersonality and confusion of hospitals and physicians' offices, the reason some people fail to utilize medical services is very clear.[30]

Knowlton, in writing of his experiences with Mexican-Americans of the Southwest, further emphasizes the cultural gap between

Anglo-American medical personnel and lower-class Mexican-Americans. "American medical schools," he says, "teach their students to be calm, rational, objective, unemotional, and Olympian in their relationships with their patients. Mexican-Americans, therefore, tend to define Anglo-American professionals as cold, heartless, hypocritical, irreligious, and unsympathetic."[31] The Mexican-American, according to his value, expects health professionals to be warm, sympathetic, communicative, reassuring, and personally interested in the welfare of the patient.

In working with migrant farm laborers, who are perhaps the most destitute poor in the United States, Gangitano also places the blame on the system. He found that inequalities in the fee-for-service system, depersonalization of the physician-patient relationship, and fragmentation of care were among the variables associated with underutilization of health services.[32] Failure to understand the medical care system is suspected as a major reason for poor utilization among migrant workers; this would apply to other low-income groups as well. Since humans function primarily on the symbolic level of interaction, behavior is largely directed by cues provided by the symbols in one's cultural environment. If a patient lacks an understanding of the symbols utilized in the health-care system, he will experience confusion and fear, and will react with resistance, hostility, withdrawal, and other similar psychological responses that fail to support utilization of medical services.

In China the delivery of medical care has been dramatically transformed under a system of decentralization and demystification. The delivery of medical care begins at the lowest possible level. Initial medical care is provided by health aides who are part of the community. From this initial point of contact a clearly organized referral system leads level by level up to a plateau of sophisticated medical specialization. The system is an efficient, low-cost one, according to investigators Sidel and Sidel.[33]

The attitudes of the poor probably have much to do with their failure to utilize medical facilities more fully. Irelan has delineated three attitudes that lead to a lower concern for health and, hence, underutilization of health services:

1. the attitude of fatalism — helplessness or lack of control over events in one's life;

2. preferences for particularistic and personalized relationships, as opposed to more businesslike, formal exchanges;

3. more materialistic, concrete modes of thinking and talking.[34] Poor people, she finds, are less articulate than the better educated, upper-class members. Their interpersonal exchanges involve smaller amounts of symbolic, linguistic behavior. Their habitual language is

centered on concrete, rather than abstract, ideas. It is therefore extremely difficult for them to understand diagnoses and treatment procedures, and so the tendency is to avoid contact with physicians and hospitals whenever possible.

This brief summary of some of the reasons for poor utilization of health services by people in the lower-income bracket of society is provided as an introduction to the in-depth studies that follow.

Of course, the ultimate question is, if our standard of living continues to rise, will social class differences in the receipt of medical care diminish? As some of the factors associated with a lower-income life style improve, will the health care orientation change from the treatment of emergencies to attempts at prevention of disease?

HEALTH AND ILLNESS BEHAVIOR MODELS

An understanding of health and illness behavior is of great importance in any study of utilization. The models presented illustrate a variety of attempts to explain why people respond the way they do when illness occurs. The reader should not infer that only these models are the most useful. They have been selected as illustrative of the variety of insights and pragmatic formulations available.

Health behavior is seen differently by the various disciplines — one definition of *illness behavior* is any behavior relevant to causing an individual to concern himself with his symptoms to seek help.[35] Kasl and Cobb define *sick role behavior* as any activity undertaken for the purpose of getting well by those who consider themselves ill.[36] *Health Behavior*, on the other hand refers to measures taken by an individual in an attempt to prevent illness from occurring.

Conditional Models

Several models emphasize the conditions that must exist before a person decides to seek care. Wirick proposes five determinants of willingness to act in the case of suspected illness: (1) physiologic need, (2) realization of need, (3) personal resources available to meet that need, (4) a specific motivation to act (pain, bleeding), and (5) availability of services.[37] The likelihood that care will be purchased is proportionate to the number of conditions met.

The decision to take action is influenced by a person's beliefs that (1) the situation is a serious one; (2) he may be directly affected by it; and (3) he can avoid it through some effort on his part. When these three conditions (perceived seriousness, perceived consequences, and perceived benefits) are present, the probability is that the ill person will be motivated to seek medical care.[38] (see Figure 1).

FIGURE 1

HYPOTHETICAL STRUCTURE OF THE DEMAND FOR MEDICAL CARE AS A MULTI-EQUATION SYSTEM

	COMPONENT OF DEMAND				
	HOSPITAL CARE	DOCTOR CARE	DENTAL CARE	PRESCRIBED MEDICINE	OTHER EXPENSES
ASPECT OF DEMAND EXPRESSED BY THE VARIABLE	(NUMBER OF DAYS IN HOSPITAL DURING THE YEAR)	(NUMBER OF VISITS, EXCLUDING THOSE FOR INJECTIONS ONLY)	(TOTAL NUMBER OF VISITS DURING THE YEAR)	(TOTAL AMOUNT OF EXPENDITURES ON PRESCRIBED MEDICINE)	(TOTAL EXPENSES, INCLUDING THOSE FOR PRESCRIBED MEDICINE)
PHYSIOLOGIC NEED	AGE SEX	AGE SEX	AGE SEX	AGE SEX	AGE SEX
REALIZATION OF NEED	HOME CARE PRESCRIBED MEDICINE	ATTITUDE TO EARLY CARE HOSPITAL DAYS	ATTITUDE TO EARLY CARE EDUCATION OF HEAD	ATTITUDE TO EARLY CARE	FAMILY SIZE EARLY ENVIRONMENT OF FAMILY HEAD
RESOURCES	INSURANCE LIQUID ASSETS	ADJ. INCOME INST. DEBT	FAMILY INCOME LIQUID ASSETS	FAMILY INCOME INST. DEBT	INSURANCE ADJ. INCOME
MOTIVATION	DOCTOR VISITS	UNMET NEEDS	FAMILY SIZE DOCTOR VISITS	DOCTOR VISITS	HOSPITAL DAYS
AVAILABILITY OF SERVICE	INDEX	INDEX	COMMUNITY INCOME LEVEL		

Source: Wirick, G. C., Jr. A Multiple Equation Model of Demand for Health Care. Health Services Research, 1,3:301-46, Winter, 1966. Reproduced by permission of author and publisher.

Another model describes five "timing-triggers" necessary in a person's decision to seek medical care:

1. an inner, personal crisis, such that the situation calls attention to the symptoms in such a way that the patient dwells on them;

2. social interference — the symptoms begin to threaten a valued social activity;

3. other people begin telling him to seek care;

4. the threat of the consequences of not seeking help is perceived;

5. the nature and quality of the symptoms themselves (pain, severity, duration, etc.) cause action.[39]

These triggers affect various social strata and ethnic groups differently, as Zola reports. Lower-income groups are much slower to be motivated than are the more affluent.

Another model by Kasl and Cobb describes the two variables having the greatest influence on health and illness behavior (Figure 2). The probability that an individual will exhibit a particular kind of illness behavior is a function of two variables: (1) the perceived amount of threat, and (2) the attractiveness or value of the behavior.[40] The extent of the threat perceived depends on (1) the importance the individual attaches to health matters; (2) his perceived susceptibility to the disease; and (3) his perceived consequences if he fails to take action. The value of the preventive action he contemplates depends on: (1) the expectation that the action will lead to the desired results, and (2) the "cost" of taking the action, as opposed to taking no action and suffering the consequences.

A person's willingness, or reluctance, to adopt the sick role is the basis for Talcott Parson's model to explain why some people fail to seek medical help.[41] Individuals vary in their tendency to adopt the sick role when not feeling well. Being sick carries with it certain rights and certain obligations: the rights include some exemptions from certain normal roles and freedom from responsibility for the illness. That is, a person cannot be blamed because he is ill and, while he is ill, he should be relieved of his regular responsibilities. However, the duties of being ill entail the obligation to want to get well, to seek competent help, and to cooperate in attempting to get well. If the sick person is entitled to the rights and privileges of the role, he must also fulfill the obligations of seeking medical care and attempting to get well as quickly as possible. Some people resist adopting the sick role even when definite symptoms are present; they practice denial and continue regular roles as long as possible. When people look upon being ill as a sign of weakness, they are not very likely to adopt the sick role, and consequently not likely to seek competent help. Thus, a cultural value acts as a constraint on utilization.

FIGURE 2

THE SUCHMAN MODEL

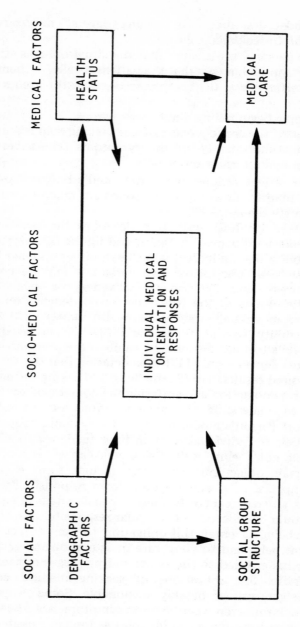

SOCIAL FACTORS   SOCIO-MEDICAL FACTORS   MEDICAL FACTORS

Source: Suchman, E. A., Social Factors in Medical Deprivation. American Journal of Public Health, 55, 2:1725-33, Nov., 1965. Reproduced by permission of author and publisher.

SOCIOCULTURAL MODELS

A sociocultural model is based on the assumption that illness behavior can be classified as (1) a product of social and cultural conditions, (2) a part of a coping repertoire, and (3) a means of achieving secondary gains.[42] Illness behavior as a response to symptoms or pain is largely, though not solely, determined by cultural definitions and social support or pressures. Thus an individual seeks, or fails to seek, medical advice depending upon his definition of the situation (which has been socially learned) and/or the influence of those around him.

Suchman constructed a model to test his hypothesis that the more parochial an ethnic group, the more likely its members will adhere to a popular or nonscientific health orientation.[43] Studying the social factors among medically deprived persons of lower-class backgrounds, he found that the more someone lacks an objective understanding about disease, the more dependent he will be upon his own group for support during illness, and the less likely he will be to seek professional help (Figure 3). His study revealed that lower socioeconomic groups are more likely to have a negative health orientation to a significantly greater degree than do upper-class socioeconomic groups. Lower socioeconomic status was related to a lower level of understanding about disease, unfavorable attitudes toward medical care, and a dependency upon lay support during illness. He concludes:

> These findings underscore the widening gap between modern medicine . . . and large segments of the lay public, especially among the lower socio-economic and minority groups, who cling to a more personal folk orientation. It is possible that the sheer bureaucratic complexity of modern medical care is a major barrier for those lower socio-economic groups to overcome. Resistance may be due more to confusion than to antagonism.[44]

Overutilization of physician services may occur when a patient uses illness as a means of seeking reassurance and support; the illness represents a socially acceptable complaint. In this instance, the symptoms are either psychosomatic or are masking another problem of an emotional nature. Frequently a patient will seek the services of a number of physicians while attempting to find relief.

In other situations, persons may adopt the patient role to make claims on others, to get attention and care, to distract attention from some other socially inappropriate behavior of which he may be guilty, or to provide an acceptable reason for academic, physical, or

FIGURE 3

THE "HEALTH BELIEF MODEL" AS PREDICTOR OF PREVENTIVE HEALTH BEHAVIOR

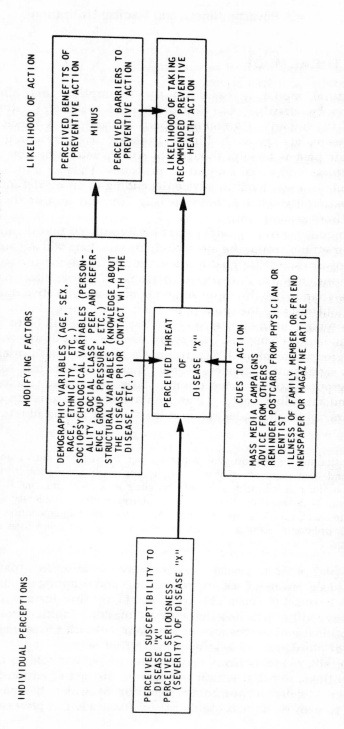

Source: Becker, M. H., Drachman, R. H., and J. P. Kirscht. A New Approach to Explaining Sick Role Behavior in Low Income Populations. American Journal of Public Health, 64,3:205-16, Mar., 1974, reproduced by permission of author and publisher.

social failure. This type of illness behavior is less likely to lead to a real effort in seeking medical services because of a fear of discovery that the motivation is fraudulent.

According to Kassebaum and Baumann, *normative expectations* pertaining to the sick role are influenced by the sociocultural and demographic attributes of patients, and by the medical attributes of the illness.[45] People adopt, or fail to adopt, the sick role because of their psychological attributes, their cultural background, and their social situation.

The subculture in which an individual finds himself (composed of values, norms, definitions, beliefs, and modes of behavior) is one of two major determinants of the utilization patterns in another model; the other determinant is the type and organization of health services provided. McKinlay bases his theory on the utilization patterns of maternity and child welfare services in Aberdeen, Scotland.[46] McKinlay states that certain subcultural elements are significant determinants of maternity and child health services utilization in pregnancy and child health situations.

Another model, that of Kriesberg and Treiman, states that attitudes follow behavior, rather than precede it.[47] In studying dental utilization behavior, Rayner developed a causal model of adult behavior, which provides guidance for changing children's behavior.[48] Her hypothesis is that beliefs and attitudes among adults follow, rather than motivate, the practice of going to the dentist for preventive care. For example, as a child you brush your teeth because your mother insists, and you then develop the attitude that tooth brushing is appropriate behavior. Figure 4 represents her model showing that attitudes are causally related to practice and that dental health practices correspond to perceptions of the normative health values.

Systems Model

A systems-oriented formulation, development by Fabrega, visualizes the individual seeking treatment for illness as directed by four systems: (1) the biological system, including his chemical and physiological processes; (2) the social system, which involves a person's relationships with others; (3) the phenomenologic system, which includes an individual's self-awareness and self-definition; and (4) the memory system, his attitudes and beliefs, earlier illnesses, and experiences with illness.[49] Nine stages of illness behavior are described:

1. recognizing and labeling the illness;
2. recognizing the undesirable characteristics associated with an illness (pain, discomfort);

FIGURE 4

DENTAL HEALTH PRACTICES OF MOTHERS--CAUSAL MODEL FOR TOTAL SAMPLE

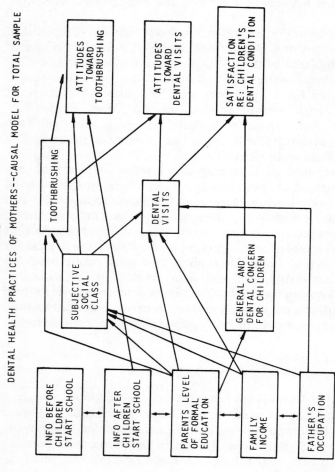

THE MODEL IS READ IN THE DIRECTION OF THE PATHS (ARROWS) AND VARIABLES TO THE RIGHT ARE CAUSALLY DEPENDENT ON THOSE TO THE LEFT.

Source: Rayner, J. F. Socioeconomic Status and Factors Influencing the Dental Health Practices of Mothers. American Journal of Public Health, 60,7:1250-58, July, 1970. Reproduced by permission of author and publisher.

3. planning some kind of treatment to combat the illness;
4. assessing various treatment plans;
5. computing the potential benefits that would accrue from the various treatment plans;
6. computing the costs associated with the treatment plans;
7. net benefits-costs of treatment subtracted from potential benefits for each plan;
8. selecting a treatment plan on the basis of information from stages 5, 6, and 7;
9. recycling the output from stage 8 (updating the history of the person and feeding it into the memory system for subsequent input in preparation for a new cycle).

SUMMARY OF MODELS

Three approaches to health behavior have been illustrated: the conditional, the sociocultural, and the systematic. All assume that most people consider illness as an undesirable state.

The conditional models state various conditions as prerequisites to the individual's seeking medical care. One model (Rosenstock and others) considers three beliefs as necessary forces to prod an individual to action: a belief that the problem is a serious one, a belief that he may be affected by it personally, and a belief that he can avoid being affected by it by some effort on his part. Another model (Zola) sees illness behavior as a process in which triggers are necessary to overcome the barriers to utilization. Parson's sick role includes various privileges and obligations. Two of the obligations are to seek competent medical care and cooperate in attempting to get well.

In his sociocultural model, Suchman sees the individual's understanding of disease, his attitudes toward medical care and general cultural responses to illness as the key factors in the decision to seek care. Mechanic suggests that an individual's definition of a situation is socially learned.

Subcultural norms, beliefs, values, and modes of behavior are viewed by McKinlay as impediments to, or facilitators of, the decision to seek medical care. In a slightly different approach (Rayner), health behavior is viewed as following the health-illness norms of one's social class. One follows the norms and acts, and then internalizes the attitudes.

The systems model (Fabrega) utilizes an elaborate, multifactorial system that is cyclical.

Currently, models are usually developed and used as guides for the development of medical innovations. A critical review of these models suggests that, while most have merit, each is limited by a singular focus on a limited facet of health and illness behavior. It seems apparent that no single model is yet comprehensive enough to explain all of the variations in response to illness and to provide a basis upon which an optimum medical care delivery system can be developed. Nonetheless, these observations in no way detract from the importance of the models available today. The point to be emphasized is that they provide only a limited function because of the selective emphasis they place on one or two aspects of health behavior.

APPLYING THE MODELS

The major purpose of this volume is to examine the problem of underutilization of health resources by the poor. Our increasingly affluent society will, we hope, devote some of its potential to a more equitable distribution of health services to bring lower-income and other disadvantaged populations up to national standards.

Contemporary writers on the distribution of health services and facilities vary considerably in their assessment of the situation. All agree there is a health crisis in America, but there is less consensus about the prognosis.[50] There are several reasons for not expecting an immediate improvement in health-care distribution: health care is not free, it must be purchased from providers at steadily increasing prices. "The poor man usually does not know where to go if he is ill," says the Ehrenreichs, "and even after he finally arrives, he must chop his way through the tangled morass of medical specialization."[51] The crisis, they believe, can be traced directly to the fact that patient care is not the primary aim of the medical care system.

But even if the currently available health-care system were available to all, some feel that the poor would not use it; they view the problem of underutilization as a hopeless one: "What has become clear is that no carpet of money, even if there were enough to subsidize an efficient system, will transport the poor to the doctor's office. A whole new approach is needed."[52]

Thus, the problems of underutilization by the poor are being actively discussed. The situation challenges those responsible for the health-care delivery system to decide whether the present system should continue as it is, be augmented — or undergo a complete reformation.

The readings presented here should help to stimulate thinking about the reasons for low utilization among low-income groups and the ways in which the poor can be motivated to take appropriate health action. Perhaps it will be necessary to change the medical care system radically. In addition, great strides may also be required to educate and change the attitudes of the poor. Both the providers and the consumers will probably need to participate.

NOTES

1. U.S. Department of Commerce, Bureau of the Census, *Pocket Data Book, U.S.A.* (Washington, D.C.: U.S. Government Printing Office, 1973).

2. C.O.Dummett, Understanding the underprivileged patient, *Journal of the American Dental Association* 79 (October-December 1969): 1363–67.

3. J.M. McLachlan, Cultural factors in health and disease, in *Patients, Physicians, and Illness*, ed. E. Gartly Jaco (New York: Free Press, 1958), pp. 94–105.

4. M. Jahoda, Current Concepts of Positive Mental Health, Joint Commission on Mental Illness and Health, Monograph No. 1 (New York: Basic Books, 1958).

5. L.M. Irelan, ed., *Low-income Life Styles*, U.S. Department of HEW, Social and Rehabilitation Service (Washington, D.C.: U.S. Government Printing Office, 1972).

6. H.E. Sigerist, The Special Position of the Sick, in *Henry E. Sigerist on the Sociology of Medicine*, ed. M.I. Roemer (New York: M.D. Publications, 1960), p. 12.

7 C.W. Stiles, *The Rockefeller Sanitary Commission for the Eradication of Hookworm Disease* (Washington, D.C.: Judd and Detweiler, 1911).

8. Irelan, *Low-income Life Styles* pp. 56–57.

9. M. Cherkasky, The Montefiore Hospital Home Care Program, *American Journal of Public Health* 39 (February 1949): 163–66.

10. E.L. Koos, *The Health of Regionville: What the People Thought and Did About It* (New York: Hafner, 1967).

11. Irelan, *Low-income Life Styles*, p. 57.

12. J.T. English, The dimensions of poverty, *American Journal of Nursing* 69 (November 1969): 2424–27.

13. C.R. Greene, Medical care for underprivileged populations, *New England Journal of Medicine* 282 (May 1970): 1187–93.

14. E.L. White, A graphic presentation on age and income differentials in selected aspects of morbidity, disability, and utilization of health services, *Inquiry* 5 (March 1968): 18–30; U.S. Department of HEW, Public Health Service, "Limitations of Activities Due to Chronic Conditions, United States, 1969 and 1970," Vital and Health Statistics, Series 10, No. 80 (Wasington, D.C.: U.S. Government Printing Office, 1973).

15. H.F. Dorn and S.J. Cutler, *Morbidity from Cencer in the United States* Public Health Service Publication No. 590 (Washington, D.C.: U.S. Government Printing Office, 1959).

16. J.M. Ellis, Socio-economic differentials in mortality from chronic diseases, in *Patients, Physicians, and Illness*, ed. E. Gartly Jaco (New York: Free Press, 1958), pp. 30–37.

17. U.S. Department of HEW, *Human Investment Program: Delivery of Health Services For the Poor* (Washington, D.C.: U.S. Government Printing Office, 1968).

18. J.H. Knowles, The quantity and quality of medical manpower: A review of medicine's current efforts, *Journal of Medical Education* 44 (January 1969): 81–119.

19. U.S. Department of HEW, Public Health Service, *Prevalence of Selected Chronic Digestive Conditions*, data from the National Health Survey, 1968, Vital and Health Statistics Series 10, No. 83 (Washington, D.C.: U.S. Government Printing Office, 1973).

20. U.S. Department of HEW, Public Health Service, *Prevalence of Selected Chronic Respiratory Conditions*, data from the National Health Survey, 1970, Vital and Health Statistics Series 10, No. 84 (Washington, D.C.: U.S. Government Printing Office, 1973).

21. U.S. Department of HEW, Public Health Service, *Impairments Due to Injury: United States, 1971*, data from the National Health Survey, Vital and Health Statistics Series 10, No. 87 (Washington, D.C.: U.S. Government Printing Office, 1973).

22. U.S. Department of HEW, Public Health Service, *Mortality Trends: Age, Color, and Sex, United States*, 1950–69, data from the National Health Survey, Vital and Health Statistics Series 20, No. 15 (Washington, D.C.: U.S. Government Printing Office, 1973).

23. M. J. Lefcowitz, Poverty and health: A re-examination, *Inquiry* 10 (March 1973): 3—4.

24. J.A. Ross, Social class and medical care, *Journal of Health and Human Behavior* 3 (Spring 1962): 35–40.

25. B. Stein, The crisis in services to the poor: How we got into the mess, and some suggestions for getting out of it, *American Journal of Orthopsychiatry 42* (October 1972): 755–60.

26. A.L. Strauss, Medical organization, medical care, and lower income groups, *Social Science and Medicine* 3 (August 1969): 143–77.

27. G.E. Garrison et al., Migration of urbanites to small towns for medical care, *Journal of the American Medical Association* 227 (February 18, 1974): 770–73.

28. L.H. Andrus and M. Fenley, Health science schools and rural health manpower, *Medical Care* 8 (March 1974): 274–78.

29. Irelan, *Low-income Life Styles*.

30. W. Madsen, *Society and Health in the Lower Rio Grande Valley* (Austin, Texas: The Hogg Foundation, 1961).

31. C.S. Knowlton, Cultural factors in the non-delivery of medical services to Southwestern Mexican Americans, in *Health Related Problems in Arid Lands*, ed. M.L. Riedesel (Tempe, Ariz.: Arizona State University, 1971), pp. 64–65.

32. J.L. Gangitano, Health and the low income family, *California Medicine* 116 (June 1972): 89–92.

33. V. Sidel and R. Sidel, The delivery of medical care in China, *Scientific American* 230 (April 1974): 19–27.

34. Irelan, *Low-income Life Styles*

35. D. Mechanic, *Medical Sociology: A Selective View* (New York: Free Press, 1968).

36. S.V. Kasl and S. Cobb, Health behavior, illness behavior, and sick role behavior: I. Health and Illness behavior, *Archives of Environmental Health* 12 (February 1966): 246–66.

37. G.C. Wirick, Jr., A multiple equation model of demand for health care, *Health Services Research* (Winter 1966): 301–46

38. See: S.S. Kegeles, Why people seek dental care: A test of a conceptual formulation, *Journal of Health and Human Behavior* 4 (1963) 166–73; H. Leventhal and P.N. Kafes, The effectiveness of fear-arousing movies in motivating preventive health measures, *New York State Journal of Medicine 63* (March 15, 1963); 867–74; J. Wakefield and L. Baric, Public and professional attitudes to a screening program of cancer of the uterine cervix: A preliminary study, *British Journal of Preventive Social Medicine* 19 (1965): 151–58; I.M. Rosenstock, Why people use health services, *Milbank Memorial Fund Quarterly* 44 (July 1966): 94–127. M.H. Becker, R.H. Drachman, and J.P. Kirscht, A new approach to explaining sick role behavior in low income populations, *American Journal of Public Health*, 64 (March 1974): 205–16.

39. I.K. Zola, Illness behavior of the working class: Implications and recommendations, in *Blue-Collar World: Studies of the American Worker* ed. A.B. Shostak and W. Gomberg (Englewood Cliffs, N.J.: Prentice-Hall, 1964).

40. Kasl and Cobb, "Health Behavior . . . ,"

41. T. Parsons, Illness and the role of the physician: A sociological perspective, *American Journal of Orthopsychiatry* 21 (July 1951): 452–60.

42. A. Strauss, The medical ghetto, *Transaction* 4 (May 1967): 12.

43. E.A. Suchman, Sociomedical variations among ethnic groups, *American Journal of Sociology* 70 (November 1964): 319–31. See also his Social patterns of illness and medical care, *Journal of Health and Human Behavior* 6 (Spring 1965): 2–16, and note 44.

44. E.A. Suchman, Social factors in medical deprivation, *American Journal of Public Health* 55 (November 1965): 1731.

45. G.C. Kassebaum and B.O. Baumann, Dimensions of the sick in chronic illness, *Journal of Health and Human Behavior* 6 (Spring 1965): 16–27.

46. J.B. McKinlay, A brief description of a study on the utilization of maternity and child welfare services by a lower working class subculture, *Social Science and Medicine* 4 (December 1970): 551–56.

47. L. Kriesberg and B.R. Treiman, Preventive utilization of dentists' services among teenagers, *Journal of the American College of Dentists* 29 (March 1962): 28–45.

48. J.F. Rayner, Socioeconomic status and factors influencing the dental health practices of mothers, *American Journal of Public Health* 60 (July 1970): 1250–58.

49. H. Fabrega, Jr., Toward a model of illness behavior, *Medical Care* 11 (November-December 1973): 470–84.

50. W. McNerney, The national health scene, *Journal of the American College Health Association* 22 (December 1973): 75–79; R. Kunnes, *Your Money or Your Life: Rx For the Medical Market Place* (New York: Dodd, Mead, 1971); R. Tunley, *The American Health Scandal* (New York: Harper & Row, 1966); R. Smith, Family medicine and the health care crisis in the United States, *International Journal of Health Services* 2 (May 1972): 207–15; and E. Kennedy, The responsibility of government for leadership in health care, in *Medicine in the Ghetto* ed. J.C. Norman (New York: Appleton-Century-Crofts, 1969), pp. 269–77.

51. B. Ehrenreich and J. Enrenreich, *The American Health Empire: Power, Profits, and Politics* (New York: Vintage, 1971), p. 6.

52. D. Schorr, *Don't Get Sick in America* (London: Aurora, 1970), p. 136.

The reader interested in further information on this subject may refer to the following references listed in the annotated bibliography:

Anderson and Anderson, 1967
Anderson, 1963
Hulka et al., 1970
Kosa et al., 1969

Mechanic, 1966
National Health Council, 1970
Pond, 1961
Pratt, 1971

Shannon et al., 1969
Stephens, 1970
Stockwell, 1962
Urvant, 1969

Part II

UTILIZATION OF HEALTH SERVICES AND LIFE STYLES OF THE POOR

The papers presented here provide contrasting overviews of the problems underlying the failure of low-income people to utilize health care services. Writing from the perspective of years of experience in public health work, Bergner and Yerby use data from the National Center for Vital Statistics and the National Health Survey to describe the differences in health utilization patterns of various income groups.

Lefcowitz, from his background in the social sciences, challenges the assumption that poverty produces either less utilization of medical care or more ill health. Since much of our recent health policy for the poor is rooted in this belief, this assumption warrants closer examination.

Elliott compares the effects of demographic and cultural variables on the perceptions and behavior of rural and urban poor in three communities. This report illustrates not only the variation in behavior among equally poor populations, but also the potential pitfall of ascribing similar findings to similar causes.

If health care is to be considered a right rather than a privilege, efforts must be made to overcome the barriers established by both providers and recipients. If education is established as the major deficiency, it follows that remedial action should be taken to improve the educational level of the target population (the indirect approach) or to develop ways of attracting the less educated to use the health-care services they need.

The reader interested in further information on this subject may refer to the following references listed in the annotated bibliography:

Adler et al., 1963
Aledort and Grunebaum, 1969
Alexander, 1969
Alpert et al., 1967
Andersen et al., 1970
Antonovsky, 1972
Baca, 1969
Baumgartner, 1961
Becker et al., 1972
Berkanovir and Reeder, 1974
Berle, 1958
Bice and White, 1969, 1971
Bice et al., 1973
Breslow, 1970
Brinton, 1972
Brown, 1968
Bugbee, 1968
Bugbee et al., 1968
Cauffman et al., 1967a, 1967b
Cervantes, 1972
Cherkasky, 1969
Clark, 1959
Clausen, 1963
Clifford, 1969
Cobb et al., 1954
Collver et al., 1967
Cons and Leatherwood, 1970
Cornely et al., 1962
Curry, 1969
Davidson, 1970
Deas, 1968
Donabedian and Rosenfeld, 1961
Dummett, 1969
Elling et al., 1960
English, 1969
Fabrega and Roberts, 1972a, 1972b
Feldstein, 1966
Flora et al., 1966
Freidson, 1961
Gans, 1962
Geiger, 1969

Ginzberg, 1969
Gornick et al., 1969
Graham, 1957
Greenlick et al., 1968
Harper, 1969
Haynes, 1969
Herman, 1972
Irvine, 1970
James, 1965
Kegeles et al., 1965
Keibuman, 1969
Kessel and Shepherd, 1965
Knowlton, 1971
Koos, 1954, 1955
Kriesberg, 1963
Kriesberg and Treiman, 1962
Laughton, 1958
Lavenhar et al., 1968
Lerner and Anderson, 1963
Lerner et al., 1969
Leveson, 1972
Leverett and Jong, 1970
Lowry et al., 1958
Ludwig and Gibson, 1969
McBroom, 1970
McKinlay, 1970a, 1970b
MacGregor, 1967
Martinez and Martin, 1966
Mechanic, 1962, 1964, 1972
Michal et al., 1973
Milone, 1973
Moody and Gray, 1972
Nall and Speilberg, 1967
Nikias, 1968
Nolan et al., 1967
Notkin et al., 1958
Olendzki et al., 1963
Parsons, 1958
Paul, 1955
Pearman, 1970
Perkins, 1972

Plaja et al., 1968
Podell, 1969
Pomeroy, 1969
Pratt, 1971
Rabin et al., 1974
Rayner, 1970
Read, 1971
Rein, 1969
Richardson, 1969, 1970
Riessman et al., 1964
Roghmann et al., 1967
Rosenblatt and Suchman, 1964a, 1964b, 1969
Rosengren, 1964
Samora et al., 1961
Saunders, 1958
Schulman and Smith, 1963
Sheatsley, 1957
Sills and Gill, 1958
Simmons, 1957
Sparer and Okada, 1974
Stoeckle et al., 1963
Strauss, 1967
Suchman, 1964, 1965a, 1965b, 1969a, 1969b
Tiven, 1971
Torrens and Yedvab, 1970
Tyroler et al., 1965
U.S. Department of HEW, 1968, 1972a, 1972b
Wan and Soifer, 1974
Watkins, 1968
Watts, 1966
Weinerman et al., 1966
Weiss and Greenlick, 1970
Weiss et al., 1973
Welch et al., 1973
White et al., 1967
Wingert et al., 1969
Wolfe and Falik, 1970
Yamamoto et al., 1967
Yankauer et al., 1953
Zola, 1964, 1966

1. Low Income and Barriers to Use of Health Services

LAWRENCE BERGNER AND ALONZO S. YERBY

In 1967 Americans made an estimated 850,000,000 visits to physicians — approximately 4½ visits per person for the civilian, noninstitutional population of the United States.* The cost of these visits, it is estimated, accounted for 25 to 30 percent of the $48,000,000,000 (6.2 percent of the Gross National Product) spent on medical care. How can we determine whether this number of visits is adequate or too high or too low?

The funds expended on medical care may be viewed as the result of direct competition with other needs. On a national scale the share of funds allocated to support a large military effort reduces the portion that can be spent on health and welfare programs. On a more modest scale, individual or family allocation of funds for medical care is a response to other sets of needs and priorities. In view of the multiple and varying pressures that determine expenditures, it is noteworthy that except for periods of epidemic disease, the annual number of physician visits has remained stable at around 4.5 per person for at least a decade.[1]

Does this mean that the proper frequency of physician visits has been attained? Would additional visits improve the health status of the American people? Could we get by with fewer services without a

---

* Our estimate, based on projection of current data from the National Office of Vital Statistics. Subsequent data on physician visits are from the published reports of the National Health Survey and refer to the civilian, noninstitutionalized population. Definitions of the units of medical care are those employed by the Survey unless otherwise indicated.

From *The New England Journal of Medicine* 278 (1968), pp. 541–45, reprinted by permission of the authors and publisher.
Presented in part at the State-wide Conference on Barriers to Utilization of Health Services, March 1967, Albany, New York. Jointly sponsored by the New York State Public Health Association and the Public Health Association of New York City.

deterioration in our present situation? Comparisons with other affluent industrialized countries are inconclusive. Nations with the same or fewer per capita visits, different physician-to-population ratios and different patterns of delivery of care have similar health records.[2]

The national average of 4.5 physician visits per person per year masks a broad range of behavior. In the United States population under forty-five years of age — before the onset of the multiplicity of chronic conditions associated with aging — the number of such visits when the family income is under $3,000 is 3.2; when the family income is $10,000 or over the number is 5.0.[3]

The proportion of persons of all ages who have had a physician visit within a year is 59.2 percent when the family income is under $2,000 and rises to 72.8 percent when the income is $10,000 or above.[4]

Where family incomes are under $4,000, 4.6 percent of the population will have seen an ophthalmologist during a one-year period, and that proportion increases to 6.9 percent where family incomes are $4,000 or more. Similarly, for optometrists, 7.5 percent of persons will make a visit during one year where family income is less than $4,000, and 9.3 percent where it is above that level.[5]

The proportion of the female population with obstetric or gynecologic visits in a one-year period increases sharply with increasing family income. Where family incomes are below $2,000 only 2.8 percent have made such visits. At $2,000 to $3,999, 5.5 percent, and so on up to 12.5 percent at family incomes of $10,000 and above.[5]

For visits to a pediatrician the story is similar. At family incomes of under $2,000, only 7.5 percent of the population under seventeen made such a visit in a one-year period. At $10,000 and above the proportion was 33.0 percent.[5]

And finally the pattern of visits to a dentist is no different. Where family income was under $4,000 the number of visits per person per year was 0.8. Between $4,000 and $7,000 it was 1.4 and so on up to 2.8 visits per person per year at family incomes of $10,000 and over. A striking additional finding is the distribution according to type of service obtained when people do come for care. In the group under $4,000, 26 percent of the visits that were made were for extractions and other surgery. This fraction decreased with increasing income until at incomes of $10,000 and above, only 8.5 percent of the visits were for this purpose. Conversely, the higher-income groups had a greater proportion of their visits devoted to cleaning of teeth and examination — activities usually associated with prevention.[6]

This relatively low figure of use by low-income families is not due to fewer disease problems. The number of chronic conditions and the annual experience of days per person of restricted activity, bed disability and time lost from work are markedly greater for persons with low family incomes.[7] At the same time members of families with high incomes have the lowest rate of hospital discharges, with the highest rate occurring near the low end of the income scale. The average length of stay is longer among the lower-income groups.[8] The differences in hospital-discharge experience may be partly explained by the upper-income-group substitution of other types of medical care such as visits to physicians and specialists. The excess length of stay for lower-income groups could be related to delay in obtaining treatment or difficulties in arranging post-hospital care. In any case it does not seem reasonable to relate the lower use of ambulatory services by the poor to less morbidity.

THE NEW YORK CITY EXPERIENCE

Will the new programs of Medicare and Medicaid make a significant difference? In any attempt to assess the importance of direct cost to the patient as the most significant barrier to the use of care it is instructive to consider the experience of New York City. An extensive system of municipal hospitals, outpatient clinics and health-department programs have been available at no cost to the medically indigent for many years. This has been supplemented by free or token-charge services by voluntary hospitals and philanthropic organizations. In 1966, 600,000 persons receiving public assistance were eligible to have their medical bills paid for by the welfare agency.*

In a 1961-1963 special study of health problems associated with poverty in neighborhoods of New York City, sixteen poverty areas were identified on the basis of low income and high frequency of social problems. Table 1 shows some of the health problems of these areas relative to the rest of the city: births out-of-wedlock, 3.8 times as high; too little or too late prenatal care, coupled with maternal mortality, more than twice as high; and "low-birth-weight" babies and infant death rate, 1.6 times as high. The excess mortality in poverty areas from a variety of causes is included. These are crude rates obtained by use of the deaths at all ages as the numerator and the population at all ages as the denominator. The sixteen poverty areas have a smaller proportion of their population in the older age groups than the population of the rest of the city. This tends to lower the crude rates in the poverty areas and thus to reduce the apparent differences.

*By December, 1967, there were 780,000 persons on the welfare rolls, all automatically enrolled for Medicaid.

TABLE 1. *New York City — Health or Social Problems in Poverty Areas, 1961-1963.**

PROBLEM	TOTAL	16 POVERTY AREAS	REST OF CITY	PERCENTAGE EXCESS OF POVERTY AREAS OVER OTHER AREAS
Infant death rate/1,000 live births	26.2	34.8	21.8	60
Maternal mortality/ 10,000 live births	7.3	11.8	5.0	136
Percentage of mothers receiving late or no prenatal care	22.3	38.4	14.0	174
Percentage of live-born infants weighing 2,500 gm or less	9.7	12.7	8.2	55
Percentage of births out-of-wedlock	10.5	20.3	5.3	283
Cases of infectious syphilis/100,000 population	95.6	206.7	51.8	299
Crude death rate/ 100,000 population:				
Tuberculosis	9.3	15.3	6.9	121
Diabetes	22.6	23.4	22.3	5
Pneumonia & influenza	44.5	53.5	41.0	30
Home accidents	12.3	13.7	11.8	16

*Source: Statistical Division, Department of Health, City of New York.

Immunization is a primary preventive measure and the foundation of our present programs for the control of communicable disease. In New York City in 1964 a special study revealed the immunization status of children in the group one to four years of age. The wide differences by family income may be seen in Table 2.

These immunizations have been widely available at no cost as part of the routine program of well-baby clinics and at regularly scheduled sessions at district health centers.

A study conducted in Erie County, New York, in March, 1966, revealed strikingly similar data for measles immunization. For the city, the suburbs and the rural areas a similar pattern was demonstrated.

Among the susceptible children, the higher economic groups had considerably higher levels of measles vaccination.[9] The overall cover-

TABLE 2. *Full Immunization of Children One to Four Years of Age According to Family Income and Type of Immunization (New York, 1964).**

FAMILY INCOME	PERCENTAGE FULLY IMMUNIZED		
	DIPHTHERIA PERTUSSIS & TETANUS	POLIOMYELITIS	SMALLPOX
$0 — 1,999	50.7	23.9	44.8
$2,000 — 3,999	64.5	40.1	69.1
$4,000 — 5,999	77.7	55.4	85.1
$6,000 — 7,999	82.5	63.1	87.8
$8,000 — or more	90.6	66.0	92.6

*Adapted from: Immunization status of New York City population under 30 yr of age, 1964 (New York City Department of Health).

age of 50 percent of all susceptible children under the age of 10 masked the fact that substantial differences existed among the various geographic and economic subdivisions. In the city of Buffalo among children five to nine years of age 73 percent of the susceptible children in the upper class gave a history of vaccination as compared to 19 percent in the lower economic stratum. (The vaccine has been available through private physicians since March, 1963, and Health Department clinics since January, 1964.)

The New York City experience is compatible with what the English have learned after fifteen years of experience with the National Health Service: the higher-income groups make better use of the Service; receive more specialist attention; occupy more of the beds in better equipped and staffed hospitals; receive more elective surgery; get better maternity care; and are more likely to seek psychiatric help than low-income groups, particularly the unskilled.[10,11]

Similar or even more dramatic examples of the discrepencies in the United States and New York City cited above can be provided by listing data for white and nonwhite groups. Since so many Negroes are poor and so many of the poor are Negro, we would be talking about the same problem under different headings.

The poor behave differently from the middle class and the affluent across a wide spectrum related to health care. Illness is defined differently. There is less accurate health information. The poor are less inclined to take preventive measures, and delay longer in seeking medical care. When they do approach health practitioners, they are more likely to select subprofessionals or the marginal practitioners often found in their neighborhoods. It appears that the people most in need of medical services are the ones who least often obtain them.[12]

The statistics cited and other data that are available provide only a narrow and restricted glimpse at the end result of a long chain of historic events and human behavior. But neither inability to pay nor discrimination on racial or other grounds (nor the simplistic phrase, "life styles of the poor") is an adequate explanation of the existing discrepancies. The advent of Medicare and Medicaid and the enforcement of Title VI of the Civil Rights Act of 1964 will not be sufficient to erase these inequities.

THE INFORMATION BARRIER

An elaborate array of services of the highest quality is not truly available if those who are most in need are unaware of their existence and availability.[13]

Although we are most anxious and concerned with the *health* problems of the poor, we know that these problems are so intertwined with social and welfare problems that provision of accurate information in one area to a multiproblem family is likely to be meaningless and can actually serve to reinforce feelings of frustration and resignation to the status quo. Broad-purpose neighborhood information and service centers may be a means of attacking these problems in communication.[14]

The family that does not use medical services because of a lack of knowledge is likely to be among the "hard to reach" who do not expose themselves to scientific and health information as usually transmitted through the mass media. They may not come to or call any type of center. We need to search out and reach out to these people. They *can* be reached if the effort is made.[15]

The use of community health aides is one approach to this problem. Recently, the New York City Department of Health assigned a small group of untrained women to go out and ring doorbells as medical missionaries in parts of the Bedford Stuyvesant section of Brooklyn. Their job is to find people who need care, to persuade them to use available services and to try to find out why they do not. These women, who live in the community, know first hand about poverty and ghetto life. They have been briefed on the services available, but they have been intentionally left untrained. It has been found that trained community-health aides become too professional and too direct in their inquiries. They become part of existing institutional authority, and their effectiveness is thereby diminished.

The culture of poverty is pervasive, involving all aspects of the life of the poor — not solely health beliefs and behavior. But if we believe that certain health practices and services are of vital importance, we must find the means of getting our message across to the poor. We must work to place our product in a situation where it will be wanted and can be obtained.

In a very interesting book, *The Poor Pay More*,[16] we are presented with a documented description of how the poor can be maneuvered into wanting and contracting to buy certain goods that are beyond their means and that, in many cases, they have no use for or do not want to buy. Door-to-door salesmen overcome distance barriers, easy credit overcomes financial barriers, and approach in the buyer's native tongue overcomes language barriers. The author describes how group pressures to buy needless goods can be brought to bear through the "demonstration party," which is very popular among low-income families. It is interesting that the author uses an example relevant to public health and preventive medicine to describe this practice.

> The entire affair is exotically like the "smallpox parties," popular before Jenner's discovery of the smallpox vaccine, in which people would be brought together with a victim of the dreaded disease so that after exposure to a mild case they could become immune. The "demonstration parties" are designed for contagion of another sort; under the skilled guidance of a genial salesman, the itch to buy presumably spreads by example and mutual stimulation.

Perhaps it is time for public health to reclaim such a useful device from the hucksters and see if group pressures can be brought to bear for the benefit of the individual's health and the health of the community. In even the areas with the least effective use of services, there are some individuals who do use services, and we should attempt to involve these people in efforts to influence others. We must discover and establish effective working relations with the influential people in the neighborhoods and get them involved — and this does not always mean the people with a designated title or public position.

PHYSICAL AND PROGRAM BARRIERS

When we do succeed in reaching out, the properly informed potential patient may still need to overcome a series of physical and jurisdictional barriers before he can obtain care. The location of services, the availability of transportation and the hours at which the services are offered all affect the true availability of the services. Too often these arrangements reflect that which is convenient for the provider of service and quite inconvenient for the patient. Some arrangements have been hallowed by tradition but serve the interest of neither provider nor user.

The type of inquiry that is made into family finances and other criteria of eligibility can be not only demeaning but so complicated that the patient is unable to provide what is required without returning home for additional records — perhaps more than once. New York plans to insist upon repeating the cumbersome registration procedure for Medicaid each year.

The patient who is persistent enough to survive these hurdles is ready to receive the best of modern scientific professional attention. Although the circumstances are not universally applicable, in many places it may be several weeks before he can be fit into the schedule. In many clinics he faces the prospect of long waits in dingy surroundings. He may be addressed in a manner that clearly indicates that the system regards him as just another burden with no personal dignity. He is all too likely to receive a cursory inspection or a single injection and noncommunicative word or two and be sent on his way. Examinations may be performed without a modicum of privacy, and his problems discussed in a casual manner within easy hearing of other patients. If a course of treatment is prescribed, too little consideration may be given to whether he can possibly carry it out — physically, emotionally or financially. Too often he is not encouraged to ask questions or to describe his problems in his terms rather than ours. The patient's needs, expectations and priorities are not allowed to interfere with the functioning of the system. The very act of coming forward to receive care may thus serve to emphasize and reinforce social and cultural barriers and results in premature termination of treatment.[17] It will be difficult for the patient to communicate to others something positive about obtaining professional health care.

Patients will respond to evidence of personal interest. When physicians take time to explain examination and treatment in simple language, when the patient is involved in deciding what to do about his condition, and when adequate assistance is provided to help him to cope with the social problems that regularly accompany his medical problems, patients will follow through[18] — and perhaps reverse the image we sometimes form of their unwillingness to co-operate.

We certainly have much to learn about the beliefs and attitudes with which the poor adapt to a deprived existence, and which at the same time act to pertuate deprivation. However, study of motivations, perceptions, beliefs and patterns of thought cannot do much good if well motivated professionals permit outmoded physical facilities and archaic program arrangements to dictate a pattern of care that would be offensive to anyone regardless of his socioeconomic status. We must somehow escape from our tradition of "poor-law" medicine for the poor that has been our inheritance from colonial days.

In speaking of the barriers that exist in our present services for the poor Geiger[19] has said:

> These barriers are real. In this system, care is almost inevitably episodic, symptomatic, piecemeal and uncoordinated; it is certainly not patient-centered, even more certainly not family-centered, and still more certainly not community-based. And most of all, it does not truly intervene, either into the health of the poor or into the poverty syndrome itself. To treat symptoms, and then to send the patients back, unchanged in knowledge, attitude or behavior, to the same physical and social environment — also unchanged — that overwhelmingly helped to produce their illnesses and will do so again, is to provide antibiotics for cholera and then to send the patients back to drink again from the Broad Street pump.

This chaotic and extravagantly wasteful system must be ended. It must be replaced by a system based on planned comprehensive visits by appointment at which all the necessary and appropriate services that can be given at one time are provided.

Unfortunately, the widely heralded and expensive Medicaid program does nothing to ensure that comprehensive care becomes the standard care. There are lists of services that can be provided and the payments that will be made for each of them. The custom of episodic care and the separation of preventive and therapeutic medicine are maintained, although clearly no longer reasonable or acceptable. Each state may include any kind of practitioner it licenses, and so we find several states including the services of chiropractors in their Medicaid programs. Thus, we find in New York State that instead of improving medical care for those in poverty, the relatively liberal eligibility standards encourage the extension of fragmented and inadequate care up toward the middle-income range.

Although the need for comprehensive services is emphasized here, a rather special service illustrates the point that the manner in which a service is provided is vitally important. The idea that "the rich get rich and the poor get children" had been repeated so many times over the years it had become an influence on public policy. The notion that the poor would not bother to help themselves to limit their excess fertility was an accepted truism in many places and incorporated in the rationalizations offered for not initiating family-planning services for the poor. Yet when these ideas were put to a reasonable test what was the outcome?

In 1965, in New York City, it was estimated that there were 165,000 medically indigent women who at any given time were potential clients for subsidized contraceptive services. Investigation revealed that at least 73,000 (44 percent) were actually being served at sixty-seven family planning clinics.[20] And this was before the ruling by the New York State Board of Social Welfare permitting welfare workers to raise the topic of family planning with their clients who did not spontaneously request information:

> The New York City experience has demonstrated conclusively that large numbers of impoverished parents in all ethnic groups are prepared to utilize modern family-planning services if they are provided with even modest amounts of dignity, compassion, and skill. This should set to rest, once and for all, the spurious notion, held by far too many administrators and professionals, that there is little point in initiating family-planning services for the poor because "they won't use it anyway." To be sure, they will not use it if the service is so organized as to be virtually inaccessible, if its policies and atmosphere are such as to challenge the patient's integrity and subject her to threatening and insulting inquiries, or if the patient must spend hours in a dingy waiting room before being seen for a couple of minutes by a harassed and often hostile physician. But the poor will respond in large numbers to services that are genuinely accessible, dignified, and properly organized to protect the patient's privacy.

The current decline in births in New York City may be an indication of the success of this service program and the wider dissemination of information now allowed.

PROFESSIONAL ATTITUDES AND TRAINING

If comprehensive programs in excellent facilities were to become available now, where would we find the professional personnel who could function in such settings and make use of the facilities and programs? Which of our students are presently receiving didactic or practical instruction for the provision of comprehensive health care? Do they have any notion of working as part of a health team? The failure of most of our medical, dental, nursing and other schools to move ahead in these areas may turn out to be more important than all the other factors in the health-care equation. Most of our schools are still teaching in terms of ill patients who come forward for care. All eyes are on the diseased organ or cells. Where the patient came from and where he is going are shunted to the side. Prevention and rehabilitation are for someone else to worry about. Many of our medical schools are as out of step with contemporary problems and understanding of the social mechanism and impact of disease as they were out of step with modern scientific medicine at the time of the Flexner Report.

Professionals in public health and private practice are not immune to the common tendency to place people in categories and label them accordingly, especially when they differ from the social, educational or ethnic group of the professional worker.[21] This leads to stereotyping and makes communication impossible. The patient is not insensitive to the health workers' attitude and may respond with the fatalistic unco-operative behavior appropriate to the role he has been assigned. Our largely middle class professionals may actually be influenced in their diagnosis and treatment of patients from other socioeconomic backgrounds. For the same condition there may be one treatment for one group of patients and another treatment for another group of patients. This subtle discrimination may insinuate itself into the practices of the most well meaning professionals completely without their knowledge.[22,23]

Much remains to be learned about the behavior of the users and providers of health services. Investigation and experimentation are required so that we can rid ourselves of some of the useless and even harmful habits we have fallen into over the years. One must insist, however, on avoiding "demonstrations or projects which, once terminated, reinforce the alienation of the poor and their sense of an uncommitted social order.[24]

The means of overcoming some of the barriers to use of health services lie beyond the province of health professionals. But it is incumbent upon us to search out the possibilities for removing barriers — and improving the public health — that do rest within our professional competence. There are many. We cannot wait until general socioeconomic improvement leads to change in patterns of aspirations and behavior among the poor.

CONCLUSIONS

The poor in the United States receive a disproportionately low share of health services. The barrier of direct cost is not sufficient to explain this underuse, and the advent of Medicare and Medicaid will not erase the existing discrepancies.

The failure to inform adequately potential clients of the existence and availability of services is a significant barrier. The organization, administration and conduct of services can be important deterrents to use. The professional health worker must be trained to be able to provide effectively his services in comprehensive programs for the poor and uneducated.

NOTES

1. U.S. Department of Health, Education, and Welfare, Public Health Service, National Office of Vital Statistics, *Vital and Health Statistics: Volume of physician visits by place of visit and type of service, United States, July 1963–June 1964 (by Carolanne H Hoffmann).* Washington, D.C.: Government Printing Office, 1965. (Series 10, No. 18.)

2. Peterson, O.L., et al. What is value for money in medical care? Experiences in England and Wales, Sweden and U.S.A. *Lancet 1:771–776,* 1967.

3. United States Department of Health, Education, and Welfare, Public Health Service, National Office of Vital Statistics, *Vital and Health Statistics: Age patterns in medical care, illness and disability, United States, July 1963–June 1965 (by Geraldine A Gleeson).* Washington, D.C.: Government Printing Office, 1966. (Series 10, No. 32.)

4. *Idem. Vital and Health Statistics: Physicians visits, interval of visits and children's routine check-up, United States, July 1963–June 1964 (by Charles S. Wilder).* Washington, D.C.: Government Printing Office, 1965. (Series 10, No. 19.)

5. *Idem. Vital and Health Statistics: Charactersitics of patients of selected types of medical specialists and practitioners, United States, July 1963–June 1964 (by Mary M. Hannaford).* Washington, D.C.: Government Printing Office, 1966. (Series 10, No. 28.)

6. *Idem. Vital and Health Statistics: Volume of dental visits, United States, July 1963–1964 (by Alice J. Alderman),* Washington, D.C.: Government Printing Office, 1965. (Series 10, No. 23.)

7. *Idem. Vital and Health Statistics: Medical care, health status, and family income, United States: (Prepared by Philip S. Lawrence and others.)* Washington, D.C.: Government Printing Office, 1964. (Series 10, No. 9.)

8. *Idem. Vital and Health Statistics: Hospital discharges and length of stay: Short stay hospitals, United States, July 1963–June 1964: (By Charles S. Wilder).* Washington, D.C.: Government Printing Office, 1966. (Series 10, No. 30.)

9. Lennon, R.G., Turnball, C.D., Elsea, W.R., Karzon, D.T., and Winkelstein, W. Measles immunization in metropolitan county. *J.A.M.A. 200:815–819, 1967.*

10. Morris, J.N. *Uses of Epidemiology.* Edinburgh: Livingstone, 1957.

11. Titmuss, R.M., Role of redistribution in social policy. *Social Sec. Bull.,* Vol. 28, No. 6, pp. 14–20, June, 1965.

12. United States Department of Health, Education, and Welfare, Welfare Administration. In Low-Income Life Styles, Lola M. Irelan, editor, Washington, D.C.: Government Printing Office, 1966.

13. Cornely, P.B. and Bingman, S.K., Acquaintance with municipal

government health services in low-income urban population. *Am. J. Pub. Health* 52:1877–1886, 1962.

14. Columbia University, School of Social Work. *Neighborhood Information Centers: A Study and some proposals.* Alfred J. Kahn et al., New York: The School, 1966.

15. White, M.K., Alpert, J.J., and Kosa, J., Hard-to-reach families in comprehensive care program *J.A.M.A.* 201:801–806, 1967.

16. Caplovitz, D. *The Poor Pay More: Consumer practices of low-income families.* New York: Free Press, 1963. (Columbia University, Bureau of Applied Social Research Report.)

17. Zola, I.K. Problems of communication, diagnosis, and patient care: Interplay of patient, physician and clinic organization. *J. M. Educ.* 38:829–838, 1963.

18. Watts, D.D., Factors related to acceptance of modern medicine, *Am. J. Pub. Health* 56:1205–1212, 1966.

19. Geiger, H.J. Poor and professional: Who takes handle off Broad Street Pump? Presented at ninety-fourth annual meeting of American Public Health Association, San Francisco, California, November 1, 1966.

20. Yerby, A.S., Public policy in regard to birth-control services. *New Eng. J. Med.* 275:824–826, 1966.

21. Hoff, W., Why health programs are not reaching unresponsive in our communities., *Pub. Health Rep.* 81:654–658, 1966.

22. Hollingshead, A.B., and Redlich, F.C., *Social Class and Mental Illness: A community study*, New York: Wiley, 1958.

23. Susser, M.W., and Watson, W., *Sociology in Medicine.* London: Oxford, 1962.

24. Miller, C., Income and receipt of medical care, *Am. J. Pub. Health* 55:510–521, 1965.

2. Poverty and Health

A Reexamination

MYRON J. LEFCOWITZ

Current discussions of health policies for the poor typically assume that poverty is a cause of medical deprivation. In these discussions there is much controversy over whether financial or structural barriers are more important in restricting availability and utilization of adequate health services by low-income populations. Whichever side of the argument is taken, two "facts" are accepted as true: (1) poverty leads to less medical care; and (2) poverty results in diminished health.

In this paper available information that casts doubt on these two statements has been brought together. In addition to making the relationship of income to health problematic, the evidence at times suggests that level of education is a causal factor in individual health status and medical care utilization. When education is taken into account in analyzing the income-health relationship, the correlation is considerably diminished, usually to the point of disappearance. Education, within income levels, however, remains as a factor in health status and behavior. Hence, the observed correlation between income and medical deprivation appears to be a consequence of education's relationship with both variables. Unfortunately, the published data provide only a few instances—although they are strategic—having to do with medical care for children and infant mortality.

Some possible implications of this evidence for the current health policy debate are suggested. The major objective of the paper, how-

From *Inquiry* 10 (March 1973), pp. 3–13, reprinted by permission of the author and publisher.

The research reported here was supported by funds granted to the Institute by the Office of Economic Opportunity pursuant to the provisions of the Economic Opportunity Act of 1964. The author wishes to thank Burton Weisbrod, David Elesh, Robinson Hollister, Robert Lampman and Ray Munts for their comments on earlier drafts. However, the conclusions drawn in this paper are solely the responsibility of the author.

ever, is to clear away some of the myths which have heretofore befogged that debate. Before beginning, two points need to be made. Although some of the material to be presented are recomputations of the available data, the following is primarily a discussion of information as it has been published in various reports of the U.S. National Center for Health Statistics.[1] We do not pretend, therefore, any originality in data analysis. Since the line being pursued is different from the prevailing—or, at least, published—consensus, the use of data well known to professionals in the field would appear to be particularly appropriate.

Second, we do not want to debate the definition of poverty. Whatever it is, there is agreement that in general economic terms it is at least some minimum access to a bundle of goods and services.[2] One indicator of poverty in that sense is family income. Thus, we shall be using poverty, low income, plus equivalent adjectives synonymously.

MEDICAL CARE

There has been almost universal agreement that the poor receive less than the non-poor in the way of actual medical care—both in quantity and quality. The Neighborhood Health Center programs sponsored by OEO and then HEW were designed, at least in part, to redress the imbalance. This inequity in medical care, moreover, is apparently observable.[3]

Quantity of Care

The most recent data, however, suggest that there is little correlation between average number of physician visits per person per year and family income. Based on information gathered from household interviews in 1969, the average number of physician visits was 4.8 for persons in families with less than $3,000 income, and 4.3 for persons whose income was over $10,000.[4] But, these averages mask a strong relationship for children under 15 years of age. When family income is under $3,000, the average number of physician visits from July, 1966 to June, 1967 was 4.4 for children under five, and 1.5 for those five to fourteen years of age. When income is over $10,000, the averages for the corresponding ages were 7.2 and 3.5.[5] Taking education of the head of the family income account, however, the correlation between family income and average annual number of physician visits among children disappears (Table 1). This finding suggests that education of the family head is an important factor in medical care utilization for the young.

Table 1. Number of physician visits per person per year by education of head of family and family income for persons under 15 years of age, July 1966-June 1967

Family income	Education of head of family			
	Under 5 years	5-8 years	9-12 years	13+ years
Under $5,000	2.1	2.2	3.2	5.4
$5,000 and over	1.4	2.6	4.1	5.0

Source: National Center for Health Statistics. *Volume of Physician Visits, 1966-1967*, Series 10-49 (1968) p. 23.

However, averages may not reflect the spread of utilization. Perhaps low-income persons visit the physician both less and more often than high-income persons; hence, the similarity in averages. There is little evidence, however, to support that suggestion. Although low-income persons are somewhat more likely than the high-income population *not* to have seen a physician, income is not related to a high frequency (five or more) of visits.[6]

Quality of Care

But what about the quality of that care? Unfortunately, the problem of medical care quality in general has barely been touched. It is an obviously complicated question in definition and in measurement.[7] Hence, we ought to be wary of categorical statements on the relative inferiority of health care received by the poor.

One indicator of quality, however, is use of medical specialists. Specialists relative to other physicians deal more frequently with the diseases which come to their attention and are best equipped to bring to bear the practices appropriate to mangement of the disease.[8] The three special services most frequently used, and for which information is available, are pediatrics, obstetrics-gynecology and eye care. In Table 2, the percent of the relevant population using those specialists from July, 1963 to June, 1964 is presented by family income and education of family head. In general, higher income persons had used these services more frequently than the population with incomes less than $4,000. Education also has an impact—one which appears to be sharper than income given the gross categories in Table 2. In almost all instances persons in families where the head had some college education were at least twice as likely to have used the service than when the head had less than nine years of education, regardless of income. These data, then, are consistent with the data reported on

Table 2. Percent of population using selected types of medical specialists and practitioners by family income and education of head of family, July 1963-June 1964

Type of visit Income	Education of head of family		
	Under 9 years	9-12 years	13+ years
Pediatric			
Under $4,000	4	15	30
$4,000 and over	10	20	38
Obstetrics-gynecology			
Under $4,000	2	7	11
$4,000 and over	4	10	16
Ophthalmologic			
Under $4,000	4	5	10
$4,000 and over	5	6	11
Optometric			
Under $4,000	7	7	13
$4,000 and over	9	10	9

Source: National Center for Health Statistics. *Characteristics of Patients of Selected Types of Medical Specialists and Practitioners, July 1963-June 1964*, Series 10-28 (1966).

physician visits in general; which is, that education seems more strongly related to medical care utilization than income.

Another indicator of quality medical care is the use of private practitioners relative to public clinics. The poor are depicted as relying largely on public clinics and therefore are considered deprived in the quality of their health care compared to the non-poor.[9] In fact, low-income persons are more likely to go to a hospital clinic or an emergency room than higher income persons—14 percent of physician visits from July, 1966–June, 1967 when family income is under $3,000 compared with 6 percent when income is over $10,000. More important, however, 75 percent of the physician visits of low-income persons involved either a home or office visit with a private physician. This proportion, moreover, is the same for persons with higher income.[10] Thus, the image that the poor are at the mercy of public clinics for their medical care is a bit overdrawn.

This is not to argue that quality medicine is indeed distributed equitably across income classes. But, the little evidence available does suggest that an open mind on the issue is in order. Moreover, the data do suggest that when medical care varies by socioeconomic status, it is more across education levels than by family income.

HEALTH OF THE POOR

But what about the health of the poor? If they are not as healthy as the non-poor, then similarity in medical care utilization would indicate that the poor are relatively deprived given their greater need. Assuming a corresponding demand, equal utilization may be a consequence of a relatively scarce supply of medical care in low-income areas.

Morbidity

Taking age into account, however, there appears to be very little relationship between income and the presence of chronic diseases.[11] This information is based on interviews—and fewer people report ailments than are detected by clinical examination. For example, 6.2 million persons had heart conditions in 1963–1965 according to household interviews.[12] Based on the Health Examination Survey from 1960-1962, however, 14.6 million adults had definite heart disease.[13] This discrepancy might be proportionately larger at lower income levels where people may be less informed about the presence of less obvious chronic conditions. Consequently in an actual clinical examination many more unsuspected ailments could be discovered among low-income persons than among high-income ones. Thus, the correlation between morbidity and income would be increased.

With this possibility in mind, information from the National Health Examination Survey on heart and arthritic conditions, the two leading causes of activity limitation,[14] has been summarized in Table 3. The data presented are the differences between the actual rate per 100 adults, as diagnosed through the Health Examination, and the rate that would have been expected given the age composition of the subgroup. (See the appendixes of the various Health Examination Survey reports for a technical description of the derivation of the expected value.) Thus, a *negative* value indicate *less* actual disease than might be expected from that population and a positive value denotes more. The closer the value is to zero, the closer together are the actual and expected rates.

Looking first at hypertensive heart disease, we can see that there is no apparent relationship between family income and the differences between the actual and expected rates per 100 adults. For example, white men with under $4,000 family income have less definite hypertensive heart disease than expected; the next highest income category has more; the next less; those adults with incomes over $10,000 have more. For white women the pattern is quite dif-

Table 3. Differences between actual and expected* prevalence rates per 100 adults of selected disease conditions by family income, sex and race, 1960-1962

Disease conditions	Family income				
	Under $2,000	$2,000-3,999	$4,000-6,999	$7,000-9,999	$10,000 and over
Definite hypertensive heart disease					
White men	—0.5	—0.8	0.7	—1.8	1.4
White women	3.8	—0.3	—0.7	—2.1	0.1
Black men	8.2	—6.6	—2.2	—6.9	11.9
Black women	2.7	—1.2	0.8	—6.4	—2.9
Definite hypertension					
White men	—1.6	0.4	1.0	—0.5	—1.6
White women	4.9	—0.7	—1.2	—0.7	—1.6
Black men	7.3	—5.4	—3.4	—13.8	6.5
Black women	4.3	1.9	—6.0	—0.4	—5.6
Definite coronary heart disease					
Men	—0.8	0.2	0.9	0.2	—1.7
Women	0.6	0.3	0.2	0.2	—1.2
Osteoarthritis					
Men	—2.8	0.3	—0.4	1.5	0.5
Women	0.5	0.0	—0.2	—1.0	2.0
Rheumatoid arthritis					
Men	3.0	—0.5	—0.6	—0.2	—0.1
Women	0.0	—0.5	0.7	—0.5	—0.5

*Standardized for age.

Sources: NCHS. *Hypertension and Hypertensive Heart Disease in Adults, 1960-1962*, Series 11-13 (1966) p. 24.

NCHS. *Coronary Heart Disease in Adults, 1960-1962*, Series 11-10 (1965) p. 23.

NCHS. *Osteoarthritis in Adults by Selected Demographic Characteristics, 1960-1962*, Series 11-20 (1966) p. 11.

NCHS. *Rheumatoid Arthritis in Adults, 1960-1962*, Series 11-17 (1966) p. 22.

ferent—the difference between the actual and expected rates decreases with income from 3.8 to —2.1 in the $7,000-$10,000 category and then increases to 0.1 for the highest income category. Black men exhibit a similar curvilinear pattern as white women—positive in the extreme income categories and negative in the middle categories. Among black women, however, there is no apparent relationship.

For hypertension, the curvilinear pattern appears for both white and black men, but in opposite directions. For women, however, the difference between actual and expected prevalence of hypertension does decrease as income increases (Table 3).

The general relationship is not clear, therefore, between income and hypertension, or income and hypertensive heart disease. Hypertension and hypertensive heart disease can stand for all the disease conditions reported in Table 3—that is, the negative relationship between income and these diseases is problematic. Given the relative importance of heart and arthritic conditions in limiting the activities of people, this conclusion would seem to be significant.

What about other impairments or conditions? The clinical data on diabetes,[15] anemia,[16] vision[17] and hearing[18] are generally consistent with the above conclusion. The available evidence from the Health Examination Survey, then, is consistent with data obtained from household interviews. The only conclusion is that the relationship between health and poverty—as indicated by morbidity—is not proven.

Mortality Rates

Some persons have argued, however, that mortality rates, particularly infant mortality, are a better indicator than morbidity rates of the health status of a population.[19] In general, past research has supported the generalization that these rates decrease with increased socioeconomic status. Nevertheless, the findings have not been unambiguous.[20] Data, however, are now available which permit us to obtain a fix on the variation in infant mortality rates by family income and parents' education. The necessary information was obtained by a follow-back survey of national samples of births and infant deaths for 1964-1966. The data presented suggest that for white births, family income has no consistent relationship with infant mortality when parents' education is taken into account. At all income levels, however, education, whether mother's or father's, is negatively related. For blacks, the patterns are not as clear although both income and education appear to have an impact on infant mortality rates.[21]

This evidence again forces us to be more skeptical about the presumed relationship between poverty and health even when the index of the latter is infant mortality. Rather, as our thesis contends, education appears to be the socioeconomic variable most closely related.

EDUCATION AND MEDICAL DEPRIVATION

The policy implications of the apparent effect of education on medical deprivation and the concomitant diminution of the income-health correlation when education is taken into account are not readily apparent. In this section a general interpretation of the relationship of education to health will be presented; on the basis of that framework some policy directives are suggested.

Weber[22] pointed out that people are distributed in society along three dimensions—class, status and power. Class refers to economic positions, status to life styles (prestige), and power to control of others. Since persons are distributed with reference to each, policies can be directed to redistributing the values which locate people on each dimension; or, at least by producing enough of the values, we can attempt to move all members of society above some minimum level. Hence, powerty is reduced by increasing family income—and hopefully, the poor's share of total income is increased.

In this context, our hypothesis is that health-related and health-oriented behaviors are primarily a function of valued life styles and that education is a primary agent in the development of such tastes. Put somewhat differently, every family—within reasonable limits—has access to any part of the market bundle of goods and services available. How it selects, given its income, from that bundle is the family's life style. Education is a primary determinant in the ordering of those priorities.

What are the dynamics which link education and health? We start with the assumption that reduction of illness and prolongation of life are desired states. Education, in the first instance, is a process that increases the level of information about factors related to those desirable states. It does so directly through what is taught, at least up through the secondary level, but more probably through the acquisition of skills which enable the person to be both more sensitive and more alert to relevant information. Thus, for example, we expect that the more educated a person is, the more likely he is to be aware of the relationship between health and diet or physical exercise, topics much discussed in the mass media. Therefore, we would hypothesize that: The more educated a person is the more likely he is to have the opportunity to be exposed to, to expose himself to, and to be influenced by, health information. His opportunities are greater because the mass media to which he is exposed is more likely to provide that information. He is more likely to expose himself because he is more alert to such information. Moreover, he is more influenced because he is more accepting of the claims of science in matters affecting day-to-day life.

Also, through education, the individual develops a life style which may have a greater impact on health status than what he or she may do directly. Diet, for example, may be more a consequence of food preferences or of physical aesthetics than concern about its apparent relationship to health.

This function of education is not explicit in that preferred choices are taught at each level, but rather that the level of education provides the basis for entry into social statuses; and during the distributional process different life stypes are acquired—consciously or unconsciously.

More concretely, our educational system is directed toward fitting people into urban society. In that society, for instance, small families are apparently preferred—possibly because the costs for children are larger in cities. Therefore, we should expect that birth rates are related to residential background and education. And, that is indeed the case. Low rates are found for women of nonfarm origin and nonfarm residence. On the other hand, women with a farm background rapidly approach the birth rate for women who have a nonfarm background as farm women's educational level increases.[23] Moreover, family income is unrelated to birth rates in urbanized areas.[24] Whatever the primary social or economic function of small family size, it probably has the additional consequence of affecting the health status of the offspring. Evidence indicates that, in general, infant mortality increases with parity,[25] and moreover, this relationship remains even when socioeconomic status as measured by occupational categories is taken into account.[26] Thus, we can infer that the decreasing number of children per family which flows from increased education has the secondary consequence of reducing infant mortality and, hence, improving the health status of the population concomitantly, albeit indirectly.

One more example of the possible indirect effects of education on health status relates to accidents. The accident rate for a population is in some degree a consequence of the potentiality for injury inherent in that population's physical location and movement within a social environment. Presumably, this location and movement is a function of life style. Therefore, it is interesting to note that although income, controlling for age, is only slightly related to the current injury rate, education, again taking age into account, is strongly and negatively related in general. Thus, for persons 25-44 years of age, the current injury rate per 100 persons per year drops from 35.2 for persons with only some high school to 20.5 for persons with a college degree.[27]

One explanation is that education is also negatively related to the accident potential in occupations. Some evidence for this hypothesis is that men have higher injury rates than women at all age levels up to 65. This difference is largely attributable to the much greater incidence of work injuries among men. Following the same reasoning, we would also expect that nonwhites would have a higher accident rate than whites; that is, they are more likely to be in accident-risking situations—particularly at work. On the contrary, the nonwhite accident rate is two-thirds the white one for persons under 45 and about the same for persons over 45. These data at least bring into question occupation as an explanation for the relationship between education and injury rate. We would suggest that differential life styles may be the explanation.

Consumption Patterns and Permanent Income

An alternative explanation for the analytic importance of education relative to income for health status and health care is that consumption patterns are more directly tied to permanent income, for which level of education is a proxy. There is no way using available data, however, to test directly the permanent income hypothesis. Presumably, the relationship of education to family consumption of medical care and to infant mortality rates might be explained in part by the permanent income hypothesis. However, since most physician visits are a direct response to an illness and injury—only about 20 percent of the visits by children under fifteen are for a general check-up or immunization and vaccination[28] — permanent income might be less important in the consumption of medical care than in expenditures for durable consumer goods.

Unfortunately, the above is only supposition. Efforts to find published data which could provide a more direct test was, with one exception, largely unavailing. The exception relates to cigarette smoking. We would expect in that case that average number of cigarettes smoked per day by men would increase with income—and indeed it does among present smokers. What we also find is that income is positively related to the age-adjusted percentage of men who have *never* smoked and who are former smokers. The same relationship holds for education.[29] It would be difficult to predict the fact that higher income is positively associated with not smoking cigarettes from a permanent income hypothesis. Actually, we would be more likely to predict the opposite in keeping with the generally positive relationship between income and the consumption of other goods and services.

Given the current state of our knowledge, however, the permanent income hypothesis is not so easily disproven. The above data do bring it into question, while leaving the life-style hypothesis untouched. Probably both mechanisms are in operation so that the main issue is their relative importance.

If our contention is correct that preferences (life styles) are of more moment in health behavior than access to a market basket of goods and services, what does this hypothesis have to say about whether to emphasize a financial or structural approach in our health policy? If the hypothesized lower preferences for health care among the less educated is correct, the price elasticity with respect to health care is small. Moreover, our data suggest that the income elasticity is also small (see Table 1). Although reduction in cost would clearly increase utilization (we assume, of course, that supply increases correspondingly or is already sufficient to handle the increased demand), the change would be small if the elasticities are as predicted. Whether the magnitude of that effect is optimum from society's viewpoint—that is, whether the consumption of medical services by the lower educated will move up to some level of adequacy—is problematic given the hypothesis.

The problem, then, is to increase the preference for health care and other health-inducing behaviors among the lower educated. This guideline suggests that alterations in the structure of the delivery system, as it relates to the less well-educated, be considered the appropriate policy direction. Most discussions of structural reform focus on increased supply and/or proximity of services, none of which addresses the heart of the problem as here stated. What is needed are changes that will decrease the psychic distance and that will enhance the significance of modern health practices for the medically deprived. Such programs as outreach workers sensitive to the life styles of the low-educated, medical translators to facilitate communication between the practitioner and client, reinforcement of preferred behaviors which are causally linked to health (e.g., making available at low cost preferred food which provides an adequate diet) appear to be mechanisms which in the short-range policy horizon would be more conducive to improving the health and medical care of the population concerned. An examination of the social-anthropological literature on the introduction of modern health technology among underdeveloped groups might be most instructive for our own society. If programs of this type were directed toward the low-income population, they would, by their nature, scoop in a large part of that subset which is deprived as a result of their life patterns.

HEALTH AND POVERTY RESTATED

But what about the consequences of illness? It is our contention that illness and medical care have more serious consequences for lower income populations than for the affluent. In economic terms, the costs of illness are inequitably distributed among the income categories and hence may cause or increase impoverishment. We claim no originality for this idea for which the supportive data are generally known. What we do assert is that incorrect policy implications have been drawn.

First, even though the prevalence of persons with one or more chronic ailments is unrelated to income, persons whose chronic conditions limit their major activity are much more likely to have incomes under $3,000 than where the ailment is less restrictive (Table 4). This relationship is particularly true for nonaged adults. In the 17–44 age group, among those who have no chronic conditions, one out of every eight or nine has a family income under $3,000; in the same group among those unable to carry on their major activity two out of every five have family incomes under $3,000 (Table 4). The pattern is similar for 45–64 year olds. Among the aged, where advanced years restrict activity in any case, low income is much less related to the limitations imposed by chronic conditions.

This finding is not surprising. Income and the physical demands of occupational activity are, in general, negatively related. Among persons with similar ailments, moreover, we would expect those engaged in physical labor to be more restricted in their work activity than persons in nonmanual occupations.

Some evidence for this hypothesis is presented in Table 5. Among the current employed persons over 44 years of age who report one or more chronic conditions, those in farm and nonfarm labor occupations are most likely to say that their condition limited their major activity. Alternatively, professional, technical, and clerical workers are least likely to report such restrictions (see Table 5). Haber[30] presents corroborating data from the Social Security Disability Survey. The occupations in which the workers are most limited are also somewhat more likely to include workers having one or more chronic conditions (Table 5). Thus, it is possible that the chronic condition may be a consequence of work, particularly farm work,

Table 4. Percent of adults with family incomes under $3,000 by their chronic condition and activity limitation status, 1965-1966

| | | Percent under $3,000 income | | | |
| | | | Persons with 1+ chronic conditions | | |
Age	Persons with no chronic conditions	No limitation of activity	Limitation, but not in major activity	Limitation in amount or kind of major activity*	Unable to carry on major activity
17-44	12	11	16	24	41
45-64	12	13	21	36	51
65+	43	47	54	55	57

*Major activity refers to ability to work, keep house, or engage in school or preschool activities.

Source: NCHS. *Limitation of Activity and Mobility Due to Chronic Conditions, 1965-1966*, Series 10-45 (1968) p. 26.

Table 5. Chronic conditions and limitation of major activity by occupation of currently employed persons over 44 years of age, 1965-1966

Occupation	Of all in occupation, percent with chronic conditions	Of all with 1+ chronic conditions, percent with limitation of major activity
Professional, technical	68	7
Managers, officials proprietors (nonfarm)	69	15
Clerical	68	9
Sales	72	15
Craftsmen and foremen	67	14
Operative	66	13
Service, except private household	69	15
Private household	77	24
Laborers, except farm and mine	69	24
Farm laborers and foremen	72	33
Farmers and farm managers	77	33

Source: NCHS. *Limitation of Activity and Mobility Due to Chronic Conditions, 1965-1966,* Series 10-45 (1968) pp. 48-49.

itself. That possibility aside, however, the data are consistent with, but do not confirm our thesis that the economic consequences of poor health are more serious for persons in more physically demanding occupations.

Income and Work Days Lost

Unfortunately, these data are not available for employment status and income. However, we do have, by income, the average number of days lost from work during 1968–1969 for currently employed persons. What is instructive to note is that income is correlated with work days lost for men between 25 and 64 years of age. Moreover, the relationship is quite strong. Men 25–44 years old lose twice as much time from work if their income is less than $3,000 than if it is over $10,000. Among men 45–64 years old, those with less than

$3,000 income lose more than twice as many days as men with more than $10,000 family income. Thus, precisely among primary wage earners, the differential cost of illness is greatest.[31]

Lower income families, then, lose a greater proportion of their income as a result of illness than do more affluent persons. This conclusion assumes that days lost from work means wages lost for everyone. But, it is plausible that persons in higher paying jobs are more likely to have sick leave benefits, formal or informal, and therefore, are less likely to lose any income as a result of illness. In fact, that is the case. The higher the family income, the more likely are currently employed persons to report that they are reimbursed for work time lost through illness.[32] Thus, the impact on income for wage earners in the lower income categories is even greater relative to high-income persons than just missing more days at work.

Costs of illness, obviously, can also mean direct out-of-pocket expenses for the necessary treatment and care. Such out-of-pocket costs are proportionately greater for lower income families.[33] In 1961, families with less than $4,000 money income after taxes spent between 7.5 and 10 percent of it on medical care compared to 6 to 7 percent for higher income families.[34] Family income was negatively and sharply related to coverage by hospital and surgical insurance.[35] Since the proportion of persons hospitalized in a given year does not vary by income,[36] we can assume that lower income persons are more likely to be confronted with a large medical bill than are persons with higher incomes. For example, of those persons hospitalized for surgical treatment, where family income was under $2,000, about one-third of the discharges had some part of the surgeon's bill paid for by insurance compared with four-fifths when the income was over $7,000.[37] The threat of a catastrophic medical bill is underlined by the fact that hospitalized lower income persons tend to be in the hospital somewhat longer than their higher income counterparts.[38]

The conclusion that illness has a greater financial impact on the poor than the more affluent is hardly surprising. After all, Medicare and Medicaid are attempts to correct this inequity—at least insofar as direct out-of-pocket costs are concerned—as are the various health bills currently in the Congressional hopper. What the data point to, however, is that vocational rehabilitation and cash transfer programs may be more productive in ameliorating the consequences of poor health than are health programs.

CONCLUSION

This paper has attempted to focus the available, mostly published data about income and health on the public debate over whether financial barriers or structural barriers are more important in restricting availability and utilization of adequate health services to lower income populations. This debate has assumed in part that medical deprivation is caused by poverty. Through reviewing the data, however, that assumption has been questioned. Hence, insofar as the policy controversy has been based on poverty as a causal factor in poor health and inadequate medical care, the demarcation of alternative approaches to improving health standards and increasing medical care utilization has rested on an unstable assumption. Instead, the evidence presented indicates that education is negatively related to health and health care.

Policy Directions

The policy directions for intervention between education and health status and care are not immediately apparent. We have suggested that education functions to distribute the population by valued life styles (preferences, in economic terms) and that these styles include elements which directly or indirectly affect health and utilization of health services. Presumably, as the educational level increases, the health status of the population will improve in response to the hypothesized change in life styles. At the same time, effective demand for health care will also increase. It is very difficult, of course, to demonstrate both trends as well as their causal relationship to education. If the general hypothesis is correct, however, it does suggest that policies designed to reduce medical deprivation on the basis of poverty as a cause are misguided. In this framework the current policy issue may be reformulated: What changes in health policy—financial and/or structural—will increase utilization among the less educated given their relatively lower preference for health care?

A policy explicitly for the less educated does not appear reasonable. We would hardly want to add a taste test as an analog to the means test. Since education and income are highly correlated, a health policy directed toward the poor would cover a large portion of the low-educated population. But, which type of remedy— financial or structural—should be emphasized?

The argument is presented that the effect of a financial policy would lead to only a small increase in health care utilization and/or health-improving behavior among the low-educated. The basis for that hypothesis is that both income elasticity and price elasticity with respect to such behavior are small. Thus, if we are interested in the medically deprived, policies directed to changing the preferences and/or to reinforcing existing health-inducing preference patterns are required. This conclusion suggests, then, that structural changes be given central consideration over financial changes in the health arena.

But, can we then ignore the poor as such in our development of policy? The evidence presented in the paper does support the notion that a loss of health and the use of medical care are more costly to the poor than non-poor. This cost is twofold. First, the share of income required for medical care is greater for the poor. Any policy which picks up the tab for services can to that extent redress the inequity. Clearly, however, this objective is more income-distributional than health-improving. Second, poor health can drastically affect earnings, making poor out of previously non-poor and creating a barrier to movement out of poverty for those persons already there. Policies designed to reduce the income consequences of ill health would focus on transfer payments during an illness or disability period (e.g., broader disability insurance both in coverage of working population and to other than work-related disabilities) and/or an expansion of our vocational rehabilitation programs.

To a large extent, then, a serious attempt to deal with the health and poverty issue would involve only in part what is typically considered a health program and would address itself to the relative cost inequities between poor and non-poor.

NOTES

1. See the following National Center for Health Statistics (NCHS) publication for a more detailed description of their surveys: *Origin, Program, and Operation of the U.S. National Health Survey*, Series 1-1 (1963); *Cycle 1 of the Health Examination Survey: Sample and Response*, Series 11-1 (1963); and *Plan and Initial Program of the Health Examination Survey*, Series 1-4 (Washington, D.C.: GPO, 1964).

Since the Government Printing Office is the publisher for all NCHS publications, that information will not be repeated.

2. Watts, Harold. "An Economic Definition of Poverty." In: Moynihan, D. P. (ed.) *On Understanding Poverty* (New York: Basic Books, 1969) pp. 316–329.

3. White, Elijah L. "A Graphic Presentation on Age and Income Differentials in Selected Aspects of Morbidity, Disability and Utilization of Health Services," *Inquiry* 5:18–30 (March 1968).

4. NCHS. *Age Patterns in Medical Care, Illness, and Disability, 1968–1969*, Series 10-70 (1972) p. 10.

5. NCHS. *Volume of Physician Visits, 1966–1967*, Series 10–49 (1968) p. 19.

6. *Ibid.*, p. 39.

7. Roth, Julius. "The Treatment of the Sick." In: Kosa, John, *et al.* (eds.) *Poverty and Health* (Cambridge: Harvard University Press, 1969) pp. 222–226.

8. Mechanic, David. *Medical Sociology* (New York: The Free Press, 1968) p. 354.

9. Roth, *op. cit.*, pp. 217–218.

10. NCHS. Series 10-49, *op. cit.*, p. 30.

11. NCHS. *Limitation of Activity and Mobility Due to Chronic Conditions, 1965–1966*, Series 10-45 (1968).

12. NCHS. *Age Patterns in Medical Care, Illness and Disability, 1963–1965*, Series 10-32 (1966) p. 55.

13. NCHS. *Heart Disease in Adults, 1960–1962*, Series 11-6 (1964) p. 7.

14. NCHS. Series 10–45, *op. cit.*, p. 6.

15. NCHS. *Blood Glucose Levels in Adults, 1960–1962*, Series 11-18 (1966).

16. NCHS. *Mean Blood Hematocrit of Adults, 1960–1962*, Series 11-24 (1967).

17. NCHS. *Binocular Visual Acuity of Adults, by Region and Selected Demographic Characteristics, 1960–1962*, Series 11-25 (1967).

18. NCHS. *Hearing Level of Adults by Education, Income, and Occupation, 1960–1962* Series 11-31 (1968).

19. Lerner, Monroe, "Social Differences in Physical Health." In: Kosa, *et al.* (eds.) *Poverty and Health, op. cit.* p. 91.

20. Mechanic, *op. cit.*, pp. 244–257.

21. NCHS. *Infant Mortality Rates: Socioeconomic Factors*, Series 22-14 (1972) pp. 13–14.

22. Weber, Max. "Class, Status, Party." In: Gerth, H. H., and Mills, C. Wright, (trs.) *From Max Weber: Essays in Sociology* (New York: Oxford University Press, 1946) pp. 180–195.

23. Duncan, Otis Dudley. "Farm Background and Differential Fertility," *Demography* 2:240–249 (1965).

24. Sweet, James. "Some Deomgraphic Aspects of Income Maintenance Policy." In: Orr, Larry L.; Hollister, Robinson G.; and Lefcowitz, Myron J. (eds.) *Income Maintenance: Interdisciplinary Approaches to Research* (Chicago: Markham Press, 1971).

25. Illsley, Raymond. "The Sociological Study of Reproduction and Its Outcome." In: Richardson, Stephen A., and Guttmacher, Alan F. (eds.) *Childbearing: Its Social and Psychological Aspects* (Baltimore: Williams and Wilkins, 1967) pp. 96–98.

26. Chase, Helen C. "Infant Mortality and Weight at Birth: 1960 United States Birth Cohort," *American Journal of Public Health* 59:1618–1628 (September 1969).

27. NCHS. *Types of Injuries: Incidence and Associated Disability, 1965–1967*, Series 10-57 (1969) p. 7.

28. NCHS. *Volume of Physician Visits by Place of Visit and Type of Service, 1963–1964*, Series 10-18 (1965) p. 26.

29. Hedrick, James L. *Facts on Smoking, Tobacco and Health* (National

Clearinghouse for Smoking and Health, 1968) pp. 10–11.

30. Haber, Lawrence D. "Disability and Social Planning: Implications of The Social Security Disability Survey." Paper presented at the annual meeting of the National Conference on Social Welfare, June 3, 1970, Chicago, Illinois.

31. NCHS. *Time Lost From Work Among the Currently Employed Population, 1968*, Series 10-71 (1972) p. 15.

32. *Ibid.*, p. 23.

33. Tucker, Murray A. "Effect of Heavy Medical Expenditures on Low Income Families." *Public Health Reports* 85:419–425 (May 1970).

34. U.S. Bureau of Labor Statistics. *Consumer Expenditure Survey Report, 1960-1961*, Report 237-93 (Washington, D.C.: GPO, 1965) p. 16.

35. NCHS. *Family Hospital and Surgical Insurance Coverage, 1962–1963*, Series 10-42 (1967) pp. 13–17.

36. NCHS. *Persons Hospitalized by Numbers of Hospital Episodes and Days in a Year, 1965–1966.* Series 10-50 (1969).

37. NCHS. *Proportion of Surgical Bill Paid by Insurance, 1963–1964*, Series 10-31 (1966), p. 8.

38. NCHS. Series 10-50, *op. cit.*, p. 14.

3. Cultural Barriers to the Utilization of Health Services

JEAN LEONARD ELLIOTT

When new health plans are implemented at no direct cost to the consumer, it is usually assumed that their success or failure depends upon the medical resources available, and the ways in which these resources are organized and distributed. Although the importance of such considerations should not be minimized, the anthropologist knows that a whole host of cultural factors must be considered in order to determine why some people participate and others do not.[1,2]

The medical program considered here is Nova Scotia Medical Services Insurance (MSI),[3] which has been in effect in Nova Scotia since April, 1969. The program is financed directly from federal and provincial taxes. The physician files claims with MSI in accord with a fee-for-service payment schedule. Unlike Great Britain,[4] Nova Scotia has made no attempt to redistribute medical resources, or to organize the medical system so as to reach out effectively to low-income and rural populations and insure their participation. Nevertheless, the financial barrier per se has been substantially reduced in Nova Scotia.[5] Problems concerning the distribution and organization of medical care have potentially clear-cut solutions if a society has adequate resources and a mandate to institute social change. However, cultural barriers such as illness definitions at odds with the

From *Inquiry* 9 (December 1972), pp. 28—34, reprinted by permission of the author and publisher.

This paper is a revised version of one presented to the American Anthropological Association, San Diego, California, November 22, 1970. The research was supported by a National Health Grant, Project #602-7-115, Ottawa, Canada.

larger society,[6] and alienation from the medical bureaucracy[7] may lead to underutilization of the health facilities provided.

If the object of health insurance schemes, in general, is to raise the health level of the population or provide treatment for those in need, these then are the kinds of criteria which could be drawn upon when health plans are evaluated. That is, before investigating "cultural barriers," it is appropriate to establish to what extent a medical care scheme has been able to meet health needs. If the health level of a population is high or higher than before the advent of a program, then an attempt to identify the presence of cultural barriers would become a somewhat futile and meaningless exercise. If, on the other hand, groups in a population can be identified which are in need of medical care and are not receiving it in spite of a substantial reduction in the financial barrier, such evidence of medical deprivation may have, in part, a cultural explanation.

In this research we set about the twofold task of first assessing health levels in three community populations in order to determine indirectly the extent to which medical services have been utilized; and second, examining whether or not cultural factors may be operating as barriers to participation.

In selecting the three target communities reported here,[8] care was given to include those with: (1) a history of medical deprivation; (2) a definitive ecological boundary; and (3) a distinctive ethnic base. Each community is either culturally or geographically isolated from the core society, but is *not* necessarily representative of a larger population.

THE COMMUNITIES

Tancook Islands

The two Tancook Islands are seven miles off the coast of Chester, Nova Scotia, forty-five miles from Halifax Although Tancook is primarily a fishing community, some farming, predominantly subsistence, is carried on.

Sixty-nine percent of the respondents (42) report a household income of $3,000 or under. There is no doctor or nurse on the islands. As for most goods and services, the islanders are obliged to travel to the mainland for their medical services or pay the doctor's ferry transportation to their home. However, there are doctors and dentists in Chester, and a hospital in Bridgewater twenty-five miles distant.

In-migration to the islands has been minimal since the initial settlement in the 1790s by German and French farmers and New

England fishermen. The French population are descendants of French Huguenots. There are no Roman Catholic families on the islands.

Out-migration, of course, does occur because of the limited land and job opportunities on Tancook. Exogamous marriage patterns may be more common for females, however, than for males. There are seven surnames occurring repeatedly in most of the households.

A rich folk medicine tradition has been noted by Creighton[9] for this island group. Senna, for example, is grown locally on the island and is used as a laxative, but not necessarily to the exclusion of the usual commercially prepared drugstore remedies.

Upper Hammonds Plains

The inhabitants of Upper Hammonds Plains are the descendants of early nineteenth century black slaves who emigrated to Canada from the northern coast of the United States, often with their British masters, in the decades prior to the U.S. Civil War.

Upper Hammonds Plains is a semi-rural community located beyond Halifax's urban fringe. It is without immediate medical facilities. Doctors' offices are located in middle-class suburban Bedford about seven miles away, and the Halifax medical center is about fifteen miles distant. Prior to MSI, only 20 percent of the families were covered by a prepaid medical insurance plan. The extreme poverty in this community is evidenced by the fact that 21 percent of the homes (53) do not have indoor plumbing.

Forty-six percent of the household heads (37) have an eighth grade education or less. The men in this community are largely un-skilled seasonal laborers (51 percent). At the time of the survey, 18 percent of the households (51) reported their primary income as being derived from "welfare" at some point in time during the past year. An additional 14 percent (40) were unemployed, disabled or retired.

Mulgrave Park

Mulgrave Park is a public housing project in the North End of Halifax. Major medical facilities are located in the South End. Thus, for the most part, Mulgrave Park residents find it necessary to take public transportation (only 17 percent own a motor vehicle) in order to secure medical treatment. Since the collection of the data on which this paper is based, a community clinic has been opened in the North End.

Although residing in a metropolitan area containing a middle class and wealthy elite, the residents of Mulgrave Park are socially distant from much of the life around them. Many are unemployed recent migrants from Maritime rural areas. Much of the life in the housing project is stigmatized because it is associated with "welfare," even though only 43 percent of the residents claimed to have received welfare in the past year.

METHOD

An adult respondent in each household was interviewed in the months between April, 1969 and March, 1970. Most questions were precoded to permit response standardization and to facilitate machine analysis. Taking into account "call backs," the refusal rates in the two rural communities were negligible, below 2 percent. All households on the Tancook Islands and Upper Hammonds Plains were surveyed. Cooperation and rapport in the urban housing project, Mulgrave Park, however, was not as high. A one-third sampling strategy was used, as the community was sufficiently large to warrant sampling. Although actual refusals were low, it is felt that many residents fearing "bill collectors" would not open their doors, and call backs were to no avail; thus substitution of cases occurred in the selection of the sample. If there is a bias, however, in the Mulgrave Park data, it may be in the direction of the wealthier, less alienated group.

In each community, most respondents—approximately 80 percent—were female. There were 68 respondents on the Tancook Islands, 136 in Mulgrave Park, and 53 in Upper Hammonds Plains. The 257 respondents supplied health data for a total of 1,177 community residents.

The Measurement of Health

Lower social class members are less likely to recognize disease symptoms and are more likely to delay seeking treatment than those from the upper social classes.[10] Therefore, in poor communities the occurrence of untreated symptoms may serve as an appropriate index of community health; whereas in a wealthy area, another index might be appropriate.[11]

An adult member in each household was asked if he or any member of his family were currently experiencing any in a list of common disease symptoms.[12] If respondents replied affirmatively, they were then asked if they had or were seeking a doctor concerning the symptom. The dependent variable in this study is untreated symptoms, or symptoms which currently are not under medical surveillance by a practicing physician. Thus, respondents who reported symptoms and sought no medical attention will be compared with those who fall into the remaining categories.

Central concern is *not* with the medical reliability and validity of the measures nor with the incidence or prevalance of morbidity per se, but with the health patterns of those individuals reporting symptoms for which they have not sought treatment.

The frequency distribution of untreated symptoms for each community is presented in Table 1. From Table 1 we see that Upper Hammonds Plains leads the communities in the number of untreated symptoms reported. Only 36 percent are either symptom-free or have their symptoms under the surveillance of a physician. Thus, by this gross measurement of health, Upper Hammonds Plains has the lowest health level of the three communities. There is no difference, however, in the percentage of people in each community who report their health as "very good"—44 percent in Upper Hammonds Plains and the Tancook Islands, and 51 percent in Mulgrave Park. Thus the three communities are comparable with respect to their own subjective self-perceptions of good health.

Table 1. Percentage distribution of untreated symptoms by community

Untreated symptoms	Tancook Islands	Mulgrave Park	Upper Hammonds Plains
0	60	56	36
1	21	16	17
2	06	10	19
3	05	07	17
4+	08	11	11
Total	100	100	100
(N)	(68)	(136)	(53)

CULTURAL BARRIERS

Education and Age

One's education and age may be barriers to the intelligent use of medical facilities. Lack of formal education may result in the inability to correctly identify disease symptoms or may influence the course of subsequent health action.[13] The education level in the target communities is low relative to the median education level in

Nova Scotia. Education may be viewed as one component in the generally low socioeconomic status and cultural isolation characteristic of the communities. Nevertheless, variation with respect to education does exist in the study communities. For purposes of analysis, those with less than an eighth grade education, and those with eighth grade or more may be thought to form a dichotomy which may be examined with respect to its relationship to the number of untreated symptoms that characterize each group (Table 2). Are those with less than an eighth grade education also overrepresented with respect to the number of untreated symptoms they report?

On the Tancock Islands, the education level of the inhabitants is not helpful in identifying a potential cultural barrier to medical care. Those with less than eighth grade education are slightly overrepresented with respect to the percentage of untreated symptoms reported, but the difference is only 2 percent above the baseline figure reported for the community as a whole.

The same pattern occurs in Mulgrave Park, but the difference is more notable. Among those with less than an eighth grade education, 50 percent have at least one untreated symptom. The baseline for this community as a whole is 44 percent. A reversal in this pattern occurs in Upper Hammonds Plains.

The bivariate frequency distribution of age and untreated symptoms in each community may explain why education level is not consistently related to the reporting of untreated symptoms. If it is assumed that the formal education level in North America has increased over time, the younger adults in a community may be expected to have a higher education level than their elders. If the older people have a higher proportion of untreated symptoms in a community, we would expect to find those in the lower education category also overrepresented. Just such is the case. In Upper Hammonds Plains, for example, the under-thirty age group reports proportionately more untreated symptoms (83 percent) than those in other age groups; those with more than an eighth grade education are also overrepresented by 9 percentage points above the baseline. Thus, it appears to be important to consider age and education concurrently if one is positing one or the other as a potential cultural barrier.

Illness Behavior

The way one behaves when ill is in part culturally determined and may in some instances act as a barrier to the procurement of modern medical care. We are limited to three aspects of health action: (1)

Table 2. Education and age as related to the frequency of untreated symptoms: Percent reporting one or more untreated symptoms

Education and age	Tancook Islands			Upper Hammonds Plains			Mulgrave Park		
	Percent	(N)	P.D.*	Percent	(N)	P.D.*	Percent	(N)	P.D.*
Education									
Less than Grade 8	42	(26)	+ 2	60	(20)	– 4	50	(36)	+ 6
Grade 8 or more	38	(40)	– 2	73	(30)	+ 9	42	(100)	– 2
Age									
Under 30	17	(12)	–23	83	(12)	+19	42	(38)	– 2
30-45	44	(18)	+ 4	65	(17)	+ 1	55	(51)	+11
46-60	33	(21)	– 7	61	(18)	– 3	41	(32)	– 3
Over 60	65	(17)	+25	40	(5)	–24	14	(14)	–30

*The percentage difference (P.D.) is the reported percentage in each subcategory relative to the community baseline percentage. The untreated symptom baseline for the Tancook Islands is 40 percent; for Upper Hammonds Plains, 64 percent; and for Mulgrave Park, 44 percent (see Table 1).

home remedy usage, primarily the natural or vegetable kind—such as raw potato, catnip tea, or senna; (2) self-treatment, as evidenced by a reluctance to consult a physician except when "everything I try fails;" and (3) the initial source of help outside of the family that one turns to when ill.

Both those who name "the doctor" as the first person they consult when ill and those who admit that they go to a doctor before everything they try fails tend to be underrepresented in their reporting of untreated medical symptoms (Table 3). This pattern is evidenced in each community, but is relatively weakest in Mulgrave Park. Perhaps this is because the geographic isolation experienced here is not as great as in the rural areas.

An urban/rural difference is also evidenced with respect to home remedy usage. In both Upper Hammonds Plains and on the Tancook Islands those who do not claim to use home remedies are greatly underrepresented in the reporting of untreated symptoms. It seems that higher home remedy usage in the rural areas tends to retard the speed with which modern medical attention is sought. Since many of the ingredients in home remedies are plants, one would expect the effect of home remedy usage to be more dramatic in rural than urban communities.

Evaluation of Physicians

Next let us consider the possible effect that our respondents' evaluation of doctors' services may have on differential reporting of untreated symptoms. Evaluation is confined to skepticism concerning what "doctors say they can do," and satisfaction with treatment received in the past.

Although the absolute number of people in each community reporting skepticism is low (a total of 42), those with untreated symptoms are overrepresented in the more highly skeptical group in each community (Table 4). Similarly, while only a small absolute number of people (a total of 25) are dissatisfied with treatment received from doctors in the past, the dissatisfied groups, with the exception of the Tancook Islands, are overrepresented in their reporting of untreated symptoms.

If one is skeptical and has been dissatisfied with medical care in the past, one may be hesitant in seeking treatment in the present. However, since there is slight empirical variation in the skepticism and satisfaction variables and because of the possible instability of the findings, no further interpretation of these data will be attempted. The potential theoretical importance of these variables as cultural barriers to care remains unchallenged.

Table 3. Illness behaviors as potential barriers to medical care in three communities: Percent reporting one or more untreated symptoms

Illness behaviors	Tancook Islands			Upper Hammonds Plains			Mulgrave Park		
	Percent	(N)	P.D.*	Percent	(N)	P.D.*	Percent	(N)	P.D.*
Immediate help source[a]									
Doctor	32	(41)	− 8	53	(17)	−11	36	(63)	− 8
Other	55	(27)	+15	69	(36)	+ 5	51	(73)	+ 7
Self-treatment[b]									
High	48	(21)	+ 8	71	(34)	+ 7	47	(57)	+ 3
Low	38	(47)	− 2	53	(19)	−11	42	(79)	− 2
Home remedy usage[c]									
4 or more	61	(33)	+21	89	(9)	+25	45	(38)	+ 1
1-3	25	(20)	−15	71	(14)	+ 7	42	(59)	− 2
None	08	(13)	−32	59	(27)	− 5	46	(39)	+ 2

*The percentage difference (P.D.) is found by subtracting the percent reporting untreated symptoms in each category from the community baseline (see Table 2).

[a]Respondents were asked, "Who is the first person you go to for help outside of the family when you are sick?" In the "other" category, such responses as "friend," "neighbor," "nobody," and "God" are included. Four "nurse" responses are included in the "doctor" category.

[b]The degree of self-treatment was inferred from responses to this statement: "I see a doctor only after everything else I try fails." Those agreeing were categorized "high self-treatment"; those disagreeing as "low self-treatment."

[c]A home remedies list compiled from Creighton contained 24 items; e.g., senna, peppermint tea, salt, pumpkin seed, onion poultice, raw potato, garlic, sulphur and molasses. [See: Creighton, Helen. *Blue-Magic: Popular Beliefs and Superstitions in Nova Scotia* (Toronto: Ryerson, 1968)]. Respondents were asked if they used each, either "as medicines or for health reasons."

Table 4. The community's evaluation of the physician as a potential barrier to the receipt of medical care: Percent reporting one or more untreated symptoms

Evaluation of physician	Tancook Islands			Upper Hammonds Plains			Mulgrave Park		
	Percent	(N)	P.D.*	Percent	(N)	P.D.*	Percent	(N)	P.D.*
Skepticism[a]									
High	50	(14)	+10	100	(6)	+36	64	(22)	+20
Low	39	(54)	- 1	60	(47)	- 4	32	(114)	-12
Satisfaction[b]									
High	45	(60)	+ 5	62	(50)	- 2	41	(122)	- 3
Low	12	(8)	-28	100	(3)	+36	71	(14)	+27

*The percentage difference (P.D.) is found by subtracting the percent reporting untreated symptoms in each category from the community baseline (see Table 2).
[a]Skepticism was assessed by the following question: "Do you ever doubt what doctors say they can do for you?" Those agreeing with this statement were classified "high skepticism"; all other respondents were placed in the "low skepticism" category.
[b]The following question attempted to tap the satisfaction respondents experienced with the treatment they have received in the past: "In general, have you been satisfied with the treatment that you have received from doctors?" Those responding "yes" were labeled "high satisfaction"; the remainder, "low satisfaction."

DISCUSSION

Since there is a group in each community reporting untreated symptoms, cultural barriers to treatment may be present. The cultural barriers which emerge, however, are different for each community.

In Tancook, overrepresentation of respondents reporting untreated symptoms tends to be centered in the older age group and among the less educated. Furthermore, the overrepresentation of untreated symptoms is the most clear-cut among those reporting relatively high home remedy use and a reluctance to go to the doctor unless "everything else fails." Along with a proclivity toward self-treatment on the Tancook Islands is the tendency for those with medically untreated symptoms to report someone other than "the doctor" as the first person they see outside of the family when ill.

In Upper Hammonds Plains, the profile of the group overrepresented with respect to untreated symptoms tends to be under 30, and to fall in the upper half of the education dichotomy.

The illness behaviors parallel the ones reported for the Tancook Islands except for the fact that the tendency to go to the doctor only when "everything else fails" tends to be more clearly associated with those reporting untreated symptoms in Upper Hammonds Plains than on the Tancook Islands.

In Mulgrave Park, those between the ages of 30 and 45 tend to be overrepresented with respect to the proportion of untreated symptoms they report. The oldest group is the most solidly underrepresented.

The cultural barrier of most relevance in Mulgrave Park may be illness behavior which results in one's seeing someone outside the family other than the doctor upon first becoming ill. Perhaps one's position in a primary group network determines at what point the individual sees a physician rather than the contact with the physician being initiated on the basis of the individual's assessment of his own condition.[14,15]

CONCLUSION

The data indicate that the cultural barriers investigated are potentially more relevant in the two rural communities than in the urban housing project. Variables centering upon self-treatment tend to be more strongly associated with the overrepresentation of medically untreated symptoms in the rural communities than in the urban area.

Although self-treatment may be more prominent in the rural communities than in urban Mulgrave Park, the factors explaining the phenomenon may be quite dissimilar. One would have to have knowledge of a community's social structure and history in order to account for the presence of a particular cultural barrier. Tancook's home remedy history would appear to be the key to understanding self-treatment on these islands, while the cultural isolation of the black community, Upper Hammonds Plains, may explain the proclivity towards self-treatment there. In both communities the distance from a medical center and the absence of a resident physician would also have to be considered.

Although poor communities and poor people have poverty in common, the culture of poverty — especially in its relationship to medical deprivation — may be specific to each community. Poor rural communities may be expected to vary as well as urban ones. If such is the case, providing medical care for the poor is a task more complex than removing the financial barrier. Since distinctive patterns of health action were found for each medically deprived community, the data suggest the need for medical plans to recognize the relevance of the community's culture to the success of the medical plan. It is not enough to be aware of potential cultural barriers, but it is necessary to know which ones may be operating in which community and why.

The concept of the community health center in North America generally is increasingly being viewed as integral to the rationalization of the health care delivery system. It is "touted as the remedy for a range of divergent . . . problems such as patient alienation and the rapidly spiralling cost of medical care."[16]   Since a community health center tends to be organized on a local model, this type of health structure might be responsive to particular aspects of the health culture of the community it serves, especially if there is heavy consumer involvement in the activities and policies of the center. The community health center could help to identify indigenous cultural barriers to medical care; and when such barriers are known, the community health center might be effective in altering the barriers to medical participation.

Canada—especially in comparison with the United States—has made giant strides in the development of its health care delivery system. It indeed would be unfortunate if provinces like Nova Scotia were to think that the job of providing health care to the public is over. As long as a token financial barrier exists and as long as cultural barriers persist, poor communities will continue to be medically deprived in spite of medical reforms such as medical services insurance.

NOTES

1. Foster, George. "Problems in Intercultural Health Programs," Pamphlet 12, Social Science Research Council, New York (April 1958).

2. Paul, Benjamin D. *Health, Culture, and Community: Case Studies of Public Reactions to Health Programs* (New York: Russell Sage, 1955).

3. All provinces in Canada have a medical care scheme funded from provincial and federal sources. The cost of drugs, dental care, and medically unnecessary operations are not included in the coverage.

4. Eckstein, Harry. *The English Health Service: Its Origins, Structure and Achievements* (Cambridge, Mass.: Harvard University Press, 1958).

5. Some physicians bill their patients 15 percent above the amount allowed on the governmental fee schedule, claiming that the full cost of their services has not been met. Also, there are potential costs which the patient must meet, such as transportation, time lost from work, child care, medicines, and special diets.

6. Rosenblatt, Daniel, and Suchman, E. A. "The Underutilization of Medical Care Services by Blue-Collarites." In: Shostak, A. B., and Gomberg, William. (eds.) *Blue-Collar World: Studies of the American Worker* (Englewood Cliffs, N. J.: Prentice-Hall, 1964).

7. Suchman, Edward A. "Social Factors in Medical Deprivation," *American Journal of Public Health* 55:11 (November 1965).

8. Six communities comprise the larger study; included are Acadian French and Mic Mac Indian. Data analysis has not been concluded for all communities.

9. Creighton, Helen. *Bluenose Magic: Popular Beliefs and Superstitions in Nova Scotia* (Toronto: Ryerson, 1968).

10. Koos, Earl L. *The Health of Regionville* (New York: Columbia University Press, 1954).

11. Non-medical household surveyors have been advised to use symptom categories rather than formal diagnostic disease categories in order to obtain a valid health assessment. See: Feldman, Jacob J. "The Household Interview Survey as a Technique for the Collection of Morbidity Date," *Journal of Chronic Diseases* 11:553 (1960).

It is recognized that by recording self-reported symptoms, however, one is focusing upon a subjective rather than an objective health status. According to the research objective, subjective health may be more relevant than objective health. There is reason to assume that an individuals's behavior is affected as much by his own subjective evaluation of his health as by a physician's objective report. See: Suchman, Edward A.; Phillips, B. S.; and Streib, G. F. "An Analysis of the Validity of Health Questionnaires," *Social Forces* 36:223 (1958).

12. Such symptoms as dizzy spells, chest pains, unusual bleeding, and sore joints are included. The total list of sixteen items was compiled with reference to similar studies; namely, Ludwig, Edward G., and Gibson, Geoffrey. "Self-perception of Sickness and the Seeking of Medical Care," *Journal of Health and Social Behavior* 10:125–133 (June 1969).

13. Polgar, Steven, "Health Action in Cross-Cultural Perspective." In: Freeman, H. E., *et al* (eds.) *Handbook of Medical Sociology* (Englewood Cliffs, N. J.: Prentice-Hall, 1963).

14. Freidson, Eliot. *Patients' Views of Medical Practice* (New York: Russell Sage, 1961).

15. Weaver, Thomas, "Use of Hypothetical Situations in a Study of Spanish American Illness Referral Systems," *Human Organization* 29:2 (Summer 1970).

16. Kisch. Arnold J. "Adapting Health Manpower to Consumer Needs and Cultural Expectations," *Inquiry* 8:40 (September 1971).

Part III

COMMUNITY INVOLVEMENT IN HEALTH-CARE DELIVERY

Consumer participation has been a watchword in health-care discussions since the early 1960s, when the Office of Economic Opportunity launched its "war on poverty." Moynihan labeled the OEO call for maximum feasible participation of consumers a case of "maximum feasible misunderstanding."* The papers that follow provide some perspective on the problems inherent in consumer involvement, at both the community and personal level.

If the consumers are poor, it is not enough to give them what they want in the way of services. They need to feel they have some control over the events in their lives, especially as they affect personal health and welfare. The demand for participation, not only in planning but in decision-making as well, must be satisfied, according to Hochbaum. On the other hand, lay members of planning bodies are not equipped to determine technical issues that require the expertise of health professionals. In this confrontation between the consumer and the provider of health services, Hochbaum places the burden of understanding and exhibiting patience and tolerance on the health professionals.

Hochbaum dissects the concept of consumer participation and raises a series of provocative and puzzling questions. Who *is* this consumer who acts as a lay member of the decision-making body? Whom does he represent? How do you know he is representative? How can he remain representative? How can consumers and providers communicate meaningfully with each other? His questions remain pertinent and challenging even after several years of experience with

*Daniel P. Moynihan, *Maximum Feasible Misunderstanding*. (New York: The Free Press, 1969).

the concept of consumer participation. We are still open to his criticism that despite our enthusiasm to embrace this idea it cannot be justified on the basis of demonstrated results.

If Hochbaum's questions dampen our enthusiasm for consumer participation, Geiger's forthright presentation does much to restore confidence in the concept. Writing on the basis of his extensive work in establishing a neighborhood health center, Geiger examines the provider's basic conflict about relinquishing psychological, as well as real, control over health care. He argues that unless the professional can make the adjustments necessary to accept problem definition from the perspective of the poor consumer, the services offered will have little impact on breaking the poverty cycle.

To surrender professional autonomy is a serious challenge. Difficult even in circumstances of relative social equality, it is even harder for those working with the poor. Yet, this transfer of responsibility is all the more crucial. Because of the vast gap in sophistication between the provider and the consumer, there is a vast difference between services of a technically high quality rendered *to* people and services organized *by* those same people. Despite the tremendous gain in effectiveness possible through such a shift in responsibility, it remains problematic whether professionals—both medical and social welfare—can be persuaded to relinquish control.

The reader interested in further information on this subject may refer to the following references listed in the annotated bibliography:

Apostle and Oder, 1967	Breslow, 1967	Gales, 1970
Bamberger, 1966	Feldman and Salber, 1969	Kent and Smith, 1967
Blum et al., 1968	Ferguson, 1970	Leveson, 1970

4. Consumer Participation In Health Planning

Toward Conceptual Clarification

G. M. HOCHBAUM

Consumer participation, which has its roots in concepts and ideas advanced and stressed for many years by behavioral scientists, health educators, and others, has suddenly become the focus of attention by the other health professions. As is the fate of many such newly discovered concepts, it is being greeted with attitudes ranging from total rejection and dubious caution to overoptimistic enthusiasm, and is embraced by some as though it were a poisonous snake, by others as though it heralded an era of social harmony and of perfect health services for all.

No careful and objective student could fail to recognize that this concept holds both great promises and many risks, and that it has to evolve through many trials and mutations before it will emerge in forms which lend themselves to any real assessment of its worth. Then, and only then, will it be possible to evaluate its strength and its weaknesses, and its ultimate contributions to the health and welfare of our communities. The final result will be either to discard it altogether, or—more likely—to adopt it with some modification as a method which under certain conditions, and for certain purposes, can help to realize at least some of the hopes we now place into it.

But it behooves us at this time of our initial and often clumsy trials with this approach not to be swayed either by exaggerated expectations or by hostile rejection—both born of emotional bias— but to observe and evaluate it rationally and with all the knowledge and tools available particularly from the behavioral sciences. It is

From the *American Journal of Public Health* 59 (September 1969), pp. 1698–1705, reprinted by permission of the author and publisher.

This paper was presented before the Public Health Education Section of the American Public Health Association at the Ninety-Sixth Annual Meeting in Detroit, Michigan, November 12, 1968.

especially important at this stage to analyze the social processes that take place in the interaction between the groups that confront one another in "consumer participation"—the representatives of the "consumers" and the representatives of the health professions—for it is in this interaction where the hazards lie, but also where help with the achievement of our goals may be found.

I would like to discuss certain problems which frequently arise in this interaction.

CHANGES IN OUR SOCIETY

We have witnessed over the past few years some radical changes in the structure and nature of our society. Segments of our population, which until recently have played a passive role, are demanding full and equal access to all the resources and services that our society is capable of providing—many of which these people have been at least partially deprived up to now. I am thinking primarily of our urban black population, of other minorities, and of the poor in general. We have been trying to respond to these demands by making more and better health services available to them, by locating health centers within their neighborhoods, and by removing economic barriers for the utilization of health resources and services.

If accessibility of sufficient high-quality health services to the disadvantaged were the only issue at stake, these steps should logically be able to satisfy the demands of these disadvantaged as long as we carried them out effectively and on a large enough scale. But accessibility is not the only issue. Indeed, it is not even the most important and urgent issue.

Behind these demands by our disadvantaged citizens, and behind their demands for better housing, for better educational and job opportunities, and for a voice in the affairs in our society—behind all of these demands lies an awakened and steadily growing need and desire to live, to feel like, and to be treated as fully equal citizens of our society.

For a person with such a need and such a desire it is not enough to be given what he wants. He feels an urge to have something to say about *what* is given, *where*, and *in what ways* it is given. He wants to know that he has at least some control over such things which, after all, affect his health and welfare and his very life.

Therefore, some kind of participation in health planning—or for that matter in planning for a variety of other community programs— is of great importance to many of these people for its own sake, as a visible symbol of their equal human rights, quite apart from the more tangible beneficial health results that may stem from such participation. But this fact tells us also that it is not enough for the authorities to patiently listen to the views and ideas expressed by the representatives of the people before the authorities reach decisions—even when these decisions take such views and ideas into account.

DEMAND FOR PARTICIPATION

To put this differently: The demand for participation in planning on the part of the disadvantaged (especially of the more vocal and militant segments) cannot be satisfied for long if we offer them merely a platform to express their views but reserve the right for final decisions for ourselves. Their demands can be satisfied only if they feel that they share in the decision-making process itself. Failure to satisfy these demands can have very serious consequences not only for health services themselves, but equally for community politics and race relations.

It is this question of sharing in the *decision-making process* (rather than of merely participating in planning discussions) which is a potential source of problems and friction. The reason is that each of the two groups which confront one another—the health professionals and the spokesmen of the consumer population—may bring different and conflicting attitudes and expectations to their joint meetings. The health professionals probably feel that *they* are the experts when it comes to people's medical care needs and to methods for meeting these needs. They may be willing to listen to the consumer spokesmen, and even to make allowances for some of their special wishes and preferences, but are often unlikely to give up their own authority to make final decisions even on these wishes.

The consumer spokesmen, on the other hand, may feel justified in claiming a far greater slice of the issues to be decided than the professionals are inclined to yield. As mentioned earlier, these spokesmen may view the confrontation with the professionals and authorities as a test for their newly won political and racial ambitions, extending far beyond their more limited desire to merely assure better health services for their people. Therefore, they may demand and expect a share even in decisions concerning aspects which they are not equipped to judge and handle, although they may be fully aware of this lack of competence. For Example, in one such actual case, consumer spokesmen insisted on certain types of medical personnel to be on duty in a planned neighborhood health center in order to be ready at any time to provide medical care for certain specific medical problems. The health professionals rejected the demand. They argued that such problems occurred only relatively rarely, that even when they did, they would not represent emergency cases, and that they could be handled more efficiently by referring patients elsewhere. These arguments fell on deaf ears despite their obvious soundness. A great deal of hostility was aroused on both sides. The health professionals were perplexed and angered by the apparent unreasonableness and stubbornness of the consumer representatives, and the latter saw the episode as evidence that so-called "consumer participation" was just a cover-up for continued refusal of equal health services for the black community.

What had actually happened was this. The consumer spokesmen honestly believed, though erroneously, that all health facilities in the more affluent white communities have such personnel and offer such medical services. As far as these spokesmen were concerned, they only demanded the same for their own clinic. In other words, the question of whether such services were actually needed was really irrelevant to them. But they attached great importance to these services as symbols of equity with the more affluent white society.

In the light of this, the strategy by the health professionals in the planning group would have been better if they had not argued against the demand only on the basis of its medical virtues or lack of virtues. An attempt should have been made to demonstrate to the consumer representatives the fact that health facilities in affluent white communities do *not* as a rule have such medical personnel and services, that those patients who require such services are usually referred elsewhere, and that therefore the demand was not justified *on the basis of the concept of equity*.

NEED FOR COOPERATION

This somewhat oversimplified example illustrates the frequent and disruptive problem that arises when two such groups look at the same issue from two quite divergent points of view without being aware of this fact. While the health professionals are usually primarily concerned with the medical care aspects and argue their own views on the basis of *medical care* considerations, the consumers are equally or more concerned with the *social, political*, and *racial* aspects and argue their case correspondingly, usually to the irritation and total consternation of the professionals in the group. Unless this fact is understood by the latter, and unless they learn to cope with it, much time can be lost, a good deal of hostility can be aroused on both sides, and the end result may be very disheartening.

The example also illustrates a second problem that should be anticipated and understood. As pointed out earlier, the spokesmen of our disadvantaged population groups, especially the more vocal and militant spokesmen of our urban black communities, demand to an increasing extent a real and substantive role in the actual decision-making process. In fact, they often demand to be *the* ones who make the decisions and regard the health professionals as persons whose job it is to meet these demands merely by making their skills and competencies available. This view is of course in conflict with the views of even those generally flexible and liberal professionals who are perfectly willing to allow the lay sector in the planning group to make all sorts of decisions on nonmedical and nontechnical matters, but who still reserve professional and technical decisions for themselves.

Alan Mayers has used "decisional territory" to describe the scope of issues on which a given group lays claim for being entitled to make the decisions. The two sectors in the planning group—the consumers and the professionals—each bring their own decisional territories to the confrontations. One can visualize these territories graphically as two overlapping circles. One encompasses all the issues for which the professionals claim the sole right to make decisions since they feel such decisions require special expertise which only they possess. The other circle contains all the issues for which the consumers claim the right to make decisions. The area formed by the overlapping of the two circles represents the potential battleground because both groups lay claim to it.

Such an overlap of the two decisional territories is probably unavoidable and must be expected. Sometimes it may be reduced if the two groups succeed in reaching some prior agreements as to the boundaries of their respective territories. But this solution is not always feasible and does not always work.

It is very important and necessary for the professionals to understand *why* lay members of the planning body insist on determining technical issues which they are clearly not equipped to judge. In this confrontation between consumers and providers of health services, the burden of understanding the other and the burden of exhibiting the skills and the often superhuman patience and tolerance necessary to cope with such conflicts, rest clearly primarily with us, the health professionals.

TRAINING CONSUMERS AND PROFESSIONALS

It is on *this* point that I slightly disagree with those who place their emphasis on needs to train merely the consumer representatives in planning skills, on certain technical aspects of the health area, and in other related matters. Without denying the need for such training, we must place still greater emphasis on the need to train the *professionals* so that they develop the understanding and skills required for resolving the conflicts inherent in such confrontations.

Let me summarize the main points made so far:

1. We must recognize and accept the fact that it is the *consumers* of health services who are the final and proper judges of what kinds of services they want, how they want them delivered, what form they should take, and in what setting they should be provided. It is only on the medical and other technical details that the health professions have any exclusive right to make decisions. This leaves, of course, the gray area of overlap which is the primary source of conflict.

The main problems arise from two facts. The first is that the health professions have traditionally usurped the absolute right to be the final arbiters on *all* issues pertaining to health and are usually unwilling or unable to surrender this right. The second fact is that because of the emotions engendered by the social and racial revolution, consumer groups are often unable or unwilling to accept even reasonable limits to *their* decisional territory and therefore demand at least symbolic rights to make decisions also on some issues beyond their competency.

2. It has long been a basic principle of health education that the people with whom we work should be involved at early stages of planning. But today's vogue of "consumer participation" has primarily grown out of political rather than educational concerns. It is seen as a means to help the disadvantaged guide their newly emerging aggressive demands for equal rights and greater power into constructive channels and to calm our restive communities.

We have learned from work in industrial psychology that participation of employees in management decisions does hold the promise of more ready acceptance of managerial innovations. Also quite plausible claims for greater utilization of health services following consumer participation in the planning of such services have been made in several instances. Yet I know of no really convincing or even persuasive evidence that such consumer participation is resulting in health services which are any better and more effective than health services that are planned by professionals who make a concerted effort to learn about, understand, and appreciate the characteristics and needs of the people to be served. In fact, I suspect, that often the opposite is true. Joint planning by consumers and providers can easily lead to compromises between conflicting opinions, to dilution of standards, and thereby to *less* adequate services. Nonetheless, we must first find ways to accommodate the political, social, and racial issues and to satisfy these reasonably well in the eyes of our target population. To the extent to which we succeed in this, we should be able to develop a better basis for constructive consumer participation in planning with diminishing conflicts on the respective decisional territories. To repeat, we must deal with the social, political, and racial issues *before* we can generate the proper attitudes on *both* sides for more effective joint health planning.

PROBLEM OF COMMUNICATION

There is still another problem which seems to arise whenever a group of people—whether they come from the consumer population or from the professional sector—get together to discuss the subject of consumer participation. This problem is one of communication and stems from the fact that the term "consumer participation" has been used freely and carelessly to describe a wide spectrum of modalities of the underlying concept. A short time ago I witnessed a rather heated and prolonged dispute over the desirability or undesirability of such consumer participation. After a while it became clear that each member of the group was talking about a different thing although all used the same term. When each person was asked to write privately on a piece of paper what his concept or mental image of "consumer participation" was, and the several responses were compared, this fact was dramatically brought home, and resulted in a much more orderly and productive discussion from then on. In fact, to everyone's surprise, there was much less real disagreement than the preceding discussions seemed to reflect.

The question, then, as to what consumer participation really means, needs constant clarification and, in turn, gives rise to other highly important questions.

For example, what is meant by "consumers"? Are consumers only those who obtain services within a given delivery system, or also those who do not, yet obtain their services from some other delivery system such as the private sector of medicine? Do we include as "consumers" even those who do not yet, but hopefully will obtain services at some later date? Does the term "consumer" apply *equally* to the individual with a broken finger who comes to a clinic into which he has never set foot so far and probably will not set foot again for a long time if ever, as well as to the individual who conscientiously comes for his yearly check-up in addition to seeking medical advice whenever appropriate reasons exist? If we include any other persons, in addition to those who *actually* obtain health services from a specified delivery system, the term "consumer" has a misleading connotation and should be dropped.

What do we mean by "participation"? If consumer representatives are permitted to express their needs, wishes, and complaints but the decisions as to what to do about these rest with the professionals, is this participation? Or does the term imply an actual sharing of decision-making power?

The term "consumer participation" implies the selection of spokesmen for the consumer population. Who are they to be and how are they to be selected? Should they be the more educated and knowledgeable members of the population, those who are likely to bring the best understanding of the issues involved to the planning? If so, can they be selected by the lay population or must they be identified on the basis of their qualifications as determined by professionals? Are the better educated and more affluent members of, say, the urban black ghetto really true representatives, or are they almost as far removed from the people for whom they are to speak as are the professionals themselves? Or should these representatives be selected from the very segments of the population which heretofore have been its most disadvantaged? If so, would they not be so uneducated, so naive about health services and about planning, and so incompetent as to be unable to contribute meaningfully to the planning? Moreover, would attempts to communicate between them and the professionals be so difficult as to be almost futile?

ANSWERS AND OBJECTIVES

These are only some of the questions with which we need to struggle. Each of them may have one best answer or it may have several answers depending on context and situation. The trouble is that in discussions on consumer participation each person carries with him a certain image of his concept of the term—an image that is a mosaic of his own private and implicit answers to these questions and one that may be different from that of some others in the group. It is not always necessary to resolve all such differences and reach complete consensus as to any one specific set of answers. But it is necessary for each person in the group to make his own "image" explicit in order to avoid the confusion of a dialogue in which similarities and differences between persons' concepts are obscured by everyone's use of the same but undefined terms, thereby giving rise to apparent but not necessarily real agreements or conflicts.

A very similar problem is often generated by the question of *why* we should advocate consumer participation in the first place. What are the objectives which we try to pursue by it, what specific purposes is it to serve? Is it to bring about more effective delivery of more appropriate and better health services through assuring their greater accessibility to those who find it difficult now to obtain such services? Is it to assure that the services provided are in accord with the needs and desires of the consumer population *as felt by them?* Or do we aim at larger goals of which the actual delivery of health services is only a part? For example, do we hope that consumer participation will lead to a greater awareness of health matters on the part of the population, to increase motivation to improve their own health status, to a spilling over of the educational effects of the services provided into the realm of people's personal health habits and practices? Do we also see consumer participation in *health* planning as an effort coordinated with participation in planning for housing, education, job training, and other community problems, and leading to the political, economic, and social motivation of population groups which have heretofore been relatively passive, naive, and helpless in the face of the community power structure? Is there also the more or less implicit hope that such participation will lead to a calming of the increasing turbulence in our restless cities?

Depending on one's views of these goals and purposes, different approaches, methods, and procedures in consumer participation will have to take prominent positions. Especially when the question of evaluation is raised, different criteria and measurements would be appropriate, and disagreements concerning these may be less a function of disagreements concerning the values of the several possible criteria and measurements than a function of disagreements concerning goals and purposes. Again, if these latter remain only implicit and are not explicitly clarified, it will be difficult if not impossible to discuss such matters rationally and to reach consensus.

SUMMARY

The problems discussed in this paper are only a few of those that must be considered. They have been selected for attention because I believe them to be fundamental and crucial to the future of consumer participation. The concept of consumer participation in the planning of consumer health and welfare programs, while not new, is only now entering into the arena where the future of our society is being forged. As we struggle with the concept itself and with ways of translating it into operations, we must be sensitive to the fact that we are treading on uncertain ground and are groping for new ways of dealing with problems as old as human history. Precipitous commitments to specific solutions can have exceedingly serious consequences. We must be willing to analyze and evaluate on a continuous basis both the concept and its various operational counterparts as they change with time and experiences; and we must do so in the light of theoretical considerations as much as against the purposefully planned accumulation of reliable observations and concrete data.

It is this last requirement—that of rigorous, factual, and objective study and evaluation—which I believe to be of paramount importance. It is here where social scientists should and can make their most significant contributions because the question is predominantly a social and not a medical one.

I do not mean to imply by this that an evaluation of biomedical results is not also needed, but the process by which such results are to be achieved is a social one of which the actual medical procedures are only a part. In fact, when we look at some of the most disturbing health problems of the disadvantaged such as, for example, infant mortality, there is considerable evidence that they have social and behavioral components that contribute more to these problems themselves than the biomedical components. Thus the effectiveness of health services dealing with such problems must be assessed against consumers' behavior as well as against such traditional measures as the number of people treated or reduction in morbidity and mortality among consumers.

Thus the importance of social science to an evaluation of consumer participation, as a means to improve health services and the welfare of our communities in general, is beyond doubt. But social science can make constructive contributions only if social scientists approach the questions raised in this paper as true scientists who are objective and nonpartisan—whatever their own personal feelings are about the disadvantaged and about the nature of the political, economic, or social issues involved. And they can make such contributions only if they are permitted to carry out objective, nonpartisan studies, and if the results are considered by the health and the political leadership—even if these results should run counter to preconceived notions and to wishful thinking.

Social scientists represent, of course, not the only professional group that can play this role, and they cannot do so without close cooperation with other professions. Nonetheless, they probably come closest to meeting the professional and technical requirements for reliable and objective investigations both of the concept of consumer participation in the planning of health services and of the various operational systems based upon it. But whoever may carry out such scientific investigations, these are desperately and urgently needed. Only with their help can we hope to learn whether, under what conditions, for what ends, to what extent, and in what forms the concept of consumer participation has real social value, or whether its continued encouragement will bring about a chain reaction which may intensify other problems or even generate new ones in our communities.

After all, it is entirely possible that out of our present, often fumbling experiments with the concept, there will emerge elements of more effective health services delivery systems. On the other hand, we must guard against welcoming the concept precipitously out of a feeling of frustration, even of futility concerning our present systems, much as a cancer patient—whose confidence in legitimate medical resources has been shaken—may turn to Krebiozen merely because it is claimed to have some special healing powers not possessed by traditional medicine.

It must be admitted that as of now the tendency to embrace consumer participation in planning and especially in decision-making is not based on much demonstrable and objective evidence as to its actual results. But too much is at stake to allow this trend to continue unchecked unless and until we have more factual knowledge on which to judge and plan a development which could irrevocably change our health care and even our entire social system.

5. Of the Poor, By the Poor, or For the Poor

The Mental Health Implications of Social Control of Poverty Programs

H. JACK GEIGER

Almost since the beginning of the "war on poverty," and our recognition that poverty is a national problem of great social consequence, we have been engaged in a running debate over the orientation and control of anti-poverty programs. Shall there be programs *for* the poor, in the classic public welfare sense? Shall there be programs *by* the poor, involving (in that wonderfully nebulous phrase) "maximum feasible participation" of the target population in the implementation of programs, in the acquisition of new jobs, in consultative or advisory roles that give (or seem to give) a share in decision-making, policy-making, choice, and management? Or shall there be programs *of* the poor, implying not merely participation but control and power—the real social power that comes from choice of programs and from control of money and jobs?

This debate, this choice between passive receptivity, participation and power, is important. It involves much more than the methods of anti-poverty programs; it contains within it real differences over the diagnosis and formulation of poverty problems, on the one hand, and over the very goals of anti-poverty programs, on the other. And, as we shall see, it has implications for those concerned with mental health, particularly the mental health of impoverished, deprived populations.

The purpose of this paper is to consider the substance of this dispute, and its relationship to mental health, by drawing on our own experience with the Tufts Comprehensive Community Health Action Program in Boston. This is an intensive program involving both the

From *Psychiatric Research Reports* 21 (April 1967), pp. 55–65, reprinted by permission of author and the American Psychiatric Association.

provision of comprehensive health services and the formation of a new community organization in a participating *and* policy-making role in one well-defined community.

First, however, it might be well to review the three positions briefly, beginning with poor old *"for* the poor," the public welfare formulation. It doesn't get a great deal of attention these days. The very existence of the "war on poverty" is in part a statement that the existing assistance mechanisms are failures, mere palliatives that institutionalize dependency—and inadequate palliatives, at that. Whether or not this statement is accurate, it is widely believed. Yet it should be noted that the welfare-public assistance system is still the *major* system in the United States, far larger in the amount of money it spends, the services it provides and pays for, the number of lives it touches, and the impact it has on those lives than any other system. It should also be noted that while most of us readily accept the hypothesis that money and services alone cannot eliminate poverty, particularly hard-core, three-generation, multi-problem poverty, we have never tested it. As Levitan points out, the resources of the system are concentrated on providing a substandard income, thereby leaving most recipients in abject poverty. The average income paid by the government to AFDC recipients, for example, is about $1.00 a day.[1] One reason for the continuation in poverty of most people on public assistance is simply that the level of public assistance keeps them there, struggling for the very essentials of existence. Finally, it must be noted that many public welfare officials have responded with panic and hostility to the threat of new kinds of programs, to the idea of doing things with people rather than for them, and to the suggestion that control and power be taken from their hands and given to their clients. Consider, for example, this recent public statement by a Chicago welfare official: "The leadership has formed . . . to mobilize public and private agencies whose experience can assure victory. Some demagogues screech that they would turn the job and the accompanying millions of dollars over to a planless, self-appointed spokesman who asserts that he represents the poor."

At the other extreme are the organizations *of* the poor, emphasizing what Haggstrom calls "the psychology of the powerlessness of the poor.[2] Most of the poor, he adds, are "heavily dependent on outside forces . . . enforced dependence gives them little scope for action under their own control . . . being powerless, with needs that must be met, leads to dependence on organizations meeting those needs . . . dependency relationships become institutionalized and perpetuated. The dominant community must provide the poor with participation in the decision-making process. Joint initiative by the poor on their own behalf can be most effectively exercised by powerful conflict organizations based in these neighborhoods." The argument is that indigenous, locally-based and locally-led conflict and protest organizations, fighting for power and control over jobs, services, money and programs, involve the uninvolved; that they are in themselves educational, provide the necessary first step for other and later kinds of involvement with the larger social order, train leadership, and at once provide and fight for an end to alienation, institutionalized dependency, failure, withdrawal, and frustration. By implication, any other system is a sellout, an opiate, or the same old hand-me-down welfare system in a shiny new package. These organizations have roots and parallels in the civil rights movement, with which they are closely allied; and indeed, there is evidence that the civil rights movement has involved the previously uninvolved, and has psychosocial consequences beyond civil rights—for example, Fishman and Solomon's finding that crimes of violence decrease as direct civil rights action increases in a community.[3]

Somewhere in between are the proponents of programs *by* the poor, emphasizing "maximum feasible participation" of the target population in the implementation of programs and services, oriented toward doing things with people rather than for them, sometimes providing a *share* of control, policy- and decision-making for the poor, but usually leaving safely in the dominant community's hands all decisions as to what is "maximum," what is "feasible," and what constitutes "participation." These proponents agree with the protest-and-conflict supporters that there is a subculture of poverty, a poverty cycle or syndrome that extends far beyond mere economic level, and a range of associated psychological or psycho-social characteristics; but where one group sees powerlessness and lack of control as central and primary issues, and responds by saying, "march!", the other sees participation, involvement, and the acquisition of new skills and experiences as more important than control, and asks, "What do we do when the marching stops?"

Our experiences in the Tufts Comprehensive Community Health Action Program at Columbia Point in Boston relate to all three points of view. Very briefly, under an Office of Economic Opportunity research and demonstration grant, our Department of Preventive Medicine undertook to design, build, equip, organize, and staff a comprehensive, twenty-four-hour-a-day neighborhood health center, providing the full range of both preventive and curative ambulatory services: emergency, sick child and well child, sick adult and adult health screening, home medical care and home nursing, health education, psychiatric services, social work, community organization, laboratory, pharmacy, ambulance and patient transportation, specialty consultation, prenatal care, and close ties with teaching hospitals and consultants for hospitalization or specialty needs. Our goals were, and are, to provide the full range of ambulatory health services *in* the community with all the usual barriers to access removed: distance, time, cost, fragmentation, impersonality; to provide new patterns of organization of service through family health teams comprising physicians, community health nurses, nurse's aides, social workers, and indigenous community health aides or "patient's agents"; and to have maximum *social* impact.

It is worth digressing briefly to note some other features of this project, which is the model and prototype for at least fifteen other planned OEO-financed neighborhood health centers across the nation. The Columbia Point Housing Development is an exquisitely defined community; its 6,000 residents live in relative isolation on a peninsula jutting out into Boston Harbor, cut off from central Boston by two expressways, limited public transportation, and a very real psychological distance; the project was built on landfill previously used as a city dump. For once, in this research and demonstration project, we have reached out to work with the "defined population," the "measurable universe," and the "community as laboratory" which have for so long been the favorite (but usually empty) phrases of social epidemiologists. We have accomplished a 100 per cent census of this population, which we keep continually updated, and for every resident of Columbia Point (whether he becomes a patient or not) we know age, race, sex, family structure, position in family, education, income, source of income, occupation, birthplace, length of residence at Columbia Point, in Boston, and in other settings, and a considerable number of other significant demographic and social variables. We have interviewed a random stratified sample of Columbia Point's families at length not merely with regard to health knowledge, attitudes, behavior, and previous utilization of health services but also concerning attitudes toward the community, social mobility, educational and other aspirations, participation in formal and informal social networks, and the like. Finally, we have devised an ongoing computerized data-recording and analysis system that couples all this data with every instance of contact between health-center staff and a Columbia Point resident, and every kind of utilization of our services.

Thus we will be able to determine *rates*—not merely of the distribution of illness or the utilization of services, but also of social mobility, attitude change, and a variety of behavioral indices—by relevant social characteristics. And since we are oriented toward longitudinal study, we should be able to measure change in both individuals and in the total community over time.

As our concern with *social* impact implies, our goals extend well beyond the mere provision of health services to an attempt to use these services as a means of inducing or facilitating other and broader types of social change—as a route in, so to speak, to the poverty cycle. For this and many other reasons, including our belief that our technical skills *had* to be joined with the recipient's knowledge of his own community and his own needs, and that *involvement* was as important as access, we began with community organization. Our first efforts, therefore, went into a series of some forty livingroom meetings in the community to discuss current health problems, views, and attitudes toward health and health services, the services needed from a neighborhood health center, and the planning and policies of the center. From these meetings there emerged, partly at the initiative of our community organizers and partly at the initiative of the community, an *ad hoc* or planning committee for a Columbia Point Health Association to represent the residents. This committee of some thirty residents undertook to share in the physical design of the health center (by intensively reviewing the floor plans), in the selection of nontechnical equipment (*i.e.*, decor, waiting-room and other furniture, etc.), and in planning methods of payment; to form a permanent Health Association, conduct a membership drive, set Health Association dues and policies, and conduct a community-wide election for its directors; and to join with Tufts in planning and conducting the Health Center's opening ceremonies.

Now this was clearly a mixed situation. The money, the "ultimate responsibility," and the policy- and decision-making power initially rested with Tufts; but we were offering to share them, in varying degree, with the community—*not* because we were required to do so (community action agency rules that the poor be represented did not apply to us automatically as a research and demonstration project), but because it was an intrinsic part of our program and goals to do so.

What happened? The Ad Hoc Committee met with us regularly. It had some excellent changes to suggest in the floor plans, the decor, and the furniture, including the extremely sensible suggestion of big and little (mother- and child-sized) rocking chairs instead of modern cribs for the sick-child waiting area. It conducted a highly successful membership drive, involving parades by the local drum and bugle corps, inventive health exhibits, and free flu shots, and signed up 500 of Columbia Point's 1,200 families. It agreed to take major responsibility for health education programs. It planned and ran an extremely successful opening ceremony, which brought to Columbia Point such figures as House Speaker McCormack and the national director of Operation Headstart. And it conducted an election for permanent directors in which 40 per cent of the eligible population participated.

But this is only one side of the coin. By the ninth or tenth meeting with us, there emerged, as we had anticipated, a powerful current of suspicion, anger, and mistrust. Over and over again we were asked, and tested, as to whether we *really meant it* when we offered a "significant voice" in policy- and decision-making. A critical decision won by the health association that all subprofessional jobs would be open to community residents, without regard to the confidentiality of health center records, only led, predictably, to further testing, and a request for close examination of our total budget. Temporary frustration and delays often produced the comment that the committee was merely "a bunch of puppets on a string, and Tufts is going to run everything in its own way anyway." On a number of occasions we were cordially invited to "just go build your health center and leave us alone."

Certain problems, particularly those involving the dominant community, produced noticeable ambivalence. For example, the decision to purchase special waiting-room furniture led to a decision to attempt to raise money from stores, industrial firms, or foundations in the "outside world" for the extra costs involved. A fund-raising letter was written. Then it was decided that personal visits should be made. Fear was expressed that the committee would be seen as beggars; it was decided that all visits would be made by teams of at least two residents. Next it was decided that the committee should have an honorary chairman: the Governor of Massachusetts. This decision was reversed, on the grounds that the money should be forthcoming on its merits and not because the Governor asked for it. At this point the committee decided to seek professional fund-raising advice from Tufts; some 150 letters were mailed out, and many drew enthusiastic invitations for a follow-up visit, but very few visits have been made.

In short, predictably, the shorter-term and more discrete tasks have been successfully accomplished. There *is* a community organization; the health center is open; it is a significant source of employment as well as service for local residents; a community-wide opening ceremony was held; an election was conducted; some policies have been made; large numbers of people have been involved in varying degree; new and powerful leadership, extending well beyond the community's elite, has appeared, in some cases to stay, in others to withdraw in frustration, boredom, or anger.

Direct utilization of our health and health-related services, at the health center and in the home, has been sufficient to shatter forever (at least in this instance) the myth that the poor don't care about or value health services. In the first six weeks, we saw more than 1,200 of Columbia Point's 6,000 residents. Currently we are seeing more than 100 patients every twenty-four hours, a rate that we had not anticipated for at least a year.

On longer-term or more abstract issues, there are problems: no health education program has emerged; negotiation over payment mechanisms has stalled; though utilization of health center services is extremely high, and still growing, there is constant suspicion that it will turn out to be "just like the City Hospital," impersonal and unyielding; and the Health Association has become, at least for the moment, a stage for the expression of a major community conflict over racial balance.

We remain extremely confident over the long-range prospects of effective joint Tufts-and-community action; we have, at least, had the wisdom to become thoroughly involved with the community, in discussion and joint programming and debate and occasionally open anger, as a basis for trust. But how are we to interpret events thus far?

We can only do so, I think, by reference to the major *existing* poverty program in the community, the public welfare system which has been a dominant feature of residents' lives for years. What characterizes this system, and the interactions of residents with it? Listen to the residents:

First, lack of resources. One resident says:

"We don't think of the power structure as people. We look at things as being dollars and cents, in our ADC check, or relief, or what we can get out of the welly worker. I have enough just day-to-day problems. Should I buy Christmas presents for the kids or pay the rent? Should I buy food for lunch or take the money for carfare and take my son to the dentist? Well, we have lunch and we pay rent and we wait until we have an abscess and the police department takes us to the dentist."

Second, lack of choice and control. Another resident says:

"Very often, what happens is, there's no choice—you have to take that which is free, because that's the one thing that is available. A while ago a social worker from public welfare walked in and said, 'I'm your new welly worker and I came down to find out if you want to be eligible for ADC.' Did you hear that? Not if I *am* eligible but if I want to be. For the first time I realized I didn't have to take ADC if I didn't want it. I had been given a choice."

And she adds:

"Now, like the medical center. I figured it would be the usual deal—you were going to let me provide the illnesses and you are going to run the services."

Third, as a kind of ignominious bargain: You give me your psychodynamics and I'll give you the rent. A resident told us:

"The social service people come in here and think of it in terms of being a hard-core community with multiproblem people living in it. Well, there are two sides to a glass window and we are able to look out as well as you looking in—we see you as being hard-core social workers. You're insulting with your belief that you have everything to give me. You forget that I not only know how to take but I can give, too."

Finally, and most important, the system is *seen* as a system— hostile and controlling—a system that you have to beat, though it ultimately beats you.

A resident told us in a taped interview:

"I work very hard at beating the system you work for. Many times it takes 3 or 4 days for me to figure out a way to beat the system . . . some of us can do it best with tears, others with tantrums, others do it with hysteria, and others just by appearing to be terribly well informed."

And again:

"I know how to get families to get clothing—the extra clothes you need, like boots for the kids when winter comes in but the clothes allowance is the same as for the summer. I know how to get money for all kinds of special diets. I know the names of more diets than the doctors who are giving them. I even know how much money they give for each type of diet—so, depending on the economic problem in the family, this is the type of diet we strike out for."

So much for apathy! So much for the professional's belief that he has unilateral control of the system. So much for those who ignore the importance of informal social networks and the recognition that in almost every community there is already a powerful peer organization. Our task is not to create such a network, but rather to identify the existing one and use it for understanding, for teaching, and for accomplishing social change.

One final quote is in order. Of OEO, a resident says:

"In fact I was really planning to spend next year looking for a husband— but what happened to me is I find I have to start beating OEO's system. It's very hard to keep taking time out to beat systems."

Against this background, it is a little easier to identify the need to define the new health center and health association as another system to beat or be beaten by, the need to feel the injured person, the victim. This is *both* reality and projection. It is easier to identify the pain and the risks, in view of past experience, involved in trusting and working with the power structure or the professionals, in deciding that reality isn't relentlessly hostile and that temporary frustrations don't mean a sell-out or total failure. It is easier to see the ambiguity, from the residents' point of view, of *sharing* power, when past experience is predominantly with having none or having it all. Finally, in view of the day-to-day emergencies of sheer survival, it is possible to understand why shorter-term and more specific goals are easier to deal with successfully than longer-term or more abstract ones.

It seems to us in review, that either/or choices as to the diagnosis and formulation of the poverty problem are foolish at our present level of knowledge. It is not *either* a matter of material deprivation, unemployability, lack of education, and lack of opportunity, *or* a matter of powerlessness, alienation, institutionalized dependency, or withdrawal; it is all of these, in varying degree, for different communities, different individuals, and different programs. In Mississippi, as Jencks has recently pointed out, the significance of last year's Operation Headstart was much more in the control and power it gave Negro communities than in its substantive content or material change; in other communities the opposite may be true.

By the same token, we do not have an either/or choice of goals. We must act both to change the material circumstances of the impoverished (as public assistance has never done to a sufficient degree) and to create *multiple* routes for the involvement of the poor: *first* through protest-and-conflict organizations demanding increased power, money, and programs, and likely to be particularly effective in obtaining such short-term goals as more playgrounds, real enforcement of housing codes, increased garbage collection, lower rents, fewer rates, and restraints on the police; *second* via co-determination models, in which the poor and the affluent more nearly share power, and the organizations of the poor negotiate with the power structure, in the classic political model, for a piece of the action; and *third* via organizations that provide participation in programs, through new jobs and middle-level roles, without real power.

All three approaches—of, by, and for the poor—are needed. We suspect that each has its constituency among the deprived, its corps of individuals who by past experience and individual personality are most responsive to that particular model. Each is particularly useful for particular goals—material or psychosocial, short or long-term—in particular environments: Alabama or Bedford-Stuyvesant, Appalachia or Watts. And each has its political role: without protest-and-conflict groups, we would never have had a poverty program at all;

without varying models of accommodation, we would never get past the marching.

Finally, what are the mental health implications of this multiple choice? Certainly our own experience, thus far, is too limited to give more than crude and qualitative answers, including the obvious recognition that different individuals in a community are ready for different types of involvement at any one point in time, and that the same individual may move from one kind of involvement to another, over time. We need to know a great deal more, and we have been attempting to find out, while remembering that poverty is *not* primarily a mental-health problem, any more than we in preventive medicine think it is primarily a health problem. We have no desire to trade someone's psychodynamics for a flu shot and begin the system all over again. We *do* have to specify operational goals. We have to decide what we mean by social impact, and how we shall attempt to measure it. We have the enormously difficult task of defining measurable outcome variables, measuring them accurately, documenting our interpretations of the things these variables represent, and identifying and measuring the effects of random or contaminating input factors. Freeman and Sherwood[4] have recently outlined some of the difficulties of these tasks in action research programs, and we are very much aware of them.

In this light, the Tufts Department of Psychiatry, while providing psychiatric services at Columbia Point, has also been deeply involved in a quite independent research program as part of the Tufts Comprehensive Community Health Action Program. Drs. Leon Shapiro and Miles Shore have conducted a series of some thirty extensive, unstructured interviews with Columbia Point residents; these have been supplemented by a number of survey instruments used by the Department of Preventive Medicine. The goal is at least a preliminary exploration of the life-styles, psychological characteristics, and character formations of a representative number of residents.

From this material has emerged, so far, hints of the usual broad range of healthy, coping, responses and neurotic or characterological problems. Particular attention has been paid to the abandoned mother, the female head of the incomplete family, and a number of patterns are suggested. A substantial number of the interviewed women seem, in their current relationships, to be endlessly reenacting a masochistic, eroticized relationship with their fathers in the painful, repetitive cycle of marriage, pregnancy, and abandonment. Others, who grew up in incomplete families and were forced into an "assistant mother" role at an early age, appear to have sought escape in adolescence by choosing a mate with the same essential characteristic as the absent father, *i.e.*, he wasn't there, or not for long. We are very aware that these are preliminary observations, without control studies.

It would be easy to generalize, to try to translate these preliminary observations of individual psychodynamics into community behaviors; for example, to say that the need to beat the system, and be ultimately beaten by it, expresses this same possible constellation in abandoned women. This would be both inappropriate and a dangerous oversimplification; what is needed is not a translation, but a search for some coherent interface between individual dynamics and group or community behavior. From the point of view of community mental health, we need all possible organizational models so that we can learn something about the individuals who are attracted to them, are involved in them, and learn from them. For these populations, *new experiences* (from the novel experience of having enough money for the children's food and the rent and the dentist, to the experience of having choices, or joining a protest group, or negotiating for power, or participating without full power) may be much more useful in intervening in the poverty cycle than cognitive insight.

I cannot close without mentioning at least one other mental health implication of this multiple choice: the implication for the professional. It is painful and stressful for the professional, too, to give up the psychodynamics-for-rent exchange; to be involved and challenged; to have his half-conscious needs for gratitude and subservience by his clients go unmet; to accept that clients have relevant skills, and that professionals are not the only (or primary) source of care [to recognize, for example, that most of the pediatric care in our society is given by "subprofessionals" called mothers, rather than by pediatricians]; to have the Protestant ethic that often motivates him seemingly violated; and to surrender control. Many professionals are saved, I think, only by the knowledge that they can always walk away; this is the very knowledge that infuriates the resident, who cannot. It is, after all, difficult to follow the wise precept of the Columbia Point resident who told us: "I just want you to show me how to get the happiness that *I* want—and damn it, will you stop insisting that I be happy?"

NOTES

1. Levitan, Sar A. Programs in Aid of the Poor, *Poverty and Human Resources Abstracts*. (Institute of Labor and Industrial Relations, Ann Arbor, Mich.) Vol. 1, No. 1, Jan.-Feb. 1966, p.21.

2. Haggstrom, Warren C. The power of the poor. In *Mental Health of the*

Poor, Riessman, Cohen, Pearl, eds. (New York: The Free Press of Glencoe, 1964), pp. 205–223.

3. Fishman, Jacob R., and Solomon, Frederic. Youth and social action. In *Mental Health of the Poor*, *op. cit.*, pp. 400–411.

4. Freeman, Howard E. and Sherwood, Clarence C. Research in large-scale intervention programs. *The Journal of Social Issues.* 21 (January 1965): 11–28.

Part IV

SOCIAL, PSYCHOLOGICAL, AND STRUCTURAL DETERMINANTS OF HEALTH CARE

The papers presented thus far have alluded to the greater likelihood of illness as well as to the physical and economic barriers to health care among the poor. The diversity of these forces often makes it difficult to sort out the specific effects of a given set of variables.

This difficulty may in part explain the frustration expressed by Coe and Wessen over the dearth of social-psychological research concerning the causes of people's medical behavior. In their review, they focus on the potential of the doctor-patient relationship, showing how the physician's approach can reinforce or obviate negative behavior patterns. Furthermore, they point out that the patient's self-image and attitudes toward illness will have a significant influence on the way she/he seeks health care.

The rising costs of health care have become an issue of national concern. Generally attention is focused on the direct costs of care, the moneys disbursed to pay for the services provided. For the poor especially, the indirect costs, which are rarely subsidized by welfare or health insurance systems, may be an even greater problem. These more subtle costs include loss of work and income, travel and babysitting costs, costly changes in diet, and so on.

The problems of availability and accessibility of medical care are relevant ones. Availability means some measure of the actual existence of services. For example, are there physicians or clinics in an area? When are they open? Accessibility refers to the likelihood of actual use of the potential service in terms of the ease of gaining entry. This may be expressed in terms of the distance to be traveled or travel time, or it may refer to other barriers to care, such as fees, waiting time (for an appointment and in the office), policies restricting admission, or general personnel attitudes that discourage entrance and compliance. These two related concepts have particular relevance to the plight of the poor. While much concern has been focused on the major impediments to care, such as financial barriers and inadequate facilities, less attention has been paid to the question of how to package the necessary care to encourage use after these major barriers have been removed.

In a provocative paper Stoeckle and Zola project us into a not-too-distant future when the bill for care may no longer be an issue. They confront us with a series of questions about the way in which services *should* be organized to make them truly accessible. They then ask to what extent and how much we are willing to invest in bringing health care to those populations we have thus far been unable to reach.

Strauss argues that the failure of the medical system to provide adequate care for the poor is inherent in its structure and advocates a series of changes that will increase both the number of patients and the quality of their experience. It is not merely a matter of pouring in more money and manpower, but of altering the style in which care is rendered. Such changes can only be brought about by combined efforts at all levels—providers, consumers, and government.

The reader interested in further information on this subject may refer to the following references listed in the annotated bibliography:

Aitken-Swan and
   Paterson, 1955
Alexander, 1967
Alpert et al., 1967(a),
   1967(b), 1969
Ambuel, et al., 1964
American Public Health
   Association Confer-
   ence Report, 1968
Andersen and Benham,
   1970
Anderson, 1973
Apple, 1960
Badgley and
   Hetherington, 1962
Banks and Keller, 1971
Bashur et al., 1971
Baum and Felzer, 1964
Beck, 1973
Becker, 1972
Berkanovic and Reeder,
   1974

Berkowitz et al., 1963
Bice et al., 1973
Blum et al., 1968
Brinton, 1972
Brooks, 1973
Brown, 1969
Bullough, 1972
Cauffman et al., 1967
Cervantes, 1972
Clausen, 1963
Coburn and Pope, 1974
Davis, 1966, 1967,
   1968
Davis and Eichhorn,
   1963
Deas, 1968
Deasy, 1956
de Vise, 1970
Dodge et al., 1970
Dummett, 1969
Elling et al., 1960
Fabrega and Roberts,

   1972
Fay et al., 1970
Feldman, 1966
Feldstein, 1966
Feldstein and Carr, 1964
Fink et al., 1968
Fishman, 1969
Flora et al., 1966
Freeman and
   Lambert, 1965
Gallagher, 1967
Gibbs et al., 1974
Glasser, 1958
Glogow, 1970
Gochman, 1972
Goldsen, 1957, 1963
Graham, 1957
Gray et al., 1966,
   1967
Gursslin et al., 1959
Hardy, 1956
Haynes, 1969

Hochbaum, 1958
Hoff, 1966, 1969
Hollingshead and
  Redlich, 1958
Holloman, 1969
Hulka et al., 1972
Irelan, 1965
Kasl and Cobb, 1966
Kassebaum and
  Bauman, 1972
Kasteler, 1970
Kegeles, 1963
Kessel and Shephard,
  1965
Kriesberg and Treiman,
  1960
Lashoff, 1968
Lurie, 1973
McAtee, 1969
MacDonald et al.,
  1963
Maloney, 1967
Montiero, 1973
Muller, 1965
Newman, 1969
Olendzki et al., 1972

Osofsky, 1968(a),
  1968(b)
O'Shea and Bissell,
  1969
Parsons, 1958
Peterson, 1969
Picken and Ireland,
  1969
Plaja et al., 1968
Rainwater, 1968
Reinhardt, 1973
Richardson and
  Neuhouser, 1968
Robinson, 1967, 1968
Roghmann et al., 1971
Rosenblatt and
  Suchman, 1969
Rosenstock, 1960,
  1966
Ross, 1962
Salber et al., 1972
Schneiderman, 1965
Schorr, 1970
Simon, 1967
Solon et al., 1958
Stein, 1972
Stoeckle et al., 1963

Stuart, 1972
Suchman, 1969(a),
  1969(b), 1972
Tagliacozzo and
  Mauksch, 1958
Tiven, 1971
Triplett, 1969
Tucker, 1969
Tucker, 1970
Walsh, 1969
Walsh and Elling,
  1968
Wan and Soifer, 1974
Watts, 1966
Weiss and Greenlick,
  1970
White, 1968
Willie, 1960
Wingert et al., 1968,
  1969
Wise, 1968
Wise et al., 1968
Wolff, 1958
Wood, 1968
Yerby, 1965, 1966
Yerby and Agress,
  1966

6. Social-Psychological Factors Influencing the Use of Community Health Resources

RODNEY M. COE AND ALBERT F. WESSEN

The purpose of this paper is to explore some social-psychological concomitants of the utilization of health services. It would probably be wise at the outset, however, to indicate that the title of this paper—"Social-psychological Factors Influencing the Use of Community Health Resources"—is somewhat misleading. At least it is misleading to the extent that the focus of these remarks will be on "social-psychological factors" rather than on "community health resources." For the purposes of this paper, it is not important to discuss separately the social-psychological factors found to be associated with the use of various clinics, hospital outpatient services, inpatient care, or even visits to the offices of physicians in private practice. Rather, we shall concentrate on an event common to all medical settings, namely, the social encounter between the patient and the therapist as a significant part of the more general process of response to illness. The term therapist is used here rather than physician to permit generalization of the social relationship to paramedical personnel and healers other than orthodox physicians, e.g., chiropractors, faith healers, and others who, after all, must be includ-

From the *American Journal of Public Health* 55 (July 1965), pp. 1024–31, reprinted by permission of the authors and publisher.

This paper was presented before a Joint Session of the Mental Health and Public Health Education Sections of the American Public Health Association at the Ninety-Second Annual Meeting in New York City, October 6, 1964. It was prepared with support of the Medical Care Research Center, an agency sponsored jointly by Washington University and the Jewish Hospital of St. Louis, under funds granted by USPHS, grant number CH-00024.

ed in the community's total health resources. We will return to this point later. First, however, it would seem appropriate to summarize briefly the results of some previous studies in utilization and to indicate some important issues raised by these studies.

In general, most of these studies make use of a host of demographic and social factors related to utilization of health resources.[1] Such investigations provide a description of trends in utilization and of the variations in important social and demographic factors associated with this use. It has been found, for example, that rates of utilization of health services are greater for females than males, and that use increases with age for both sexes.[2] It has been shown that utilization varies directly with social class standing.[3] It has been demonstrated that while upper social classes spend more for health services, the amount they spend represents a smaller proportion of their total income than the amount spent by the lower social classes.[4] It has been found that owners of various health insurance policies utilize health services more often than people without insurance.[5] It is also known that to a certain extent ecology influences the use of various health resources, especially hospitals.[6]

These studies emphasize the importance of the factors of *availability* of medical care. They are useful, timely data designed to answer specific questions about the extent or quantity of medical care received by a population. They are used as indicators of the medical behavior of certain segments of the population. They also provide administrators and others with data needed to organize and prepare their agencies or facilities for giving medical care. Although such studies describe who is treated and what treatment is received, they cannot, nor are they intended to, answer questions as to *why* people seek care, *why* some patients delay and others do not, *why* some patients go to physicians, and others go to faith healer or quacks. The answers to these questions are to be sought in motivational studies which include research into social-psychological factors.

RESEARCH ON MEDICAL BEHAVIOR

At the present time, the extent of social psychological research on why people exhibit the medical behavior they do is not very great nor is it very systematic.[7] Attempts to assess motivation of medical behavior directly have generally failed, perhaps because of the difficulties involved in obtaining objective measures of cognition or extent of knowledge, from attitudinal studies and from studies of value orientations. A classic example would be the research of Merrill and his associates.[8] In evaluating a poliomyelitis vaccination campaign in California, they found that the influence of friends, neighbors, and the family doctor was very important. Mothers who believed their friends did not like the idea of vaccination also exhibited an unfavorable attitude toward the program and were unlikely to have their children participate. Opposition to the program by husbands or family doctors also influenced the mothers not to let their children participate. Much of the negative attitude was traced to certain beliefs—such as that fostered by the Cutter incident—which led to an expression of fear and anxiety, two variables frequently found in studies of this type. On the other hand, mothers who were favorably disposed toward vaccination, but who did not participate, often gave such reasons as negligence, they did not know about it, the child was sick that day, or the child was in an age group believed to be less susceptible to the disease.[9]

Many of these same factors, and some new ones, emerge from studies on patient reaction to specific diseases, particularly cancer. Most of these studies have sought answers to the question of why patients delay in seeking treatment. Early studies, such as those by Harms et al.,[10] and by Aitken-Swan and Paterson,[11] emphasized utilitarian features, i.e., symptoms were not serious enough, negligence, ignorance, or high cost. The research by Goldson and her associates, however, has emphasized "generalized fear" and a personal reticence to submit to examinations as causes of delay in seeking treatment for cancer.[12] The interesting interpretation of this study, however, is that patients who seek treatment for cancer symptoms early do so to the extent that they seek treatment for any symptoms early. In other words, an attempt was made here to relate behavior with respect to symptoms of a specific disease to a generalized response to illness on the part of the patient. This ties in with other research which demonstrates that response to illness varies with age, sex, race, and ethnicity.[13]

These findings of response to cancer symptoms, as part of a generalized response to illness, have been challenged by Kutner and Gordan.[14] Their investigation showed that patterns of seeking care for cancer resulted from factors which are different from those involved in response to symptoms of other diseases. They go on to say that while delay in seeking treatment for any illness is greatest in the lower classes, delay is more pronounced for cancer symptoms. Likewise, while amount of education is negatively related to delay in seeking treatment for general symptoms, there is a more pronounced negative relationship between amount of education and delay in seeking treatment for cancer.[15] One may well ask if the more pronounced response to cancer might not be due to a third factor, fear. That is, the response itself is not really different from response to other disease symptoms, as Kutner and Gordan contend, but is emphasized because fear of cancer is greater than fear of symptoms of other diseases, such as poliomyelitis. Some support for this latter interpretation is offered by Levine.[16] He found that a national sample of nearly 3,000 respondents rated cancer as the disease they feared most. Moreover, he found that personal acquaintance with a cancer victim, especially a member of the family, was more important in producing fear than amount of education or degree of specific knowledge about cancer. Although interesting, these studies in themselves do not explain much of the wide variation in response to illness that has been observed in demographic studies of utilization. A more promising approach has been suggested by Suchman and his associates who have attempted to combine sociocultural and social-psychological factors in explaining medical behavior.[17]

DATA ON INTERVIEWS

From interviews with about 1,800 respondents in an ethnically heterogenous section of New York City, Suchman obtained information on demographic and social characteristics, social status, health status, attitudes toward medical care and the medical profession. These data were organized to measure the position of particular groups along several dimensions: (1) *degree of skepticism* about doctors and their abilities; (2) *cosmopolitanism-parochialism*, or the degree of orientation toward urban, "worldly" values as opposed to close-knit, traditional relationships; and (3) *ethnic exclusivity*, or degree of ethnocentrism of the group. As might be expected—and as Suchman found—these dimensions are interrelated, but each also showed highly significant relationships with medical behavior. For example, respondents who resisted or delayed seeing a physician tended to be more parochial, highly skeptical of the medical profession, and most often turned to their own ethnic group for advice and counsel.

In these dimensions one can recognize the familiar elements of cognition, attitudes, and values. For example, skepticism of the medical profession reflects, in part, the patients' degree of medical knowledge. Highly skeptical persons tended to have less factual knowledge about the medical profession and nature of disease and, therefore, utilized their services less often. This is similar to the results reported by Browning and Northcutt,[18] Anderson,[19] and Glasser,[20] all of whom found that utilization of health services inversely varied with the amount of knowledge held by the patient.

Similarly, Suchman's findings on attitudes varying along the cosmopolitan-parochial dimension and values related to ethnic exclusivity support the previous results of Freidson,[21] Bloom,[22] and many others. Here Suchman found highly "cosmopolitan" people tended to seek the services of a physician very early in the stage of illness, while those at the "parochial" end of the scale depended more on the advice and prescription of relatives and close friends, i.e., utilized what Freidson called the lay referral system. Moreover, ethnically exclusive respondents—who also tended to be more parochial—maintained many of the values of their ethnic group, and some of these values conflicted with those held by practicing physicians. For example, for some groups time is not an important element; this may lead them to be late or break appointments with the doctor. To other people preventive medicine, in the form of annual examinations or vaccination, is unheard of; they do not go to a doctor unless they are ill. Others may not maintain a dietary regimen because the food customs of their ethnic group encourage deviance.

The importance of a study such as Suchman's is that an attempt was made to examine medical behavior within the broad framework of a sociocultural setting rather than trying to identify single, specific factors associated with certain observed behavior as so many earlier studies have done. However, even Suchman, who claims a "social system" approach, has omitted one of the key elements, the therapist who provides the care. Many of the studies already mentioned, including Suchman's, allude to the influence of the physician on the medical behavior of the patient. Other studies, such as Koos's classic report on a small community in New York,[23] suggest that certain kinds of patients, especially those in the lower classes, complain most about doctors and were more likely to seek care from chiropractors and faith healers. Simon and Rabushka[24] found that impersonal treatment by clinic physicians was the chief complaint of patients in a labor union health clinic. The Sussman[25] study of attitudes toward a hospital clinic showed that patients most wanted a definite appointment time, the same physician each visit, and the possibility of home calls by physicians. What these and other studies are suggesting is that our understanding of the medical behavior of patients is incomplete if the influence of the physician is omitted from consideration. We would go a step further. The understanding of medical behavior lies in an examination of the therapist-patient relationship—the nature of their social interaction—in the context of the patient's response to his illness. Unfortunately, little empirical research has been conducted on the therapist-patient interaction except, perhaps, in the field of mental health, so that much of what follows must neccessarily be somewhat speculative. Nonetheless, it is felt that further research on the ideas suggested below will better enable us to account for the somewhat disparate factors already mentioned.

By this time, nearly everyone must be aware of the changes which are taking place in the field of medicine. Many writers have pointed to such trends as increased specialization in practice, which is accompanied by fragmention of patient care and emphasizes the therapist's interest in the disease rather than the "whole patient."[26] The trends toward group practice, partnerships, and the declining number of general practitioners, especially in urban areas, also is evident.[27] An increasing number of people are now covered by some form of health insurance. This has increased the demand for medical care services which must be provided by a declining ratio of physicians to population.[28] Although these changes are important, it is felt that the trends noted above serve only to define some of the external constraints on the interaction which takes place. Of greater importance may be the characteristics of the therapist-patient interaction itself.

We have already examined some characteristics which patients bring to the encounter. Besides certain social and demographic attributes, it has been suggested that patients exhibit a "selective attention" to symptoms[29]; that they employ a lay referral system; that, in other words, there is a wide variation in response to illness. In one of the classic studies, Barker and his associates reported that perception of symptoms of illness often constituted a threat to that person's self-conception in terms of pain, incapacitation, disfigurement, and even death.[30] They indicated also that anxiety and fear, accompanying the uncertainty over the meaning of symptoms, are not necessarily alleviated by professional treatment. They suggest that patients lack knowledge of, and therefore are frightened by, an array of unusual instruments, unfamiliar sounds and smells. While this may be true to some degree, the important point is that the social-psychological ramifications of illness—uncertainty, fear, anxiety, etc.—may be aggravated or, more technically, may be reinforced by the therapist-patient encounter. To make this point clearer, we must now look at the healer's role in the encounter.

DOCTOR-PATIENT RELATIONSHIP

Early descriptions of the doctor-patient relationship assumed that, as in the case of other kinds of social interaction, there were explicit norms governing the behavior of both parties. Parsons,[31] to take a well-known example, analyzed the roles of doctor and patient in terms of his concepts of pattern variables. The intent was to show that the role attributes which each one brought to the encounter were complementary and were understood by each party. That is, the physician held certain expectations of the patient, and the patient knew what they were and could comply and vice versa. Recently, however, some writers have begun to question the explicitness of these expectation. Zola,[32] for example, suggests that potential sources of conflict were overlooked by early analysts because treatment of acute, infectious diseases became the type for medical practice, and because such treatment was often successful after a short period. Under these conditions, the therapist-patient encounter was likely to be brief, perhaps only a one-time affair and had, as its principal component, a specific therapeutic intervention. For example, when one had a streptococcal infection, one went to a doctor, one was quickly diagnosed, and might be treated with a penicillin shot. Control of chronic diseases, however, may require many, varied treatments and medical supervision over a long period of time and, therefore, does not "fit" the earlier model.[33] Zola suggests also that sources of conflict were overlooked because of the great power differential between physician and patient.

In fact, if one looks at the amount of preparation—or socialization, if you will—by the role players, one finds enormous disparities. On the one hand, a physician has a great deal of medical knowledge learned through long years of study during which time he also learns certain attitudes and values.[34] He is a doctor by choice and as such accepts the rules and regulations, both formal and informal, designed to control his behavior. The patient, on the other hand, ordinarily does not *choose* to be ill and enters the relationship without any clear conception of what is expected of him or of the norms, if any, which are supposed to guide his behavior in that situation.

PROBLEM OF DIAGNOSIS AND TREATMENT

Superimposed on this relationship, which on the face of it places the patient in a very unfavorable position, is another factor, namely, the manner in which physicians handle the problem of uncertainty of diagnosis and treatment. Although as Scheff[35] has pointed out, uncertainty has always been a part of medical practice, it has been accentuated by the current shift in morbidity and mortality from acute to chronic diseases. The remarkable progress in medical science in reducing death rates from acute, infectious diseases has led to similar public expectations with respect to the control of chronic ailments. As yet, however, medical research has not produced the required results. Thus, practicing physicians are often confronted with problems for which they have no answers. At best, they may have available only palliative measures. Accordingly, physicians must often decide whether to treat a patient, even if the therapy has not been tested, or not to treat a patient and hope that somehow the body will heal itself. In the absence of effective ways of restoring health, the physician may either continue ineffective measures almost indefinitely and/or may come to lose interest in his patient.[36]

This situation may have unfortunate consequences for the doctor-patient relationship. Not only does it mean prolonging the relationship with repeated appointments, so that the doctor may observe the outcome of his therapy—thus increasing the cost to the patient—but the physician's uncertainty or disinterest is often communicated to the patient, thereby increasing the latter's anxiety or fear and his skepticism about the competence of physicians. More important, however, by these procedures, the physican forces the patient into a "sick role," where he more than likely does not want to be and may not really belong.[37] Indeed, if persons seeking help for a medical problem are forced into a role which they do not want, and which places them in an unfavorable position vis a vis the physician because the latter is unable to cope successfully with his problem, one can begin to see how the various disparate factors—anxiety, skepticism, complaints about expense, generalized resistance to physicians and even hostility—can arise.

IMPORTANCE OF PATIENT SELF-CONCEPT

All this leads back to an important social-psychological facet of response to illness which is reinforced by the therapist-patient encounter: the impact of the encounter on the self-concept of the role incumbents, especially the patient. According to early analysis, patients willingly gave private and personal information to the physician because (a) they *knew* he had to have that information to carry out his role and (b) their private information was safe with him. However, just as the assumption about knowledge of role expectations is being questioned, we may well question the validity of this one.

Under conditions imposed by contemporary medical practice—of extreme impersonality, of skepticism about the physician's competence, of the inability to establish the relationship stereotypically represented by the "old family doctor"—it is more likely that patients may resent and *resist* the intrusion into what Goffman dramaturgically described as the "backstage region," i.e., the area of private and personal affairs.[38] The thought of permitting access to private data, without any kind of reciprocity and without being able to control what information is discovered, as well as the dependency relationship that the therapist's advice concerning this patient's behavior may impose, is a direct assault on a person's conception of himself. There is a considerable amount of research which suggests that people tend to resist or even altogether withdraw from situations in which they occupy a disadvantaged position, or lose control over the factors which enable them to present themselves in a favorable light.[39]

From this admittedly speculative viewpoint it seems likely that most, if not all the significant factors associated with resistance to utilization of community health resources, can be traced to characteristics of response to illness. Specifically, it is suggested that the nature of the therapist-patient interaction, under conditions imposed by current medical practice, is such that it may reinforce a threat to the patient's concept of self, a threat that may make it difficult if not impossible for the patient to continue the interaction. This may account for the phenomena of "shopping" for a physician, or why patients continue to go to chiropractors or other "healers" who must, of necessity, give "personalized" service. If the hypothesized importance of the nature of the therapist-patient relationship can be demonstrated to be an empirical fact, implications for effecting changes to improve the utilization of health resources would be evident.

In fact, some studies have already shown that negative attitudes toward clinic personnel can be partially mitigated by modifying the physician's approach to the patient.[40] Essentially, physicians must be made aware of the importance of using themselves as a therapeutic tool in the encounter. This, of course, would require not only a reemphasis on sociological factors of illness in medical education, but also some changes in conduct of contemporary medical practice which would permit an increase in the therapist's commitment to patient care rather than disease treatment. These areas plus other facets of utilization, such as "over-utilizers," should be made high priority targets for future research.

NOTES

1. Cf. Anderson, O. W. The Utilization of Health Services. In Freeman, H. E.; Levine, S.; and Reeder, L. G. *Handbook of Medical Sociology.* Englewood Cliffs, N. J.: Prentice-Hall, 1963, pp. 349-367.

2. U. S. Public Health Service. National Health Survey, *Acute Conditions, Incidence and Associated Disability.* Ser. 10, No. 10. Washington, D. C.: Gov. Ptg. Office, 1964.

3. Koos, E. L. *The Health of Regionville.* New York: Columbia University Press, 1954.

4. Anderson, O. W., and Feldman, J. J. *Family Medical Costs and Voluntary Health Insurance.* New York: McGraw-Hill, 1956.

5. Anderson, O. W., and Sheatsley, P. B. *Comprehensive Medical Insurance —A Study of Costs, Use and Attitudes under Two Plans.* Chicago, Ill.: Health Information Foundation, Research Ser. No. 9, 1959. Also Roemer, M. I. and Shain, M. *Hospital Utilization under Insurance.* Chicago: American Hospital Association, Monogr. Ser. No. 6, 1959.

6. McNerney, W. J., and Riedel, D. C. *Regionalization and Rural Health Care.* Ann Arbor, Mich.: University of Michigan Press, 1962. See also Koos, *op. cit.*

7. Anderson, *op. cit.*, p. 362.

8. Merrill, M. H.; Hollister, A. C.; Gibbens, S. I.; and Haynes, A. W. Attitudes of Californians Toward Poliomyelitis Vaccination. *A.J.P.H.* 48:146-152, 1958.

9. Ibid., pp. 151-153.

10. Harms, C. R.; Plaut, J. A.; and Oughterson, A. W. Delay in Treatment of Cancer. *JAMA* 121:335-338, 1943.

11. Aitken-Swan, J., and Paterson, R. The Cancer Patient: Delay in Seeking Advice. *Brit. M. J.* 1:623-627, 1955.

12. Goldson, R. K., Gerhardt, P. R., and Handy, V. H. Some Factors Related to Patient Delay in Seeking Diagnosis for Cancer Symptoms. *Cancer* 10:1-7, 1957.

13. See for example, Zhorowski, M. Cultural Components in Response to Pain. In Jaco, E. G. *Patients, Physicians and Illness.* Glencoe, Ill.: Free Press, 1958, pp. 256-268. See also Saunders, L. *Cultural Differences and Medical Care.* New York: Russell Sage Foundation, 1954.

14. Kutner, B., and Gordan, G. Seeking Care for Cancer J. *Health & Human Behavior* 2:171-178, 1961.

15. Ibid., p. 177.

16. Levine, G. N. Anxiety about Illness: Psychological and Social Bases. Ibid. 3:30-34, 1962.

17. Suchman, E. A. Social Patterns of Health and Medical Care. Unpublished manuscript, New York City Department of Health, 1963; Suchman, E. A., Socio-Cultural Variations in Illness and Medical Care. Ibid. 1963; Suchman, E. A. Illness Behavior and Medical Care. Ibid., 1963.

18. Browning, R. H., and Northcutt, T. J. *On the Season.* Jacksonville: Florida State Board of Health, 1961.

19. Anderson, H. P. The Bracero Program in California. Los Angeles: University of California School of Public Health, 1961 (mimeo.).

20. Glasser, M. A. A Study of the Public's Acceptance of the Salk Vaccine Program. *AJPH.* 48:141-146, 1958.

21. Freidson, E. Patients' Views of Medical Practice. New York: Russell Sage Foundation, 1961.

22. Bloom, S. B. *The Doctor and His Patient.* New York: Russell Sage, 1963.

23. Koos, op. cit.

24. Simon, N., and Rabushka, S. Membership Attitudes in the Labor Health

Institute in St. Louis. *AJPH* 46:716-722, 1956.

25. Sussman, M. B. Report: Social Class and the Hospital Clinic—A Pilot Project. Cleveland: Western Reserve University, 1959 (mimeo.).

26. Steiger, W. A.; Hoffman, F. H.; Hanses, A. V.; and Niebuhr, H. A Definition of Comprehensive Medicine *J. Health & Human Behavior* 1:83-86, 1960.

27. U. S. Department of Health, Education, and Welfare. *Medical Groups in the United States*, 1959. Washington, D. C.: Gov. Ptg. Office, 1963.

28. Somers, H. M., and Somers, A. R. *Doctors, Patients and Health Insurance.* Washington, D. C.: Brookings, 1961.

29. Mechanic, D. The Concept of Illness Behavior. *J. Chronic Dis.* 15:189-194, 1962.

30. Barker, R. G.; Wright, B. A.; and Gonick, M. R. *Adjustment to Physical Handicap and Illness: A Survey of the Social Psychology of Physique and Disability.* New York: Social Science Research Council, Bull. No. 55, 1946.

31. Parsons, T. *The Social System.* Glencoe, Ill.: Free Press, 1951.

32. Zola, I. K. Needed Problems of Research. Paper read at National Tuberculosis Association Conference, Chicago, 1964.

33. Cf. Wessen, A. F. Some Sociological Characteristics of Long-Term Care. Part II., *Gerontologist* 4:7-14 (June), 1964.

34. Merton, R. K.; Reader, G. G.; and Kendall, P. L. *The Student-Physician.* Cambridge, Mass.: Harvard University Press, 1957.

35. Scheff, T. J. Decision Rules, Types of Error and Their Consequences in Medical Diagnosis. *University of Wisconsin Psychiatric Institute Bull.* 2:1-22, 1962.

36. Ibid., p. 5.

37. Ibid., p. 13.

38. Goffman, E. *Presentation of Self in Everyday Life.* New York: Doubleday, 1959.

39. Cf. Shibutani, T. *Society and Personality.* Englewood Cliffs, N. J.: Prentice-Hall, 1961.

40. Straus, R. Some Sociocultural Considerations in the Care of Patients with Myocardial Infarction *J. Health & Human Behavior* 1:119-122, 1960. See also, Walker, J. E. C. Health Education and the University Ambulatory Service. Paper presented at AHA Conference on the Hospital's Responsibility for Health Education, Chicago, 1964.

7. After Everyone Can Pay For Medical Care

Some Perspectives on Future Treatment and Practice

JOHN D. STOECKLE AND IRVING K. ZOLA

One of the most important concerns about being sick is how to pay for it. But through legislation, and the mass consumption of private insurance, largely financed by industry in exchange for wages on the job, everyone will soon become a paying patient at the doctor's office, the hospital, and nursing home and then purely economic barriers to medical care will disappear. In reality, however, financing medical care is only the top portion of an iceberg. As in so many other social, economic, and political problems (our foreign policy being a prime example), money is only a step in the solution of more basic and fundamental problems.

In medical care, even with everyone a paying patient, at least four important problems remain submerged from recognition and debate. (1) Do we want treatment to reach everybody? (2) Does everyone get the best possible treatment? (3) Do we care who treats us? (4) Do we care about the size and location of our hospitals and practices?

DO WE WANT TREATMENT TO REACH EVERYBODY?

Our treatment institutions, our hospitals, clinics, and medical practices, have traditionally viewed the public who did not seek medical aid as being relatively healthy or certainly not very sick. For, if they really were, they would come to the doctor. Similar views have been

From *Medical Care* 2 (January-May 1964), pp. 36-41, reprinted by permission of the authors and publisher.

expressed about patients who did not regularly keep their appointments, who broke off in the midst of treatment or who did not wait around in a waiting-room or on a waiting list. Yet many studies and observations of those who are not going to the doctor have revealed a high prevalence of sickness, disease, and disability. In one recent industrial survey some 90 percent of the workers were found with treatable but untreated disorders. No one knows how large is this population with unmet needs that does not seek medical aid, that is apathetic about getting treatment, that procrastinates in going to the doctor; but it has been estimated at near some 40,000,000 Americans. What is more important is the fact that this population of nonusers, slow users, treatment dropouts, is found predominantly, but not only, in our lower socioeconomic classes. The irony of unmet medical needs in a country of plenty was shown in a recent survey of one of our major cities, where it was noted that those with greatest medical care needs, for example, the elderly and other low-income and "minority" groups—have the lowest recognition of their medical needs and the longest duration of care once it is initiated.

Reasons for Nonattendance

Again and again health surveys have demonstrated that the section of our population that does not participate in immunization campaigns or take preventive action—cancer checkups, going to the doctor early, mass X-rays—is not a random one. Investigators have emphasized the potential patient's contribution to this problem and have studied the characteristics of this nonattending population. They have pointed out their lack of psychological readiness, their lack of medical knowledge, their fear of seeking medical aid, their negative views of treatment and of the doctor, clinic or hospital delivering medical services, and finally, their personal (that is, idiosyncratic) and very unscientific ideas about being sick or healthy.

Too often, however, it appears as if this delay or unwillingness to seek help is all the patient's fault. Yet some is fostered, at least indirectly, by the health professions. The reasons, of course, are manifold. One is our activistic overemphasis on dramatic "cures" fostering unrealistic expectations on the part of much of our population. Either one does not have to worry because the illness can easily be cured, or the condition is hopeless and nothing can be done. These black and white expectations have not only blinded us to the necessity and appreciation of the importance of preventive measures but have also led to considerable unwillingness to embark on any long-term course of treatment which will not lead to a "complete cure." The potential patient is often enthusiastic about continuing in a course of long-term treatment which guarantees at most only remission, control, or relief, and physicians, trained in a framework of specific techniques and skills to cure or remove certain acute conditions, may find the treatment of chronically ill patients unsatisfying and so neglect it.

Another reason treatment may not reach everyone is professional reliance on the lay decision to go to the doctor. The patients who come to see him may not be all the people who can be treated. Medical advances appear more and more capable of detecting disease or its precursors in asymptomatic populations.

To rely on testing only those coming to the doctor will not, of course, find all the treatable cases. Large-scale mass testing will be necessary. So often, too, medical seriousness of a patient's symptoms may not be the major factor getting him to the doctor. In fact, he may be unaware or ignore early symptoms of sickness.

Since there may also be a general reluctance to see a doctor, it may be necessary to reevaluate what aspects of health and illness can truly be left to individual initiative and to what extent the health professions are willing and able to assume more initiative and responsibility for the initial steps in detection and treatment. Just sitting in the office waiting for the patient will not reach all the public. In the same way as getting alcoholics into treatment, some people will have to be educated, some coaxed, some led, and some sought out.

Solutions to Problem

Today the social-welfare value of making medical services available to everyone is generally accepted. While removing financial barriers to such services will help to make them more accessible, this will not lead automatically to mass participation. As we have stressed, more attention will have to be paid to the segment of unrecognized treatable illness and the reasons for the lack of action by many of us in seeking medical aid. Such facts will provoke questions about how our treatment institutions can work better and how our population's views of sickness and seeking help might be changed. But easy solutions and answers are not at hand. They will have to encompass (1) realistic health education, particularly of children, which would result in realistic expectations of patients and their families, particularly regarding the more chronic disorders, (2) development of treatment techniques and services acceptable to and able to reach different segments of the population and illness groups who may customarily avoid treatment, and (3) improving the availability of treatment, not just for the individual patient in the doctor's office but for everybody in his group—whether at school, the company office, the factory plant, his housing project, or home—whever medical resources of detection, prevention, diagnosis, and treatment can practically be brought to bear.

DOES EVERYONE GET THE BEST POSSIBLE TREATMENT?

Up to this point our concerns have been what illnesses or potential patients do not come to the attention of a doctor when we aim that treatment should reach everyone. But what of those that do come? Does everyone get the best of our services or are there differences in treatment and services unrelated to the patient's diagnosis? We do not have to look very far for objective examples of differential treatment. A walk round our cities will often reveal how marginal are the facilities of many municipal hospitals compared to the superior facilities of private voluntary ones. Even the historical basis of our private voluntary hospitals with their built-in differential service to "charity" patients is only slowly disappearing, hastened a bit by the paying status of the consumer. What confronts the patient here may still run the gamut from shabby surroundings, detailed questioning on his "means" and resources to delays and inconvenient scheduling of diagnostic and treatment services.

Differential Treatment

Other examples of differential treatment have been documented. In a recent survey of hospital care in New York City, experts rated privately owned, proprietary, profit-making hospitals poorer in standards of care than voluntary or government hospitals. That treatment was not solely related to the patient's need based on psychiatric diagnosis but also to his social class has been documented in Hollingshead and Redlich's much quoted study of psychiatric care. With the same diagnosis higher-class patients received psychotherapy while lower-class patients were given more organic forms of treatment.

Similar observations about bias in the medical diagnosis have been made among patients from different ethnic backgrounds. Among patients seen at three medical clinics, *despite* the same objective degree of psychological difficulties, emotionally caused symptoms were diagnosed more often in Italian as compared to Irish and Anglo-Saxon patients. Such problems of communication between patient and doctor may lead to underdiagnosis of treatable medical diseases. And some observers feel that when patients are treated in any bureaucratic and institutional setting they get less treatment—that is, less personal attention—than when they are treated in a private office. All these studies demonstrate that the quality of treatment in our country is not only uneven but that it is influenced by important historical and sociological conditions.

Social-Psychological Factors

Even our legislation has a narrow orientation toward medical care, in spite of evidence to the contrary that good care and treatment is not just medical. It has become clearer, but often not an acknowledged fact, that the problems of patients presenting at medical institutions and medical practices are social and psychological in important respects. Many recent studies have shown that the patient's decision to see a doctor is rarely based only on his medical symptoms or his knowledge about diseases, but more often on important events and factors in his family situation and social relationships. Other studies have shown similar influences in the decisions to undergo surgery, to rehospitalize mental patients, and to place old people in nursing homes. Likewise, it is becoming increasingly difficult to ignore the widespread prevalence of emotional and psychological distress and disability. Whether we take the results of national opinion surveys on where people take their acknowledged personal concerns, the mental distress reported from morbidity surveys of residents in midtown Manhattan, the Jersey suburbs and rural America, or the experience of doctors in practice, social-psychological factors in illness and patient care are large. When such factors are unrecognized and untreated by the physician it prevents rational diagnosis and handicaps the patient treatment.

The scientific understanding and handling of these aspects of illness, so important for future practice in the community, are still a matter of much debate in the education and training of the doctor. The curriculum and training experiences are already crowded with medical subject matter and medical orientation for practice in the hospital. Since training for practice in the community is not in itself an acknowledged aim and since hospital clinical care and research departments play so large a role in what is taught, curriculum additions dealing with the psychosocial study of illness and patient care are, in spite of their documented need, considered unnecessary.

Solutions to differential treatment (like making sure that everyone receives treatment) will have to encompass the patient, the public, and the professions. Where education contributes to professional treatment skill there is need not only for upgrading traditional medical teaching in some schools but for greater recognition of their responsibility to the community and of the need for newer programs in the social study of illness and disease. Yet, as G. Silver argues, education alone may not be translated into an improvement of treatment unless an appropriate organization—the family medical team—is developed to apply social skills and preventive medicine.

DO WE CARE WHO TREATS US?

Our nation's professional journals carry endless definitions of professional specialization of limited and exclusive enclosures of competence, of the role of the doctor, nurse, social worker, and a host of subspecialists within the professions themselves. No role, in turn, is more discussed than that of the doctor, and that of various types of doctors. Much of our thinking and planning of patient care centers on the transfer of the doctor's functions into an institutional setting, a big clinic, or a group practice, or the division of his functions among various practitioners in the community. Complaints are frequently made that there is too much division of treatment labor among specialists, that there is no one doctor for everyone in the family, that there is no "personal doctor" to deal with the more intimate problems and concerns, that no one practitioner is available for initial medical aid, advice, and direction to other sources for help, that physicians are too busy to give "physicals" to healthy individuals or to be interested in the early detection and prevention of disease, that the doctor's office is located farther and farther away from the neighborhood and home, or that emergency round-the-clock help is no longer available. These are important caretaking and treatment functions of the family doctor, who has largely disappeared in fact but not in fancy.

To want a family doctor may no longer be a question of choice. The question that needs to be asked is how are his functions being met in our organizations and patterns of specialization. Many of these essential functions are now in several hands. Much of the public, at least in the middle-class suburbs, seems to be using multiple "specialists" for health care needs at different periods of life: the pediatrician for the children and the baby; the obstetrician-gynecologist for delivery and the mother's checkups; and the internist for the mother's, father's, and grandparents' "medical troubles." Every "specialist" may be expected to take on some of the functions of the family doctor at times, and yet their professional training and orientation does not acknowledge this and their own definition as specialists deals only with technical diagnostic questions about the patient.

This problem becomes exacerbated as medical men increasingly specialize and as the lay population becomes more medically sophisticated and so goes directly to specialists or asks to be referred. This will not be "bad" if the patient's "other problems" and concerns are recognized and he is directed to a suitable source of help. But since there will often be no family physician to whom the specialist can return such patients when these other problems arise, he will have to deal with them himself—a situation for which his medical education may have left him largely unprepared.

Ancillary Professions

While much debate is centered on how the various medical specialists should be related, a still more fundamental issue concerns the transfer and division of functions among other health professions, who may do diagnostic and therapeutic work. It is in this area that what is truly "team medicine" may develop. The expectation, however, that the doctor, as "the specialist" of the team, will deal only with the complicated medical aspects of the patient, leaving personal concerns to the nurse and social worker, and ordinary diagnostic skills to the technicians, is not a likely possibility. This might seem a rational division of the technical skills of the team, but there will be social limits. For example, the patient, in seeking help, will not always view the professions as they see themselves nor be able to diagnose his illness and choose or accept the right kind of help. Called to see a patient vomiting at night, the doctor may come upon a family quarrel and a crisis over the behavior of a child. Some would argue that the family called the wrong person, that it should have call the psychiatrist or the social worker. But since the call for help was in response to a child's vomiting, it is unlikely that anyone other than a medical man would have been called and expected to cope with such a crisis.

There is, however, another side to this coin: it concerns the limits of competence of the community practitioner. Psychosomatic complaints and physical symptoms of behavior disorders are most likely to come to the attention of physicians and may require some medical surveillance and be subject to rational psychological treatment. Yet there is no evidence that more general behavioral problems are most appropriately treated by "medical men" as they are now trained. Some would even contend that the psychological training of a Ph.D. clinical psychologist is often more extensive than that of many psychiatrists and certainly of most physicians. Whether behavioral problems such as delinquency, malingering, antisocial acts and even much of what is called neurotic should be considered "illness" and therefore under the sole dominion of the medical professions has been questioned by at least one psychiatrist, Thomas Szasz.

Public Health Nurse

A less noticeable transfer and fractionization of medical duties is taking place in still another sphere. As our professions specialize and centralize—for example, at hospitals and medical centers— as they limit the hours they work and the calls they make—for example, no house calls—and as we fail to train enough doctors or to organize health personnel for the needs of the population, makeshift solutions in treatment develop. For instance, the public health nurse is filling a doctor-gap for large segments of our lower socioeconomic classes, as well as for still larger populations abroad. She has become a sort of second-choice-doctor—giving some emergency treatment, teaching health care and prevention, and doing a considerable amount of family counselling. Since it is rarely recognized or acknowledged that she is engaged in such tasks, she is often without connecting links to any chain of medical practice and lacks the face-to-face communication with colleagues that is important in patient care. One of the dangers of being outside any network of medical practice is the lack of informal supervision of the quality of patient care which ordinarily occurs through mutual consultation and interchange among professional staffs. Whether she will ultimately become the "family doctor" of choice is inextricably entwined with the degree to which doctors will continue to withdraw from and reject such duties.

Thus, who takes care of the patient—the division of labor of medical practice—will ultimately depend on the patients' views of their illness and of the professionals they seek to treat them as well as on the internal needs of professionals themselves. Fractionization of medical care has already and inevitably taken place. Much of the current dissatisfaction is due more to ineffective communication between therapists and their lack of coordination and "teamwork" than to any inherent "badness" in a division of treatment itself. Unwillingness to recognize this phenomenon has resulted in scant attention being paid to how immediate medical aid can be organized, what treatment can and should be coordinated, who can treat personal concerns and behavioral problems, how exclusively "specialistic" should a specialist's training and education be—to what, in fact, is the appropriate use of other professions whether they be behavioral scientists, human relations experts, or public health nurses. As long as these problems are not even acknowledged, effective planning of treatment work is impossible.

DO WE CARE ABOUT THE SIZE AND LOCATION
OF OUR HOSPITALS AND PRACTICES?

Not because of "specialization" but because of rising costs, the work of hospitals has also been scrutinized. Demands are made to restrict the hospital as a sickbed institution only to the performance of technical procedures required in complicated diagnosis and treatment of acute illness. At the same time, the hospital has been taking on other functions besides bed care and maintaining a "sick room away from home." For example, all phases of illness—from the acute attack to convalescence, rehabilitation, chronic care, and terminal stages—have increasingly become hospital functions. There has also been a greater recognition of the care and treatment which can be organized for a patient without hospitalization. Certainly more medical care is possible with ambulant patients, in out-patient clinics and offices, although such functions rarely receive the public, professional, or institutional support which the bed functions do.

All these trends make the hospital a bigger and bigger "center," a diversified organization with more caretaking services on its grounds. However, the mere bringing of all caretaking services to hospital grounds does not guarantee that nursing home, chronic disease treatment, and ambulatory care will, in turn, get better facilities, better professional staff, better organization of treatment, and more investment. The hospital as an institution has its own priorities and can just as well neglect certain treatment functions as the community at large.

Process of Centralization

How the bigger hospitals grow will also determine the future existence of our small local hospitals and local practices where much general care is given and where many patients prefer to attend. It will depend on whether there is merely centralization of facilities and services and practices—witness the private practice office buildings moving to hospital grounds—or whether there is growth through more effective integration and alliance with and among smaller local community institutions and practices. The trend to add and centralize more and more activities in the hospital grounds will certainly make some of our traditional local hospitals and practices less important, but growth by cooperation and integration should not have this effect. "Regionalization" has become the shorthand for this cooperative organization of medical services in a community. Unfortunately, in some situations it has only meant dividing up clientele areas, thus limiting medical competition among big hospitals. It may, however, mean a brake on duplication, on the purchase of expensive equipment by each of several hospitals, and the selected development of expensive therapies. And it can mean even more—such as the development of working relationships among institutions and medical practices, for the management of illness and disability in an urban treatment area. An important yet intangible by-product could be the informal supervision of the quality of patient care in the community that can occur through mutual consultation and interchange among professional staffs, managers, and the lay boards alike. Now they so often work in relative isolation.

Mental Health Care

Finally, we might want our hospitals to grow in still another way. For example, a major concern of our hospital staffs, managers, and boards might be whether our traditional medical institutions, whose practices are in reality concerned as much with mental health, should include treatment departments, divisions, and even special hospital units for social and psychiatric care. Such health care has long been an implicit function of the work of the personal doctor or "GP," but as a hospital function it has developed into special mental institutions parallel to but separate from our general medical ones. Large-scale psychiatric services, particularly in inpatient care, is still a comparatively rare phenomenon in a general hospital.

Some would say that to join these traditionally separate systems is too difficult an alliance both ideologically and practically. For example, mental institutions and psychiatric care have been financed through taxes and thus have a history and background different from that of the community's general voluntary hospitals with their history of private financing. However, even these differences are disappearing. As voluntary hospitals rely more and more on patient-care receipts and government programs, they are becoming increasingly like traditional public instituions, at least in financing. Another similarity is administrative management. Mental hospitals are taking on discharge and treatment policies and practices like general hospitals, returning many chronic patients to the community. Recent studies have shown that for many psychiatric patients hospitalization in a general hospital has distinct treatment advantages and that their care can be managed with minimal disruption of hospital routine. Notwithstanding differences that still exist, if demands and needs for health care are not just medical but also psychosocial, then the integration of these parallel services is a major public concern.

Solo Practice

The question of centralization of functions in the hospital has its counterpart in the current debates about medical practice. Perhaps in fear of the growing tentacles of the hospital or medical center, there is concern about whether solo entrepreneurial practice, a more dominant style of organization in our country, is suitable for the complexities of patient care as opposed to group practice where medical specialization is formally organized for treatment. Will the solo practitioner, the individual firm, the medical small business, like the corner grocer, be swallowed up by or affiliate with a big chain like a group practice or clinic? And, if he does join, will he contract his skills to the group or entrepreneur within it?

The alternatives in organization have always been pictured as either one system or another, private practice or "government medicine," solo or contractual practice. For example, it seems clear that even individual solo practice has already done many things which make ideological views outdated—it has remained as an informal network of colleague practices, it has formed into group practice units, and even contracted for medical care of groups. Some have also located on the hospital's grounds as a big private entrepreneurial business, alongside more contractual forms of group practice and clinics. Large clinics with contractual practice have also sprung up in response to the needs of the blocks of consumers found in industry, unions, and colleges. Harvard, for example, has organized a prepaid in-plant medical service for students, faculty, and employees with contractual services of doctors.

This retail view of practice and organization may not appeal to us when we are dealing with such charged transactions as our own health, illness, and treatment. However, it may caution us against too ideological a commitment to one form of practice for everybody. It may also modify views which regard only our own consumer choice as ideal and all others as undesirable, without a real respect for other choices in the domestic scene. When it comes to actual facts about what organization is best, we often adhere to traditional concepts with little evidence as to what actually works best for whom.

But there are many other public concerns about organization of medical practice. Equally important is its location—at the hospital, the school, the plant—in addition to the traditional location in the neighborhood or downtown. Medical practices at these institutional sites, in contrast to the entrepreneurial organization of private practice, have usually been contractual, with the doctors as employees. Practitioners at these sites have always been ambivalent about the scope and depth of their medical services to their clientele. Should they provide personal and comprehensive health services or restrict themselves to job-related injuries and employment examinations? The uneasiness in deciding to do the former has been due to the fear of competing with private practice. To add to the dilemma, recent research has documented the importance of the work situation in the individual's physical and psychological health. Surely, if we hope to reach everyone, these on-the-spot sites may be realistic ways of offering personal and preventive medical services, and our traditional ambivalence about competition will have to give way to concern about availability and consumption of services.

EPILOGUE

Remembering the high prevalence of treated and untreated symptoms and disorders, cited previously, there are those who claim that we cannot treat everything. There are others who note that there is probably a great deal we should not treat such as many self-limiting disorders—for example, minor burns, some communicable childhood diseases, unnecessary tonsillectomies. The task of treatment is indeed monumental, for the very progress and development of man introduces new dangers, new agents of desease. Man experiments with synthetic products and changes his diet; he constructs cities that breed rats and infection; he builds automobiles, factories, and bombs which pollute the air. When one disease or disorder is controlled, its control mechanism may produce the breeding ground for still another disease. As René Dubos contends, the goal of complete freedom from disease and struggle is almost incompatible with the progress of living; so also with medical care. Whether we should strive to provide medical care for everything is impossible to say. Until we recognize that illness and health are more than the mere presence or absence of symptoms, that seeking medical aid is more than reactive behavior to symptoms, and the health professions' responsibility is more than to wait for patients and then to treat these symptoms, our solutions for providing medical care will only be stopgaps.

With more and more possibilities of therapeutic intervention for everything, a philosophy of medicine is needed to define what is "good medical care," comprehensive care, or the "best medical care in the world." While medical care experts can furnish us with measurements of the quality and quantity of treatment, we also need to consider our directions, for example, the other problems produced by the technical capacity to prevent death at any cost in old age, the values of genetic counselling particularly in regard to the problem of treating congenital defects, or the use of the medical services to meet personal needs—that is, as a "refuge in a storm"—as much as we need to consider utilitarian demands of keeping people healthy and on the job.

Finally, it is often complained that the government will set the policies regarding medical care and practice. The basic problems besetting medical care, however, are neither financial nor administrative but the professional and public needs and aspirations. In this commentary specific solutions have not been suggested but several important issues, often submerged from view, have been discussed. Only when such issues are recognized can solutions be found: and only then can we claim to provide not only the best medical care but the best possible medical care.

8. Medical Organization, Medical Care, and Lower Income Groups

ANSELM L. STRAUSS

INTRODUCTION[1]

The National Commitment

In a special message to Congress on January 7, 1965, President Johnson dramatically reaffirmed the nation's commitment to good health for *all* American citizens.[2] Quoting Jefferson's remark that "without health there is no happiness," President Johnson emphasized that "it is imperative that we give first attention to our opportunities—and our obligations—for advancing the nation's health."

Equally notable in President Johnson's reaffirmation of the nation's responsibility for the health of all its citizens was his explicit commentary upon the health needs of the poor. The problem of poor families rests not only on their lack of money—"Poor families," the President noted: "increasingly are forced to turn to overcrowded hospital emergency rooms and to overburdened city clinics as their only resource to meet their routine health needs."

President Johnson's message prefaced what was to be sweeping and precedent-breaking medical legislation. After many years of national and congressional debate—and massive professional and political opposition—"Medicare" was passed. Legislation for establishing centers for Heart, Stroke and Cancer also was quickly passed. The latter legislation was designed to speed up the application of medical innovation, but also to give the leading medical schools, teaching

From *Social Science and Medicine* 3(1969), pp. 143–77, reprinted by permission of the author and publisher.

This paper was commissioned by the Institute for Policy studies, Washington, under the co-directorship of Richard Barnett and Mark Raskin. My thanks for useful consultation to Eliot Freidson, Melvin Sabshin and Lee Rainwater.

126

hospitals and major medical centers a greater influence in leading the scattered medical community out of the essentially disconnected sprawl which the rural-oriented Hill-Burton hospital construction program had helped to further. Medicare represents an increasing emphasis on the hospital as the center and coordinator of medical care, and promises to lift the poorest of our aged out of the medical ghetto of charity care into the stream of voluntary and proprietary hospital care. In addition, the considerable national focus on poverty, and on the need for central city reform, and such programs as Head Start, all underline the national commitment to extend quality medical care to the most economically disadvantaged Americans. Indeed, in Johnson's 1967 budget message to Congress, he proposed a quadrupling of federal spending on health care and medical assistance for the poor in 1968.

INCOME DIFFERENTIALS AND MEDICAL CARE

Current inequities in the distribution of medical care and services have been well documented by the U.S. Department of Health, Education and Welfare in a study titled *Medical Care, Health Status and Family Income.*[3] Statistics on personal health expenditures, health insurance coverage, the use of medical and dental services, chronic illness and disability, acute illness, and disability days, all demonstrate how greatly disadvantaged are the lower income groups.[4] For instance, the percentage of persons with hospital or surgical insurance coverage "is closely related to family income ranging from 34 percent among those in families of less than $2,000 income to almost 50 percent for persons in families of $7,000 or more annual income." At the same time, lower income families are more likely to have "multiple hospital episodes" than higher income families. The differential in health insurance coverage shows up strikingly insofar as:

> Among persons who were hospitalized, insurance paid for some part of the bill for about 40 percent of patients with less than $2,000 family income, 60 percent of patients with $2,000–$3,999 family income, and 80 percent of patients with higher incomes. Insurance paid three-fourths or more of the bill for approximately 27 percent of these respective income groups. Preliminary data from the current survey year show, for the proportion of bills for surgery or delivery paid by insurance, an even more marked association with income.

Concerning the utilization of physicians' visits, the "pattern of utilization . . . is quite clear cut, showing an increase of visits . . .

with increase in family income." Taking the extremes in family income groups (under $2,000 and $7,000 and over), the utilization patterns are not only clear-cut but strikingly different. Thus, the ratio of annual physicians' visits per person are 2.8 and 3.8. (For children under fifteen years of age, the ratio is 1.6 to 5.7.) The differential use of medical facilities for physicians' visits is also indicated by the ratios for visits to hospital clinic respectively, 0.7 annual visits to 0.3. The tremendous advantage of the higher income groups in utilization of medical specialists is indicated by respective figures of 12.9 percent and 27.5 percent. (The income group between $2,000 and $3,999 is not much better off: the percentage who visit specialists is 13.9).

Concerning health expenditures themselves, this government survey showed that at each family income level, amounts spent for doctors' services comprised about a third of the total health expenditures (although the lower economic groups visit physicians less often). The highest income group averaged health expenses per person of $153, whereas all other income groups averaged as much as, respectively, $112, $116 and $119 per person annually. In other words, those who could least afford the health expenses paid annually almost as much as people who could afford most. Also, since family size tends to increase with lower family income, another health differential is not surprising: health expenses ($104) for a child living in a three-member family with an income of $7,000 and over were five times greater than the amount spent for health care of a child in a family with seven or more members and an income of less than $2,000.

The lower income groups are strikingly disadvantaged in two other important ways. The first pertains to the amount of chronic illness and disability, the second pertains to the actual loss of working days due to disability. Among the lowest income group, 57.6 percent have one or more chronic conditions compared with 42.9 of the highest income group. The figures for respective chronic limitation of activity from those diseases are 29 percent and 8 percent. Also inability to move about freely is clearly associated with family income: the figures are respectively 7 percent and 1 percent. And the percentage of persons with more than one chronic condition causing limitation is 59.8 percent compared with 24.1 percent. When these figures are translated into loss of work days, the burden falls heavily on the lower income groups: the respective figures for men are 10.2 days and 4.9 days; for women, 7.5 days and 6.5 days. The government report notes that even with respect to acute diseases among persons 45 years and older the incidence rates (as well as the rates for medically attended, activity-restricting or bed-disabling conditions) are higher for families with incomes of less than $2,000 than for any other income group.

Needed: a Radical Reorganization of Medical Services

It is patent that the lower income groups do not receive a fair share of the available health services. In the following pages, I shall show that lower income groups are disadvantaged in the medical market, not only because of fewer financial supports and less availability of services, but because of a drastic mismatch between medical organization and lower income life-styles. I shall argue that the *extension of quality care to lower income groups requires a radical reorganization of medical organization.*

In the lively public discussion and debate over the improvement of medical care and services, it is striking how little attention is paid to the mismatch of medical organization and lower income life-styles. Primarily the emphasis is placed upon how the present medical organization needs to be added to, or somewhat altered, so as *better to deliver* quality care to people who do not now get it. For instance, at the 1965 Health Conference of the New York Academy of Medicine various experts addressed themselves to the question of current and future medical organization and care. Although disagreeing on particulars, they constantly emphasized the necessity for improved outreach of medical services. Over and over, they focused on better delivery of quality care through increased facilities and manpower, or through more efficient institutional arrangements of current facilities and manpower. Thus, Dr. Robert Felix[5] (formerly of NIH, and currently Dean of the School of Medicine at St. Louis University) emphasized that now, "When facilities have become available, with new knowledge accumulating, with more professionals available to deliver services, there remains *one barrier to full opportunity for achieving the right of health.* This is *adequate financing* of health programs" (our italics).

Dr. Felix then remarked on the increasing responsibility by the federal government in the health services, predicting

1. Increased health insurance coverage to the point where no person need defer seeking medical attention because of finances.

2. An increase in ambulatory-type services.

3. Development of comprehensive regional or district health complexes.

The programs and planning of federal agencies are similarly sharply focused upon more financing and more resources and better delivery. For instance, the Children's Bureau programs are among the most advanced federal programs. In a 1963 paper, Arthur J. Lesser, Director of the Division of Health Services, Children's Bureau, remarked that a President's Panel:

> urged that a new program be established with federal funds authorized on a project basis to assist State and local health departments in meeting the costs of administering programs of comprehensive maternity and infant care for women who have problems associated with pregnancy . . . and who are unlikely to receive the care they need because of low income or for other reasons. These programs would make it possible to:
>
> 1. Increase the number of prenatal and postnatal clinics.
> 2. Bring the prenatal and postpartum clinics close to the population served.
> 3. Establish special clinics for some patients with complications of pregnancy (where more time by obstetricians, nurses, social workers, nutritioners and others can be provided.)
> 4. Pay for hospital care not only for the delivery but also during the prenatal period as needed.
> 5. Relieve overcrowding in tax-supported hospitals by paying for care in voluntary hospitals.
> 6. Pay for hospital care of premature infants and other infants needing special attention.
> 7.   Provide consultation services.[6]

Such recommendations have already become part of federal legislation. What is notable about the recommendations—which are altogether admirable—is, again, the emphasis upon additional financing, manpower and resources.   (There was also some emphasis upon education.) But the special obstacles offered by discrepancies between medical organization and lower income life-styles are *not* frontally attacked.

What this signifies is that *current planning is based on a set of quite deficient assumptions. First,* it is assumed that there is basically nothing wrong with the organization of medical care, except that organization is not extensive enough to reach everyone adequately. *Second,* it is assumed what is needed for extending the health enterprise is more financial support, more manpower, more resources of various kinds (hospitals, centers, equipment, training centers). Different planners and planning agencies give different priorities to financing, manpower, or resources, but all seem to think principally in such terms. *Third,* such reorganization of medical care as is called for—other than adding money, resources or manpower to the system—is principally in terms of improved efficiency of the medical care system. For example, a more extensive and well-wrought linkage of facilities and manpower, as in the "Heart, Stroke and Cancer" legislation. Or, a linkage of municipal and teaching hospitals, as in the New York City plan initiated by Trussel. I have no quarrel with much of the planning based on these assumptions. More money, resources, and manpower certainly with help distribute quality care more widely. So will some measures designed to improve the efficiency of present medical organization.

I contend, however, that *no amount of adding to, or tinkering with, the present system of medical organization is going to achieve medical quality or equity for all citizens.* Given the conditions outlined in the following pages, it will be difficult to maintain that a startling residue of inequity would not persist—despite all attempts to improve the delivery of medical services through measures currently suggested by medical planners. It is true that if all Americans had sufficient finances to pay for their medical care, and if the medical facilities were located so efficiently as to be equally accessible to all, and if each medical facility were manned and equipped with great efficiency, then the medical care offered Americans certainly would be greatly improved. But there would still remain a striking discrepancy between the care received by lower and higher income groups—due to exactly those factors that will be outlined below.

There are no ready means whereby my contention can be proven. (The assumptions underlying current planning cannot be proven either.) Nevertheless, we do know that when medical facilities are set up in convenient proximity to lower income housing, they do not automatically draw clientele. In one instance, a clinic located between a lower income and lower-middle income population was almost wholly used by the latter. Other clinics located in lower income areas frequently follow a typical cycle: at first the staff is enthusiastic, and its enthusiasm is conveyed to its clientele; but as the difficulties of making much of a dent on lower income illness begin to wear down the staff, enthusiasm decreases, there is turnover of personnel, and eventually the clinic is much less effective in drawing or keeping its patients. No doubt medical facilities located nearer the homes of lower income people are more likely to draw and keep patients, but their mere presence does not solve the problem of delivering effective care to most people in the nearby locale.

If the national commitment is to be met in earnest, it is necessary to reexamine certain features of health services not ordinarily discussed in the context of America's strikingly large health gap. These features include certain dominant perspectives of the health professionals, their types of training, and the ways that medical facilities, especially hospitals, are organized. Facilities and personnel need to be seen in conjunction with certain widespread characteristics of lower socioeconomic life, including: dominant styles of living, attitudes toward health, and typical experiences with health services.

In general, I shall emphasize that professional perspectives and training, and the organization of facilities are not conducive to offering quality medical care to the lower socioeconomic groups.[7] Medical training and organization evolved principally to service a clientele that could afford to pay for medical services. Those services were extended traditionally of course (in a kind of double-truck system) through municipal hospitals, outpatient clinics, and some private practices. Medical organization and attitudes, nevertheless, were (and are) less suited to the life styles of the lower income groups than those of higher income.[8]

If this is so, what reorganization of the medical and health services will be necessary in order to give quality care to these Americans also—without destroying the quality of care now available to more fortunate segments of our population? A parallel question which will be explored is this: What will happen if the nation fails to institute an efficient reorganization of medical care? In general, my answers will be that if we do not institute reorganization of medical care, then its distribution will continue to be exceedingly inequitable.[9]

THE ORGANIZATION OF MEDICAL CARE

There are two major factors—relative to medical organization—that contribute to inequities in medical care. The first consists of the current organization of medical services. This acts as a brake on giving quality care to lower income groups. The second consists of the life styles of the lower income groups, which unquestionably constitute an obstacle to their receiving quality medical care.

Negative Features of Medical Organization

Even when medical services are readily available to lower income groups, these services are characteristically underutilized. In some part this underutilization is caused by some characteristic features of medical organization itself. And these same features of medical organization tend to blunt the effectiveness of medical care when patients of lower income status are actually in treatment.

What are these inimical characteristics of medical organization? *First, there is the very massiveness of medical organization itself.* Hospitals and clinics are often large, the division of labor rather complex, the work of diagnosis and treatment involving elaborate coordination of specialized hospital services and of staff effort. As Rosenblatt and Suchman remark in their study of the underutilization of medical services in New York City, medical care requires specialization of function and specialized clinics, the whole enterprise being market by a fair degree of impersonality.[10] Even middle class patients feel this impersonality, for it is one of their chief complaints about hospital care. But lower income people are less well equipped by education and experience to understand elaborate organization, or to cope with it.[11]

Why this is so is clear enough. Their own organizational life is meagre, unlike the more typical experience of people of higher economic and educational status. As we suggest later in more detail, the life of lower income people tends to be rooted in narrow locale and in family, and is less in contact with a wider community life. They do not belong much to voluntary organizations, whether economic, political or social. They may have jobs in large organizations, but they do not run those organizations and play little part in managing organizational activities even at the lowest levels. Indeed they have not usually much grasp of organizational operations. We need not at all attribute deficiencies of intelligence to lower income people to explain why they have difficulties in understanding and coping with organization, especially when it is complex: we need only remember their lacks in education and in experience.

When a lower income person enters a clinic or hospital, he is confronted by problems of understanding how it works, what it expects of him, and how best to get around in it. These institutions are organized for getting work done, whether it be diagnosis, treatment or "comfort care." They are only infrequently set up to minimize the patient's potential confusion except in certain matters, such as those pertaining to admission, or "where to go to get examined" or to wait for examination, or which clinic is the appropriate one to attend. Otherwise the patient must figure things out for himself, except insofar as he can get someone else to explain matters he wishes or needs to know. It is not unknown for lower income patients literally to get lost when sent "just down the corridor" in what seems an incredibly big, confusing institutional world. The directions given them seem inadequate, the manner brusque. A typical situation in emergency rooms of municipal hospitals is that patients sit for many minutes, even hours, expecting to be examined by order of appearance; but they are puzzled and angered because patients who come in later are taken "out of turn." They do not understand, and the staff does not bother to explain, that there are different kinds of emergencies and therefore different priorities of medical actions.

These examples represent rather simple levels of misunderstanding or of confusion or frustration, but countless more subtle ones can be cited. For instance, hospitalized patients are often sent for diagnostic tests from one hospital service to another, with little or no explanation of what the procedures are all about. Patients can be rendered exceedingly anxious by this whole process. Their anxiety may be relevant to the diagnosis itself if it affects the diagnostic findings without staff's awareness. Another instance of how complex organization baffles and frustrates the patient who does not easily find his way within it is the frequent complaint of patients, in medical plans such as Kaiser's, that they cannot find a clinic doctor whom they really like or trust. Yet the more knowledgeable, and typically the more "middle class" patients quickly discover how to "beat the system" so as to find a trustworthy doctor and to ensure assignment to him whenever they visit the clinic. The total impact of such experiences on lower income patients is considerable. Whereas higher income patients may be angered but understand (at least somewhat) what is happening at the clinic or hospital, the lower income patients understand less what is happening regardless of their consequent reactions. It is worth emphasizing that lower income patients are much less likely to have private physicians than are the higher income patients. Therefore, they have no agent who can explain the behavior of a hospital staff to them, or who can manage the establishment so as to get seemingly important things from it.

A second feature of medical organization decreasing the quality of care they might receive is the professionalization of health workers. Training in specialized schools (medicine, nursing, social work) results in characteristic goals, perspectives toward work, and modes of working with machinery and men (including patients). The higher the level of specialized knowledge attained by the professionals, the more the clients who utilize his services must take his abilities and knowledge on trust: for the gap between their understanding of these specialized matters and his is great. Some procedures insisted on by professionals may seem senseless or even dangerous, and the professionals' manner of issuing directives—or of avoiding issues—may seem impersonal or even brutal. Yet the professionals are carrying out those actions, for the most part, with genuine concern for the patient's welfare.

Again the lower income patients and their families are at some disadvantage as compared with higher income people. Generally, the former are less able to comprehend the various professional stances and their implications. They may be quite unable to understand the nature of the prescribed treatment. They have less understanding of basic psychological processes and so understand less of the diagnoses. They are less able to sense when a professional judgment may be wrong, if only because they understand less of the medical language and the specialized perspective. Physicians may assume too much about the understanding of patients and fail to communicate the sense of treatment or a prescribed regimen. Or they may not attempt to explain much, reasoning that these patients' education is insufficient to allow real comprehension. Of course the physician may decide to withhold information for very good professional reasons. The result is that patients of all income groups typically complain a great deal about the difficulties of getting sufficient information from physicians and nurses. But lower income people are less skilled at engineering matters to get that information. They are less experienced in the tactics of forcing explanations or trapping staff members into explanations. They tend also to be less aggressive in demanding explanations. Fred Davis, in a study of polio patients and their families (mainly of lower income status), has described the situation very vividly:

> In general, the behavior of parents [is] . . . eager, deferential, and subordinate; that of hospital personnel, especially the doctors, as brusque, noncommittal, and superordinate, even at times—or so it seemed to parents—condescending or indifferent. Mrs. Short's account . . . reflects a typical experience: "Well they don't tell you anything hardly. They don't seem to want to. I mean, you start asking questions and they say, 'Well, I only have about three minutes to talk to you.' And then the things that you ask, they don't seem to want to answer you. So I don't ask them anything anymore . . ."[12]

The greater aggressive and interactional skills of higher income patients yield a far better countering of strategies of withholding information, whatever the professional's reasons for withholding. In consequence, lower income patients and their families are frequently frustrated by an inability either to understand what is happening or to control events deemed important to themselves.

The greater interactional skills of higher income patients also allow them, on the whole, to manipulate the work of professionals—the pacing and scheduling of work, for instance—and this management may lead to their improved care. Just as these patients will complain more effectively about poor food, they complain about or negotiate for "baths later," for more frequent or powerful medication, and the like. Lower income patients, as is generally recognized, tend to be more docile, less aggressive, in making such demands. When they make them, they tend also to be less effective in getting them answered. In addition, the lower income patient is less likely to make direct requests of his private physician. Since he is also less likely to have a private physician at all, he has less opportunity to call upon him to intervene with the hospital staff for correcting possible deficiencies of care.[13]

There is a more subtle disadvantage, stemming from professional stances, which lower income patients suffer. The treatments deemed useful may vary somewhat in accordance with the professional's view of his patient's socioeconomic status. By this, we do not mean the expensiveness of drugs ordered or the number of days of treatment that the physician judges his patient can afford. Thus, concerning psychiatric treatment Frank Riessman and Sylvia Scribner summarize that "middle class patients are preferred by most treatment agents, and are seen as more treatable. Psychotherapy is more frequently recommended as the treatment of choice, and diagnoses are more hopeful with symptomology held constant."[14] In other words, there may be a distinct bias expressed against the lower income patient, based honestly on professional conceptions.

More usually, however, the professional makes the assumption that treatment and care should be determined by disease process. Consequently, physicians tend to prescribe the same treatments, the same regimens, for patients regardless of income status (except insofar as finances set limits). As we shall detail later, the lower income patient is thereby further disadvantaged for often the regimen is unsuited to his style of life, or the medication prescribed is so inadequately explained to him that he does not take it correctly, and so on. Riessman's comment about psychotherapy for lower income patients is apposite here: "treatment as *presently organized* is not congenial to low-income clients, is not congruent with their traditions and expectations and is poorly understood by them. In essence, these clients are alienated from treatment."[15]

But mental disease is not the only area about which such statements can be made: prescribing regimens for certain cardiac patients is done without adequate awareness of how impossible they may be for the patients to carry out. Even the simple order that medication is to be taken "with each meal" may run afoul of the fact that many lower income families eat irregularly and so do not have three meals a day.

A third characteristic feature of medical organization which profoundly influences the quality of medical care received by lower income patients—is the middle class bias of most professional health workers. Typically all but the lower echelons in hospitals and clinics are of higher socioeconomic status than the lower income patients. This difference between staff and those patients results often in two striking disadvantages for the patients. One consequence of the staff members' social background is that they do not understand the perspectives, attitudes, customs and life styles of the patients; they take for granted that the patients are human like themselves! The patients have regular meals at home—just like us. Men conscientious-

ly can support their families—just like us—or have steady employment or lead regular lives, or have the same protective attitudes
toward their children, or have the same attitudes towards health as
we do. Precisely because professionals make these assumptions about
lower income people, they issue orders that are not understood or
cannot easily be followed by the patients.[16]

A much cruder aspect of the class differential is that many
professionals display genuine prejudice against lower income patients
(sometimes side by side with the assumption that "they are just like
us"). Like middle class people outside the hospital, they often think
of lower income people in stereotyped terms. The latter are "like
children," and must be treated as children. They cannot keep appointments, having little sense of time or responsibility. They are
shiftless, irresponsible. They have children out of wedlock. They are
dirty, unkempt, unclean. Sometimes these biased notions are expressed very openly by hospital personnel—notions and expressions
probably both abetted by the tensions of a busy and often harried
schedule of work. In any event, patients often comprehend or sense
what the staff thinks of them, and may either suffer through the
prejudice or choose not to return to hospital or clinic. While some of
their dislike of municipal hospitals and clinics is attributable to
overcrowding and poor service, some dislike is unquestionably due to
the class bias of the staff members. There is not much doubt that this
kind of class bias, then, profoundly affects both the quality of
medical care which these patients receive and their underutilization
of medical services.

*A fourth feature of medical organization is that a great proportion
of these patients (especially in urban areas) are serviced at municipal
and county hospitals.* These facilities typically share certain characteristics. Usually they are run on tight budgets, at lower costs per
patient than most community or proprietary hospitals. They also
service great numbers of patients. Consequently they tend to be
relatively understaffed, especially by professionals. The nursing personnel tend to remain at these installations for many years, and
consequently develop routine modes for handling and caring for
patients. Often they tend not to be quickly receptive to newer ideas
in nursing. Typically these facilities have few or no visiting staff
physicians, but are administered by residents and internes. These
men tend to be enthusiastic but are not yet very experienced in the
nuances of medical care, and certainly not in human relations.
Frequently the hospital is very large and may even be spread among
many separate buildings.[17]

These hospitals and their accompanying outpatient clinics are
easily imagined by patients to be terribly massive and complex,

crowded and busy; while the personnel seem often impersonal, brusque or even insulting. In fact, the places do tend to be massive and crowded, the staff very rushed with need for quick movement. The physicians go from patient to patient, spending brief moments with most, accompanied by a nurse. (And where the hospital is affiliated with a medical school, the busy—often disease-oriented— physician is accompanied by an absorbed group of medical students, and by one or more residents or internes.) Patients get not much opportunity to ask questions of the busy physician or nurses. In the clinics, patients may sit for long periods of time waiting to be called, without being addressed, or paid attention to, by personnel moving to and fro. In the hospitals, the nurses are frequently busy with administrative tasks so that nursing assistants spend more time near and around patients. Patients see all of this, and may simply respond fatalistically to the rush and the bustle. They may also inaccurately attribute to the staff a humiliating brusqueness when none was meant, indifference when the personnel were only busily abstracted, and class or race prejudices where none was displayed.[18] Neverthe- less, by their very characteristics these medical institutions maximize aspects of medical organization which are among the most inimical for providing quality care. Even when the staff is excellent or the facility is connected with a top-flight medical school, many if not most characteristic features of these places still persist.[19]

Medical Organization and "Medical Care"

There is another feature of medical organization worth special atten- tion: its special focus on medical and procedural aspects of care." A certain ambiguity attends the use of the term "medical care." It will be convenient here to discuss its relationship to medical organization by distinguishing grossly among "diagnosis," treatment," and a third aspect which perhaps more properly deserves the name of "care" (whether nursing or medical). In common parlance, diagnosis means the detection of disease processes. Treatment means what is done about the disease process in order to arrest the disease, improve the symptoms and so on. Medical services are superbly organized to carry out both diagnosis and treatment—that is what the health profes- sionals traditionally are trained to do, and what medical research has focused on. The virtual eradication of many acute diseases from the American population has rested upon their accurate diagnosis and effective treatment. Public health personnel, hospital personnel, and private practitioners have all shared in that success.

In general, medical organization is less successful in the diagnosis and treatment of lower income groups, in part because medical services are less available or accessible to these people, in part because generally they themselves are less concerned about health (a point we shall discuss later). Nevertheless, even for this segment of our population, the Achilles heel of medical organization is neither diagnosis nor treatment. *Its weakness lies principally in the vaguer residual area of "care," which includes much nursing care, various kinds of instructions to patients about their regimens, along with the general evaluation of—and communication about—progress or retrogression after patients leave the hospital.*

Let us focus only on post-hospital care. Whereas higher income patients can call upon private physicians for evaluations of progress, or are likely to visit their physicians if progress eventually is not apparent, the lower income patients are much less likely to have private physicians. For checkups they must return to busy outpatient clinics, where incidentally they rarely see the same doctor twice (except through union insurance plans or plans like HIP). For a short while or in emergencies, they may be attended occasionally at home by visiting nurses, or given procedural and health instructions by public health nurses. But most lower income patients are very much "on their own" after leaving the hospital or clinic. This is because hospital and community—as many critics for many years have noted —are relatively separate entities. Traditionally, most hospitals grew up either as servicing agencies for poverty-stricken patients or as places where private physicians could house their patients. Hospitals are even rather insulated from public health agencies; they are certainly quite insulated from the homes of their ex-patients. So once again the organization of medical services (of hospital and clinics especially) tends to the disadvantage of the lower income patient. He gets less "continuity of care."

Underutilization of Medical Services

Various research studies and surveys have reported medical services are underutilized by lower income groups. For instance, the Director of the Division of Health Services, Children's Bureau, has noted "Large numbers of women are receiving little or no prenatal care." And:

> In Atlanta, 23% of women delivered at the Grady Hospital had had no prenatal care; in Dallas, approximately one-third of low-income patients receive no prenatal care; at the Los Angeles County Hospital in 1958, it was 20%; at the D.C. General Hospital in Washington, it is 45%; and in the Bedford Stuyvesant section of Brooklyn, New York, it is 41% with no or little prenatal care.[20]

Some underutilization unquestionably is due to the attitudes and life styles of lower income people, which mitigate against more frequent use of medical services even when readily available. Dr. Frank McPhail,[21] in a Dallas County Youth Study, reports that such things as "cultural difference," "working mothers," "finding somebody to stay with the other children," and "seeking care too late," are among the factors which are deterrents to good (prenatal) care. We shall have more to detail about the relevance of attitudes and life styles in the next pages.

But we should note that much in preceding pages is also pertinent to the underutilization of medical services. Patients' real or imagined perceptions of class and race bias, their many hours of waiting, the seeming or actual impersonal routines of institutional care, and the like, maximize the dissatisfactions of lower income patients—and further the possibility of infrequent visits or of no visits at all. In addition, patients may feel like "charity patients," and we know from interviews that some patients are reluctant to go to such clinics and hospitals because they believe that "what is free is not much good."

Also, the distances that patients must often travel to the medical facilities and the fares that they must pay to travel there, further the underutilization of services by raising realistic questions of money and time. Some lower income people are so poor that even expenditures for carfare must be carefully calculated. In addition, if emergencies seem to demand the use of taxis, the money may not be available. The ecology of medical services can work to their disadvantage in a more general sense. These people customarily organize their lives so as not to go far for the necessities of living. They tend to shop close at hand for most things. They do not travel much about the city except to work or for the occasional visiting or entertainment. The women especially tend to stay close to their homes or neighborhoods and not infrequently are anxious about venturing farther afield.

Sometimes other obstacles to utilization derive from medical organization itself. Thus

> many patients are ineligible under too restrictive financial requirements and yet cannot afford to pay the rate many hospitals charge for ward patients . . . Some hospitals require that clinic patients have one or two pints of blood deposited in the blood bank upon admission to the clinic. Inability to meet this requirement . . . leads to the omission of prenatal care.[22]

One set of authors who have studied underutilization of services in New York City concluded that genuinely to increase the utilization of services by "blue collar" people, "modern medicine ... must adapt itself to new forms of social organization ... some adjustment will have to be made so that the relative alienation of large segments of society will be corrected."[22] The authors are quite correct in that judgment.

HEALTH AND THE LOWER INCOME GROUPS

We have asserted that contemporary medical organization is not well adapted to giving quality care to lower income people. Now, we suggest further that our *medical organization rests on several assumptions about "the patient" which constitute additional obstacles to giving quality care to lower income people.*

Assumptions about Patients

The methods whereby health professionals give quality care assume a certain kind of patient, as well as the existence of certain relationships between the patient and the professionals. First and foremost, the patient is supposed to have his own self-interest at heart—so that when he suspects he is sick he will seek professional help, and when given a regimen to follow he will attempt earnestly to follow it. He must thereby be an active agent: he has to recognize when to visit the doctor, make decisions about which doctor to visit or when to abandon one doctor for another, control his fears and anxieties when in the hospital or clinic, and suppress actively his disposition not to follow the doctor's "orders" in favor of doing as commanded. If necessary, he must organize his life so as to manage a medical regimen. He has also to take himself back to the physician when symptoms reappear or worsen. It follows that he must trust the health professionals and especially his physician; but if not, then he should seek out others whom he believes are trustworthy. In short, medical organization tends to assume a rather educated, well-motivated patient, who is interested in ensuring a reasonable level of bodily functioning and generally in preserving his own health.

Not all highly educated or personally well-financed patients fill these expectations. Yet it can safely be asserted that the higher income groups, on the average, are closer to this image of the ideal patient than are the lower income groups. In fact, health professionals often complain, or shrug their shoulders fatalistically, about how lower income patients fail on a number of counts: they come to the clinic or hospital with symptoms in advanced stages, or parents don't seem to pay any attention to children's symptoms until well advanced, they return with the same diseases when cured or temporarily arrested or with worse symptoms if told to follow given treatment, and whether from laziness or noncomprehension or environmental difficulty they often cannot follow even simple regimens; also, when they do return, they have often delayed too long. In some hospitals, the staff openly express derogatory attitudes when certain lower income patients appear month after month, especially if the fault can clearly be pinned on the patients.

It is unnecessary to assign blame to whole sectors of the population who tend not to match professional expectations! If professionals have not discovered the reasons—and built this discovery into their professional training—that is understandable also. I shall try to illuminate both issues, drawing upon rather well documented findings about the general tenor, and characteristics, of life among the lower income groups. I would underline the qualifying adjective "general," since probably not every ethnic group (and certainly not every person) of lower income conforms to my description. But the general picture that will be drawn is relatively well founded, especially as it pertains to the *lowest* income group. But it is also relevant to many persons of the next highest income bracket.

The Facts about These Patients

The lower income person's experience of himself and his world is highly distinctive, in our country. It is distinctive for its qualities of concentration on the deadly earnest present. It is also distinctive for its problematic and crisis-dominated character. (As S.M. Miller has commented about these people, their "life is a crisis-life constantly trying to make do with string where rope is needed.") This pervasive problematic character of life tends to make unreal the careful and solicitous attitude toward health held out by the health professions, and by and large subscribed to by the higher income groups. Such concerns often seem empty or minor to those who feel they confront much more pressing troubles. They will often be inclined to slight physical difficulties in attending to more immediate ones, such as making ends meet during a particular day or week. Health problems are just one crisis among many that they must try to cope with, control, or just live with. The same medical problem is likely to stand out much more sharply for the higher income person, because his energies tend to be more quickly mobilized by anything threatening his health. Even for the so-called "stable working class" of Americans, who perhaps do not so frequently face the same chronic crisis situations, life often is made up of a series of difficulties just barely coped with. Many live with a continual sense that the world holds many potentialities for pushing them down into an unstable, crisis, kind of existence.

Another very general characteristic of lower income life—especially the lowest income group—is that the households often are much more understaffed than those of higher income. The complement of family members who normally maintain and manage a household, including at least a husband and wife, is much more often absent. Thus understaffing of households means that each individual's health receives relatively little attention as far as preventive measures are concerned, and when someone is sick then it is more difficult to care for him at home; and when the main family member is sick he or she will be in a disadvantaged position in caring properly for himself or herself, or in finding time to seek medical aid. The family's attitude toward even chronic illness is apt to be fairly tolerant; people learn to live with illness, rather than using their small stock of financial and psychological resources to do something about illness.

As for the human body itself: whereas higher income people tend to think instrumentally about its ailments, believing that improvement is generally possible, lower income people seem more inclined to accept ailments fatalistically or as natural to living and aging. They are likely to accept impaired bodily functioning as inevitable earlier in life. Rosenblatt and Suchman have noted about "blue-collar" Americans that:

> The body can be seen as simply another class of objects to be worked out but not repaired. Thus, teeth are left without dental care, and later there is often small interest in dentures, whether free or not. In any event, false teeth may be little used. Corrective eye examinations, even for those people who wear glasses, is often neglected, regardless of clinic facilities. It is as though the white-collar class thinks of the body as a machine to be preserved and kept in perfect functioning condition, whether through prosthetic devices, rehabilitation, cosmetics, surgery, or perpetual treatment, whereas blue-collar groups think of the body as having a limited span of utility: to be enjoyed in youth and then to suffer with and to endure stoically with age and decrepitude.[23]

Some students have suggested lower income people are characterized by relatively low esteem. Hence, the authors of the preceding statement add that "it may be more that a more damaged self-image makes more acceptable a more damaged physical adjustment." Another researcher, Lee Rainwater, remarks that these people, especially the lowest income group, develop "a sense of being unworthy, they do not uphold the sacredness of their persons in the same way that middle class people do. Their tendency to think of themselves as of little account . . . readily generalized to their bodies. In any event, fatalism about bodily functioning is certainly characteristic of lower income people as they move toward middle age."[24]

Their attitude toward the body applies by extension to the bodies of children. Parents display greater tolerance for physical disability or malfunctioning in their children than do higher income parents; sometimes being seemingly indifferent even to obvious infections, sores and colds. This acceptance of something short of good health has implications both for the care of children already ill and for preventive regimen.

The next question is when do they tend to seek medical treatment? The answer is: only when the impairment of bodily function becomes so obvious, or great, that medical action seems needed. The pressing problems of daily existence tend to minimize the problem of illness so that "symptoms which do not incapacitate are often ignored. For the white collar groups, illness will also relate to conditions which do not incapacitate but simply by their existence call forth medical attention.[25]

Another relevant consideration is that health education is much less advanced among these income groups than among people of higher income. Since illness is not usually self-evident except in late stages, health education is of considerable importance in recognizing illness. Particularly is this so for relatively mild or episodic chronic disorders that do not fully incapacitate or do so only temporarily. It is even more true of diseases with mild symptoms that appear to go away after a period of time.

Once illness is perceived and once it is believed that something should be done about it, these people are less inclined to use specifically medical institutions that are for higher income people. They are inclined to treat themselves with folk medicine or patent medicine. And they are likely to seek out health advisors not only from kin and acquaintances (as do also the higher income people), but also the neighborhood pharmacist, the chiropractor, and, on occasion, folk-practitioners—like the curanderos among Spanish-speaking people or the sellers of charms in Negro ghettos. These advisors or healers are not only less expensive than physicians, they are less foreign and psychologically remote. To the client, they seem more like himself than those who work in medical institutions—even if their advice or care is not free.[26]

Whether the lower income person seeks medical relief from a physician or someone else, "he is more likely at an advanced stage of illness than his higher income counterpart."[27] (The government figures quoted earlier reflect this.) He is also more likely to be in a perceived or actual state of emergency. And whereas the higher income person probably will visit a private physician before any necessary hospitalization, the lower income person is considerably less likely to visit one and less likely to be referred by him to a clinic or a hospital. A very usual path is initially to visit a clinic or emergency room, and then be transferred into the associated hospital. (Sometimes the private physicians whom they visit initially are themselves so insulated from the medical care system that they do not have hospital connections, although perhaps they are able to refer patients to physicians who do. Sometimes these patients are referred to clinics and hospitals by welfare agencies.) Hence, the lower income patient is apt to enter a hospital quite unsupported by any neighborhood representative.

The difficulties of lower income people in clinics and hospitals are compounded by how they tend to behave in medical settings. As we suggested earlier, their behavior is often frustrating and annoying to medical and nursing personnel, for they frequently violate expectations about how "good" and "considerate" patients should behave. Lack of punctuality in keeping appointments, and walk-in emergency demands, irritate the personnel because their own time is carefully measured and allocated. Other matters, including personal hygiene, also irritate the staff: these patients may not wash before visiting the clinic or hospital, may not cover their mouths when told to cough. Furthermore, they are not so likely to give excellent medical histories to examining physicians; they tend not to have very precise notions about time, do not discriminate experience by conventional disease labels, and very often have very unconventional notions of anatomy and bio-physical systems.

A point especially worth emphasizing is that they do not respond well to a properly professional "impersonality" but seek personal relationships, rather than professional ones, with staff. This search is consonant with their behavior outside of medical settings, for they tend to personalize most relationships. They are, in fact, generally not familiar with, or are uncomfortable when in unaccustomed contact with, large institutional complexes. In clinic and hospitals, these patients are confronted by an elaborate division of labor. But they are accustomed to dealing with people in nonsegmentalized ways. So these patients are even more likely to be confused and frustrated by the hospital's many functionaries than are the higher income patients. Since the former have fewer opportunities to request their own physician to sort out difficulties in the medical setting, or to moderate its impersonal division of labor, they are prone to a sense of pervasive anxiety when in these settings—and especially perhaps in hospitals. This pervasive ansiety is well depicted in a study of obstetric patients by Rosengren. Contrasting "blue-collar" with "middle-class" mothers, he remarks:

> Consider the blue-collar woman: the relative personal and social isolation in which she lives . . . and the life milieu in which she lives, where illness, incapacitation, and the like abound; and also the very real, heightened chances that either she or her baby may encounter either insult or accident during pregnancy—all of these . . . combine to make the pattern of high sick-role expectations . . . particularly understandable. Considering also that the blue-collar woman is likely to be cared for in a clinic setting rather than by a private doctor it is easy to see why she might regard herself as "ill." The middle-class woman chooses her own physician . . . She appears for her prenatal care in a treatment setting which has little of the symbolism of sickness . . . in dramatic contrast to the clinic-attending woman who experiences her treatment within the confines of a hospital with . . . nurses and internes scurrying about, sometimes in apparent anxiety, with stainless steel, tile walls, and medicinal odors intermixed with medical machinery and equipment.[28]

Abetting the patient's anxiety is a feeling of isolation, sometimes furthered by the realistic difficulties facing family members when they attempt to make frequent visits. Also family ties may be so weak that relatives do not bother to visit often.

In these medical settings, the lower income patient is markedly subordinate in his relations with virtually all staff personnel. This tends to result in a blend of passive submissiveness and hostile evasiveness in his relations with them. As we noted earlier, derogation and hostility is often expressed by staff members, both covertly and overtly; so the patient's typical response is hostile withdrawal from the staff members, allied with resentful docility to their "orders,"·prescriptions and suggestions. The sociocultural subordination of the lower income patient is emphasized by his economic subordination. Often he is receiving free treatment, and so is required to be grateful, subject to the convenience and requirements of those giving services rather than able to insist on his own perceived needs. What is given to him in many hospitals and what he may choose is largely a function of routine administrative determination—with corresponding limitations on his own powers of negotiation. This is true even when he is a paying patient, for generally he has had less experience than the higher income patient in maneuvering within organizational structures. This inability is sometimes compounded by excessive shyness in such situations, especially by the women, by rather little verbal agility, and in the case of recent immigrants by not being able to handle English well. Repeated visits to clinics or hospitals may give them more skill in negotiating with staff members—but many are so frustrated by the first visits that they do not return.

To suggest that this picture is not in the least overdrawn, we offer a true case. A laborer, who had health insurance through his union, brought his ailing wife to the clinic. She was transferred to the associated hospital, operated on for a tumor, and then sent home. Her husband was told nothing about the tumor, only that his wife "would be all right in a few days." Back home in bed, his wife dripped urine continually—as she had before hospitalization—and so after "a few days" the husband complained to the surgeon, but without getting his point across. After several more days, and further complaints, he went to a neighborhood physician with his problem, but without any success. He then approached the union's social worker, but she did not really understand his problem and so she made inquiries of the hospital but did not manage to solve it. Then he gave up going "for help," but by accident a nursing student who was making a study of "difficult cases" was directed to this family by the union's social worker. The student discovered that the family's big concern was the constant urinary drip. The nursing student intervened, requested a urinary plug via the social worker, thus solving the essential medical care problem as this family saw it.

In hospitals or on hospital services devoted to the care of permanently chronic patients, one can see written large the difficulties of lower income patients. For instance, Julius Roth, in a careful study of a rehabilitation unit within one New York City municipal hospital, has shown how the staff, imbued with professional ideals, gets discouraged with attempting to rehabilitate their virtually unrehabilitable chronic patients. (They are "unrehabilitable" if only because they have few or no resources to maintain themselves outside the hospital.) The staff members adapt to this situation by understandably concentrating effort on very few patients. In consequence, the remainder are unlikely ever to leave the hospital except to enter another custodial institution, unless they have interested families who will receive them back however disabled. Regarding the patient's possibilities for negotiating either for treatment or eventual discharge, Roth observes that:

> For a patient to survive with any possibility of independent action in such a situation, he must either be able to aggressively and skilfully coordinate his own program and fight for action on many aspects of that program, or he must have an independent agent working on his behalf—an agent—independent of the entire institutional system . . . A few patients are able to act fairly effectively as their own agents. A few others have family members or other outsiders who are more or less willing and able to carry out part of this goal—especially offering an escape by providing a place to

live. The majority ... must accept whatever disposition is offered ... for example, accept a foster home placement just to get out of the hospital ... In most cases, they are simply stuck in some part of the hospital with no way of getting out.[29]

In its turn, the professional staff either suffers from rapid turnover or its members retreat into "enclaves of research, administration, and teaching."

The Gap between Assumptions and Facts

In this section of our report we have depicted the great gap between important assumptions made about lower income patients by professional staff and the realities of lower income life, attitude and behavior. While the picture of those realities may be somewhat overdrawn, being more accurate the further down the income ladder one looks, most researchers who have studied the lower income groups agree about the substantial accuracy of the picture. Yet this knowledge has not been adequately built into the training of health professionals, nor has it especially affected the organization of medical care in hospitals or clinics (or health care outside of those institutions).

IMPLICATIONS OF INCREASED MEDICAL CONSUMPTION

Four Trends and Their Consequences

If this contention is correct, then the future of medical care appears gloomy indeed. There are additional reasons for pessimism. Chief among them is the steadily increasing flow of new purchasers of medical services, including a considerable ratio in lower income brackets. The latter will be the already tremendous strain on the resources of municipal and county medical facilities. In a study of New York City hospitals, Nora Piore has estimated that municipal hospitals now service more than half of the city's families. And in "a broad sense, aggregate tax expenditures for personal health can be said to furnish low-income families with a counterpart or substitute for the institutional services purchased through voluntary health insurance by the better off members of the population." She points out that although 72 percent of the city's population has some form of health insurance, "nevertheless the pressure on the city hospital-care system has in no way diminished."[30] Significantly, she also contends that whereas state and federal services are relatively inelastic, the city's obligations for medical care are quite open-ended. In short, this means increased density of patient populations, increasingly discrepant ratios of professional staff to patients, and almost certainly further frustration for both. Of course, it means also a decreasing level of medical care. Between the pinch in resources and the varied political pressures, it is unlikely that much attention will be paid to any fundamental reform in medical organization itself. The emphasis will almost certainly again be on "resources," "Manpower," "money" and an improved "delivery system."[31]

Another important trend that makes for some pessimism about quality care is the increasing number of lower income patients who will be entering community hospitals and clinics as paying patients. (In San Francisco, for example, recently there was a debate whether to close the municipal hospital or enlarge it, because of the anticipated influx of lower income consumers into the metropolitan medical market.) Not all patients, even the indigent, were ever given medical care solely at municipal or county hospitals. But the spread of health insurance—especially when purchased through unions or at place of work—means that increased numbers of employed men and their families in the second lowest income bracket will come to medical settings as paying patients. Hospital administrators of community hospitals have shown signs of some fright over the potential number of such patients, visualizing both strained resources and "problems" with these patients. One hospital administrator of our acquaintance said in committee that if the municipal hospital were abandoned, his own community hospital would have to build a separate wing because its regular patients would never tolerate the new type of patient. His outspoken reaction is symptomatic of how many hospital personnel will react to an increased flow of these new patients. Most relations described earlier between middle class professionals and lower income patients are very likely to be exacerbated.[32] The quality of medical care given all patients cannot help but be affected in some degree.[33]

A third trend already affecting the quality of medical care given lower income patients is the continued development of such plans as Kaiser in California and HIP in New York. The plans have relied considerably upon the insurance payments of lower income patients (especially of union members in the case of Kaiser, and city employees in the case of HIP.) Despite continuing complaint by patients, often funneled through union or group representatives, these medical plans are generally rated as offering good medical care. Certainly their growth reflects general satisfaction with their performance. Yet a number of informed guesses can be made about how their medical care probably is adversely affected by a mismatching between their internal organization and the life styles of their lower income patients.

Many of those patients are regularly entering the medical care system for the first time. They have not had much, if any, experience in finding their way around within these typically complicated medical settings. "Finding their way around" includes in some medical plans, discovering a clinic doctor whom one can trust or at least like. By contrast, higher income patients in these days seem typically to have resources—including both people and strategies—that permit them to discover and hang on to the same physician.[34] There is a pervasive anxiety among new patients that they get "a good doctor," an anxiety not always relieved. Yet many lack resources for getting a doctor with whom they will feel satisfied. Since they are likely never to have had a private physician, at least not regularly, they are additionally anxious about how to find one. Another aspect of entrance into a big medical system is the difficulty many encounter when faced with large, multi-segmented clinics. Despite internal traffic systems instituted by the clinics, patients are often very confused, and this affects the whole tenor of their responses to the medical setting.

Still another complication affecting the quality of care is that unions supply patients to these plans who sometimes tend to see medical care as a labor commodity. You pay your money for services and you should get a fair return! In consequence, the clinic and hospital personnel feel these patients are "demanding," and certain union get the reputation of being "difficult." But in their turn, the patients may feel the personnel are high-handed. Union representatives do negotiate standard complaints from time to time, in meetings or over the phone with representatives of the medical establishment. Such negotiations are unquestionably useful, but both parties tend to see only the most standardized, most visible, difficulties in giving and getting good medical care. (We know this from interviews with lower income patients.) In addition, both parties are likely to be very busy with other matters, so that grievance negotiation has not the highest priority.

An official of one medical group has noted in private conversation that the bulk of complaints received are from new patients, who also reflect higher dropout rates; yet his group has done little about investigating the causes of complaint and dropout. At another group, researchers are discovering that dropouts are "new patients" who are also of lower income. There is some possibility that these medical groups will be tempted to increase their higher income clients at the expense of lower income ones, unless they look carefully at critical points where their medical organization is mismatched with lower income life styles. In any event these medical groups have *not* directly confronted that mismatching, and until they do, their medical care is subject to the same criticism which we have directed against other medical establishments.

One additional important trend that suggests a continuing pessimism about improved medical care for the lower income groups. The continued conquest of acute disease means that the patient population consists increasingly of people with chronic disease— frequently multiple chronic disease. Lower income families, of course, suffer from more chronicity but also from more multiple chronicity. Especially as their numbers reach middle age, this chronicity shows up when they themselves feel something must be done for their symptoms. By contrast with acute disease, chronicity implies more visits to clinics, longer stays in hospitals, more alert patients, more need for communication between patients and personnel, and a need for much better teaching about self-care and regimens to be carried on at home. This national trend toward chronicity will tend further to acerbate relations at medical settings between staff and the lower income patients.

A Case Study: Psychiatry

Now I wish to suggest what increased lower income consumption of medical services may mean for particular medical specialties. Psychiatry will be used as one suggestive case study.

During the last decade, psychiatry has grown enormously as an outpatient specialty, has experimented with new treatments, developed new kinds of facilities, and grown greatly both in number of practitioners and consumers.

Quite clearly the patients are going to profit from an increased attention and an increased allocation of resources. At the same time, the professionals do not focus very much, or very directly, upon the potential mismatching of the evolving medical (psychiatric) organization with the life styles of lower income patients. The same kinds of middle class bias are shown, although expressed or rationalized by psychiatric terminology. The communication gap between patients and professionals is not necessarily lessened either, just because psychiatric professionals are more sensitized to the nuances of human behavior than are most other health professionals. After all, there is a great difference in the experiences of professionals and patients, a difference compounded by the specialized training and stances of the professionals. There is distinct danger, for instance, in the community psychiatric movement, that the professionals will assume they know a great deal about the communities and family settings of lower income patients—when really they do not. Most serious of all, perhaps, is the assumption again that professionals know what is good for these patients—after all, we are the experts and they are the nonknowledgeable, and sometimes uneducated.[36]

Responsible public officials and allied professionals are planning along rather traditional lines. Committees have been instituted to deal with familiar categories: such as retardation, addiction, alcoholism, hospitalization, clinics. In many municipal psychiatric services, this organizational defect can be easily seen. Over the last decades, the typical municipal system keeps adding an alcoholic clinic there, a day-care center there, a rehabilitation center, another psychiatric service at the city hospital, and so on. Each establishment has a vested interest in supporting its own continuance. Traditionally there has not been very generous financing of this decentralized municipal system. Now with more funds flowing into the care of their lower income clientele, one can anticipate further expansion of the whole municipal system—without very much focus on how it ought to be reorganized in the light of what life is actually like for lower income people.

One further danger, especially at those locales where the lowest income group tends to flow for treatment, is that the professionals there will become decreasingly discouraged with the results of attempts at treatment. It is predictable that if they do not take carefully into account the life styles of their patients in organizaing these medical settings and the treatments given there, the results will prove disappointing to many of the professional staff. Among them will be the more adventurous and ambitious. It is entirely probable that these locales will attract increasingly less competent personnel; or like our present municipal general hospitals, become a way station for young people early in their careers and for foreign trained physicians.

It is not necessary to believe that all this will happen in psychiatric practice. We only sketch the possibilities, and the current situation, to underscore why medical organization needs to be reformed, in terms of lower income attitudes and behavior as well as in other terms. What is true of this medical specialty is surely true of other specialties.

THE LOGIC BEHIND
A SET OF RECOMMENDATIONS

The foregoing considerations lead me to believe that *more important than any list of specific recommendations (although several will be advocated) is the necessity for spelling out how such recommendations should be formulated.* A rationale for making recommendations is crucially important for at least five reasons. *First*, sets of specific recommendations can be useful, but hardly scratch the surface of the larger problem of how to destroy inequities among income groups concerning the medical care they receive. *Second*, action guided by recommendations may even aggravate the situation unless one keeps clearly in mind the larger picture of how lower income people regard health and medicine. *Third*, specific recommendations can easily be generated by innovative persons, once the general rationale for making recommendations is clearly perceived. *Fourth*, some of these latter innovations can be put into operation without additional money, resources, or manpower. *Fifth*, as additional resources of any kind become available, they will be most effective when used according to a rationale such as developed below.

It should be evident that the medical care of lower income groups is characterized by a vicious circle. It is absolutely necessary to break the cycle. Of what does it consist? These patients come into the medical system rather later than they should, principally because they come for care only when they themselves perceive a real emergency. When they enter the clinic or hospital, they have experiences there which are likely to reinforce negative attitudes toward medicine and medical facilities, and cause them either to cut down necessary revisits for care, or if that is not necessary, to make them less eager to return when next they begin to think they might need medical care. But there is another aspect of this vicious cycle. While at the clinic or hospital, there ought to be effective communications to the patient (and family) about measures he should take after he leaves for home. These measures may be medical (taking medications, for instance) or more obviously involve adjustments in daily living (resting, staying home from work). The more chronic the disease, the more likely is the patient to be on a long-term regimen, involving either medicine or daily adjustments or both. Since communication about such regimens at the clinic or hospital is glaringly ineffective, what is done by the professionals at those sites can become partly or wholly neutralized after the patient returns home. In consequence, he gets sicker again, faster; or his chronic disease gets progressively worse, faster. If he had understood his regimens, he may not have had to return at all to clinic or hospital, or at least he would have returned in better shape or after a longer time in relative health. If, in addition, the patient has developed negative attitudes against medical personnel, he dallies in returning for medical care even though his condition really necessitates treatment.

The problem, then, is how to cut into this cycle effectively. To some extent, additional financing of lower income people helps, because then they tend to enter medical care sooner; under certain conditions (union insurance) they can even be bolder in their demands of professional personnel. Additional manpower and other resources help also, by cutting down the ratio of patient to personnel, decreasing waiting time for patients, easing the rush and associated tenseness of personnel, and generally increasing the purely technical efficiency of treatment and diagnosis connected with more time and better equipment. But additional money, manpower or resources cannot by themselves really break the cycle depicted above; they only mitigate it slightly.

Logic leads to the following directives for attacking the cycle. *First*, speed up the initial visit made by the patient for medical care. *Second*, improve the experiences which the patient has in medical facilities. *Third*, improve the communication, given and received, about any forthcoming necessary regimen (usually there is one). *Fourth*, increase the likelihood that the regimen will be properly carried out at home. *Fifth*, increase the likelihood of necessary revisits to the medical establishment (that is, prevent complete defection from medical care). And *Sixth*, decrease the time between the necessary revisits for care.

Quite obviously those directives involve changes in medical organization and in professional attitudes as well as perhaps some efforts directed at changing lower income attitudes, actions, and styles. Since attitudes and styles are notably more difficult to change than organizational structure and procedure, most recommendations should be directed at changing organizational structure and procedure. Naturally, we will not wish to institute changes that will work to the detriment of contemporary medical organization. Nor would we wish to impair the medical care to higher income afforded by contemporary medical organization at the expense of slightly improving the care offered lower income patients. The problem is to improve the care of all income groups. It is worth emphasizing that the vicious cycle noted above operates although to lesser extent with higher income patients. My recommendations as given below are meant also to improve care for these patients.

Care received by lower income clientele quite possibly can be improved *without* the expenditure of additional money, and without additional manpower or other types of resource. Improvement can be brought about by rearrangement of tasks, and by reorganization of organizational structure, by inventing new organizational mechanisms and by the reallocation of expenditures. Nevertheless, some changes may require additional resources.

Even more important, whenever additional resources are put into the medical care system, planners can profit greatly by considering both the vicious cycle described above and the specific recommendations noted below. *If money, manpower, and resources are placed according to such recommendations, they will go a good deal further toward conquering that vicious cycle. Otherwise, as suggested earlier, they may be wasted.*[36]

RECOMMENDATIONS

The following recommendations are directed at destroying the vicious cycle which marks the medical care of lower income groups.

The recommendations suggested below are only a few among those required to break the cycle. Experienced medical planners and health professionals can add to this list of recommendations, or modify it for particular medical facilities. Their recommendations, however, should be directed at breaking the vicious cycle and derive from considerations of the life-style of the populations who are of particular concern.

Speeding Up the Initial Visit

Detection. (1) *We recommend that there be continued extension of extant methods for detecting illness among lower income people.* But these methods can be intensified, and added to. For instance there could be more innovative use of mobile detection units. There could be drives against particular diseases, with attending publicity, especially drives directed at categorical illnesses which are visibly incapacitating or painful to the people themselves. And representatives of the population itself should be given some initiative in planning the drive so as both to enlist support and get effective ideas from the population.

(2) *One obvious agency for detection should be vastly improved, and that is the use of the school for detecting illness.* Currently the school nurse's effectiveness depends largely upon her own initiative. A much more active commitment to the school as a detection locale is required. The age pyramid of lower income groups is more weight-

ed toward children and parents are less likely to detect illness than in the higher income groups. This makes the school a crucial detection locale for lower income illness. The detection effort requires more energy, more manpower, and certainly more and better organization. Certainly teachers could much more effectively be used.

(3) *Subprofessionals, and ordinary family members might be utilized in imaginative ways for detecting illness.* For instance, subprofessionals can quickly be taught to recognize the symptoms of certain diseases common to lower income populations. Edgar Snow has described, in a recent book, how the Chinese have utilized subprofessionals and lay family members in drives against common categories of diseases. In America, we can surely do likewise both in drives against specific diseases and in also more general detection. This is especially feasible in housing projects and other more organized communities. It is also feasible for unions, governmental agencies, and other employers to organize general or specific detection efforts. Health insurance companies should encourage these efforts which, although they might initially increase flow to medical facilities, would ultimately benefit both the insured and the insurance companies. Subprofessionals can also be used at the schools for effective detection.

Facilitating the Visit

Detection is not enough: the patient must be willing, or able, to go to a medical facility for the requisite treatment. Therefore:

(1) *Although health professionals are understandably reluctant to decentralize facilities for giving treatment, probably the total effectiveness of medical care could be much improved by some decentralization.* (The motto might be, better less perfect treatment than less or no treatment.) The more centralized are the medical facilities, the less readily lower income people use them. The numbers of treatment centers within or close to lower income housing or neighborhoods should be greatly increased. These centers would function not only to treat but to refer patients to facilities when more extensive or complicated resources are needed. (One Children's Bureau program suggests a useful pattern: prenatal diagnosis and management near lower income residence, with high-risk pregnant women referred to a central facility. Some of these decentralized centers might be manned by trained nurses (or at psychiatric centers, by social workers and psychologists), with adequate provision for referral to more fully staffed centers when necessary. For inducing competent professionals to work at such decentralized centers—mainly located in "poorer" or undesirable" neighborhoods—it may be necessary to

reward with higher salaries, or to offer comparable psychological rewards: good team relations, a "good environment" in which to practice medicine and the like.

(2) *More extensive and organized methods for making it easier to visit a distant facility are required.* (Dr. Julius Richmond of "Head Start" has described one such method used in Rochester where extensive busing of mothers to facilities is carried out.) Use of subprofessionals, and volunteers, for accompanying children from school to clinic would help to overcome the professional's common complaint that, though the school discovers dental and eyesight deficiencies, the parents fail to get the children to the clinic! The same agents could be used to "cover" for the mother at home, while she takes her sick child to the clinic.[37] In general, research such as that carried out by Hylan Lewis (on lower income Negroes) shows that mothers actually recognize such symptomology in their children—but cannot afford time, money or dare to leave their other children alone at home, in order to take the sick child to the (often distant) clinic unless his condition seems critical. Block organization, or church organization, should be encouraged also toward the goal of "covering at home" for mothers.

(3) *Organized drives to get people, and especially children, into treatment can perhaps best be developed around drives against specific illnesses.* This would link detection with treatment in relatively efficient ways, and at the same time arouse public attention in lower income neighborhoods. Unions, churches and places of work could also get involved in such drives. Subprofessionals and volunteers, especially those drawn from the same ethnic groups or social backgrounds as the potential patients, might be especially effective in facilitating visits to medical centers: recent research suggests, in fact, that people of different ethnicity are susceptible to different kinds of social pressure or inducement in seeking medical aid.[38]

We recommend that there be much more extensive institution of evening and night clinics. Given the employment patterns of lower income families, daytime hours are simply unrealistic times for their members to visit clinics. The more extensive institution of evening and night clinics would mean some drastic changes in the lives of some health professionals—and probably increased salaries as inducement—but seems well worth the effort and money. (This change would also remove some pressure on emergency services of municipal hospitals, since these tend to be used during evenings as a substitute for daytime clinics.)

(5) *Every effort should be made to bring pharmacists explicitly into the medical picture.* Lower income families are quite likely to use the neighborhood pharmacist for self-prescriptions or counsel

before they will go to a clinic or to a private physician. Unrealistically, health professionals tend to regard the pharmacist as having a very prescribed role. The pharmacist needs to be geared in more rationally with a referral system, induced to persuade patients to enter clinics when they seem to need treatment or diagnosis. This will not necessitate alteration of current medical organization; but it will involve additional organizational mechanisms, such as the contacting and rewarding of pharmacists. (Rewards need not necessarily be monetary but of prestigious kinds.) There should be some training in detection of common diseases (as dentists are now taught to recognize oral cancer). Schools of pharmacy can greatly help in this training, especially perhaps in post-degree workshops. Other types of health healers should also be regarded as potential agents for getting patients to clinics sooner, rather than, as now, only as rivals of conventional medicine. Their referral functions can also gain these rewards if the professionals and public will pay attention to the genuine value of the functions.

(6) *We recommend consideration of methods of rewarding lower income patients, providing they enter treatment early, be carefully considered.* While such rewards might work better to induce speedy revisits, they might also be effective, and financially feasible, for inducing a speedier first visit. It would be worth money to health insurance companies, and to the various federal and local governmental agencies, if patients entered treatment earlier rather than waiting until their illnesses were further along.

Improving Experiences within Medical Facilities

(1) *We recommend that the emergency services of municipal and county hospitals be radically reorganized.* Lower income people use emergency services not only for "genuine emergencies" but as a substitute for a general practitioner and for a clinic. A great many emergency services are, therefore, unrealistically and inefficiently organized. General service gets in the way of effective emergency service. Staff biases toward lower income patients are reinforced by the wear and tear of running dual medical services, side by side. Patients resent the attitudes and behavior of staff, and frequently do not understand why they are "taken out of turn." Also, they tend to flood the services during the evening, when family members are free to visit for treatment. Therefore these services should be reorganized, in accordance with the needs of specific locales and types of client; but with full realization (rather than resentful begrudgment) that if lower income people use emergency services for general medicine, then there must be a good reason for such use. Again, representatives

of the local populations might contribute greatly to instituting effective reforms.

(2) *Clinics and hospitals should assign personnel to act as agents for patients in medical establishments.* Lower income patients need those agents for a series of reasons. They need to be oriented in institutional structures that are otherwise unduly or altogether confusing. They need to be informed better about a variety of matters than is now ordinarily the case. They need more reassurance, allaying of inappropriate anxiety, and other "psychological care" than they get under current arrangements. And they need, especially, an agent who can negotiate for them with hospital or clinic personnel, since they lack the effectiveness displayed by higher income patients in negotiation. Subprofessionals might often be especially useful agents for certain patients and their families—and their use should be made central rather than peripheral in future medical organization. In-service training in such functions should be available, whether the agents are subprofessionals or professionals.

(3) *Hospitals and clinics should build additional important types of "accountability" into their organization of care.* By accountability is meant the assigning and reporting back of certain kinds of tasks and their accomplishment during the day's routine. The report includes information about the patient, of course. Much other information that the personnel now obtains, from or about a patient, is passed along to responsible authorities fortuitously—if at all. For instance, the nursing aides commonly know a great deal about hospitalized cardiac patients which would be relevant to the nurses and attending physicians, but that information is rarely requested nor are the nursing aides usually queried about it. Whether or not these personnel are trained in the deeper meanings of such information, they ought to be held accountable for reporting it. The same can be said for information possessed by all personnel about terminal patients in hospitals.[39] Indeed the nurses' aides can be taught to recognize—if not fully understand—types of symptoms and other information which otherwise is never picked up by the professional staff. Such information, of course, includes behavior and attitudes which the aides are in an especially good position to see. If the patient's background is similar to the aide's, her report may be especially valuable to the staff. This recommendation about accountability is closely related to the previous recommendation about the patient's agent. The increased range of accountability would not only directly improve medical care; it would increase the patient's appreciation of that care, so that he would feel better about his experiences when in the clinic or hospital.

(4) *Wherever possible the medical facilities which service lower*

income patients should be made more in accordance with tastes and life styles of the patients. This includes furniture and other items as well as spatial or room arrangements. Apart from their purely functional aspects, and limits placed by finances or overcrowding, the designs and atmospheres of medical facilities seem not well suited to making lower income patients feel psychologically at ease. At their worst, these facilities are really forbidding or repelling—as in one municipal hospital where a dense mass of colored patients sits daily while waiting for the individual calls, as if they were in a grim bus station. Again, representatives of patient populations can give good cues to how even old facilities can be made more comfortable and "normal."

(5) *We recommend—as an absolute necessity—attempts at training health personnel to lessen their prevalent class and professional biases against lower income patients.* Since the changing of attitudes is usually more difficult than instituting changes in organization and procedure, this recommendation implies a long-term program. In-service training will be useful, but the training received in professional schools is likely to be most effective in the long run. Such training is virtually non-existent in schools of medicine or nursing.[40] Schools of medicine need especially to face this problem, since their highly technical orientations—increasingly technical, if anything—leave little room for this kind of training, at the same time that their graduates will increasingly be in contact with lower income clientele. Teaching programs that insure greater contact with families and communities are a step in this direction, but are not enough. Social science teaching needs to be built systematically into even these programs.

(6) *In addition, medical educators need very much to innovate new organizational links between teaching hospitals and medical schools in order to ensure a more extensive contribution to lower income health.* The need for inventive—and honest—thinking about this problem is rendered even more urgent by the increasing role assigned university medical centers in the health organization of the nation.

(7) *Medical facilities should carefully consider how they might improve the lodging of complaints against their services by their patients.* The lower income patient and his family have few resources for lodging effective complaint when dissatisfied with medical services, especially after he has returned home. (Higher income clientele are much more skilled at conveying grievances and possess many more channels of effective protest.) Unions whose members have purchased health insurance currently negotiate complaints but tend to focus only on rather obvious ones, and probably many unions

wait for grievance reports from members rather than effectively seeking them out. Medical groups currently suffer the defection of new members rather than rationally attempt to organize a grievance process. It might even be feasible to build certain kinds of standards into health insurance to maximize the probability that grievances would be aired and met, when possible, by medical establishments. Again, representatives of populations served by the medical facilities might well be useful in articulating and funneling grievances. When more effective grievance processes have been organized, lower income patients will feel less helpless at clinics and hospitals—and certainly more inclined to turn to them for care.

Improved Communication about Regimens

Almost all patients who visit clinics or stay at hospitals must be put on at least some minimal regimen when they leave for home. Yet, communication about regimens tends to be ineffective with lower income patients. In busy clinics and hospitals, the professionals are focused primarily upon diagnosis and immediate treatment. This is what physicians and nurses have been trained to do with great professional skill. Explaining regimens is a far less professionalized activity. Middle class and professional biases of personnel are further obstacles to careful explanation. When good explanations are actually made, the patient may not understand either its details or its rationale because he is still too ill, or too gripped with anxiety to listen carefully.

(1) *We recommend therefore that considerable thought be given to this problem of how to convey the sense of regimen to patients.* Even a busy clinic or hospital can be somewhat reorganized so that more care is devoted to communicating regimens. In some areas, like diet, there seems to be genuine confusion over who communicates what to the patients.[41] There should be a clearer division of labor worked out in those presently confused areas. Sometimes communications are too brief because the physician is busy, when a nurse might just as well communicate the regimen. Ordinarily there is little or no attempt to follow up on whether the communication has been correctly understood: subprofessionals might usefully interview patients shortly after professionals have communicated regimens to check on whether patients understand what they have been told. With complicated regimens, nurses probably should do these interviews.

(2) *Special training should also be given to improve the ability of professionals to communicate regimens* Since they now receive little or no training in this skill, it is necessary that much more attention

be given to this problem in schools of medicine and nursing. In-service training at the interne-resident level, and for nurses, would also be useful. This training should not focus merely on how professionals should talk to patients; but also how to interview them about whether they can or care to follow those regimens, and how to listen to their questions about the regimen. Since professionals are not ordinarily trained either in interviewing or in listening to patients—and since lower income patients tend not to press their views on professionals—training in those special skills is particularly necessary. Social scientists have developed excellent interview methods but they are little used for teaching them to medical or nursing students. When patients frequently fall into certain foreign language groups, nurses at least should be asked—even paid—to learn one language at least. And there should be a full-time interpreter at the facility.

Checking upon Home Regimens

Even when the patient and his family understands his prescribed regimen, when he returns home he may not follow it correctly. He may not have understood all its details. He may be discouraged by its rigor. The family's style of life may mitigate against his following it closely. Sometimes he has not really understood the regimen because he is told about it too early, while still confused in the hospital. And, of course, very often he has not understood the regimen at all. But if he does not follow his regimen with some accuracy, he suffers the consequences—and so does the clinic or hospital, because he returns all the sooner.

(1) *We recommend therefore that clinics and hospitals attempt to organize their services to include checking on the regimens of ex-patients who have no private physician.* This reorganization might include a number of measures. Patients should be encouraged to telephone specifically assigned personnel for queries about regimens, and possibly personnel should contact patients to solicit queries. At many locales it should be possible to get closer collaboration between clinic or hospital and the public health agencies precisely around the issue of regimen checkups. Probably we also need to build in additional types of personnel responsible to agency or clinic/hospital. Subprofessionals might do certain kinds of checking upon regimens, but where the patient is sicker or the regimen more complicated (perhaps involving more equipment) specially trained nurses may be necessary to mitigate this portion of the vicious cycle in medical care. The medical care system *must* take responsibility for this kind of feedback of communication with lower income patient—and the responsibility *must* be institutionalized.

(2) *In lower income locales, the hospitals and clinics should attempt to bring the local physicians into some sort of association with the medical facility.* Many of these physicians operate without hospital connections, practice deficient or old-fashioned medicine, and yet are often in contact with patients after (and sometimes before) he goes to, or is referred, to the clinic. Often the patient prefers after leaving the clinic to go to the doctor down the block, either because of other minor ailments or because he has not really understood what the staff told him at the big establishment. Therefore a determined attempt to connect the local physicians with clinics and hospitals will not only help educate these men; it will help the patient after (and sometimes before) he leaves the clinic or hospital.

(3) *Medical establishments should make special efforts to discover something about the prevalent life-styles of their patients.* One major block to correct or persistent adherence to regimens is the family's life style. This effort will require special studies by social scientists, or at least special interviewing by responsible personnel. Too much is now assumed about the lives of patients—either they are supposed to live no differently than anyone else, or they are perceived as living so differently that they will not follow regimens correctly no matter what told. Both types of assumption are likely to be proven incorrect once the patient's life is really understood. It is necessary to understand the social backgrounds and home life of patients reasonably well, otherwise regimens cannot be communicated accurately nor followed closely at home.

(4) *Imaginative attempts should be made to create a medical technology, for use at home, of the utmost simplicity or that relies as little as possible on patients' judgment and motivation.* The long-working tranquillizers now being experimented with on mental patients are instances of such technology; so is, in its own way, the contraceptive "loop." Given some of the characteristics of lower income life and attitudes toward the body, the more such technology can be invented the less need patients be given complicated regimens (which involve repeated actions, good timing, persistence, and so on). This technology may evolve by itself, but special focus upon its benefits for lower income patients might speed its evolution.

Decreasing Defection from Care, and Decreasing the Intervals between Necessary Revisits

I shall not offer special recommendations for these two, final, segments of the vicious cycle in medical care. The preceding recommendations bear quite directly on both these segments. Innovative reorganization of medical services need only extend or add to those recommendations to affect defection or decrease intervals between necessary revisits to clinic or hospital.[42]

FOUR LEVELS OF RESPONSIBILITY

Obviously some of the above recommendations are not original, and various medical facilities have been experimenting in similar directions.[43] What makes these recommendations different is that they are related to each other through the guiding idea of the "vicious cycle." A principal argument of this paper is that equity of health care cannot be obtained unless all portions of the vicious cycle are attacked simultaneously. A scattered, piecemeal attack will simply not do the job.

To insure sufficiently broad action to begin genuinely to break this cycle, one further, very general, recommendation is necessary. This recommendation involves four levels of responsibility: professional, institutional (clinic/hospital, etc.), lay, and governmental.

(1) *The professional societies and schools must take responsibility for certain reforms bearing on the total vicious cycle.* For instance, vigorous and imaginative steps should be taken by schools of medicine and nursing in order to counteract the prevailing class bias of their students, and to teach them how to communicate much better with lower income patients. Surely they need to attack more seriously the problem of relating schools and teaching hospitals to community realities. Professional societies like the National League for Nursing and the American Nursing Association can be instrumental in furthering subprofessional training and in instituting better use of the nursing aide on nursing services. The more aware of the total difficult cycle are the associations and the professional schools, the more effective can they be in attacking it across the board.

(2) *Likewise, specific medical institutions* might act on specific recommendations offered above as well as on recommendations they have thought of themselves—but they should also consider how broadly across the total cycle they can spread their action. They bear the responsibility for attacking all six segments of the cycle, not just bits and pieces of one or two segments. Most programs of reform are relatively ineffective, it is safe to say, because they are based on such partial attacks. At the very least if a hospital, for instance, cannot take responsibility for surveying the patient's regimens when he is at home, then vigorous attempts to gear its programs with those of public health, and other community agencies, should be made.[44]

(3) *It would seem absolutely foolhardy not to enlist the respon-*

sible efforts of lower income people toward the goal of getting them better health care. Many of the recommendations listed above involve the use of subprofessionals drawn from the same income groups as the patients who are being serviced. Other recommendations urge the cooperation of "community" representatives, for example in instituting grievance procedures and improving detection of disease. Some lower income populations constitute relatively genuine communities or neighborhoods (especially ethnic groups, like the Polish-Americans who tend to live in parishes), and they could be effective contributory agents in improving health care. Some populations, however, in no sense whatever constitute "communities"—entire city blocks being composed of isolated families (or fragments of families). Getting lay representation for the latter people is a much more difficult problem. Each medical facility must make special efforts to determine what kind of representation its patient populations can manage—and the facility must help in organizing that representation. But not so rigidly, or with so much authority that lay representatives meekly follow directives. It should even be possible, and useful, to get lower income representation on advisory boards for those clinics and hospitals which service mainly lower income patients. Also, wherever there are genuinely indigenous community organizations, medical facilities should seek to urge and get their cooperation in the common enterprise, without getting captured by particular perspectives often characteristic of specific community organizations.[45]

(4) *Finally, governments (at varying levels, from city up through federal) have an immense responsibility* for persuading, inducing, or pressuring medical institutions and health personnel toward reforming our system of medical care. If governmental agencies were guided by the concept of "the vicious cycle," their influence on reforming medical organization would be measurably greater. While our citizens wish a great amount of "free choice" and "free enterprise," these are not of course incompatible with the institution of regulatory mechanisms by responsible governmental agencies. My argument is that without such regulatory mechanisms—directed according to some such conception as "the vicious cycle"—much of the money spent on improving medical care will be wasted, and even on occasion harmful. The so-called "trickle down" approach—with moneys funneled out by governments for additional equipment, manpower, beds, research and construction—must be anchored in an appropriate organization at the local level. This problem is all the more pressing, as indicated earlier, because influence is shifting rapidly to the elite medical centers, which in some instances are far removed from lower income concerns and perspectives.[46]

EPILOGUE—THE CONVERSION OF
LOWER CLASS STYLES

In closing this paper, I wish to counter one type of potential criticism based on unwarranted optimism about changes in the life and attitudes of the lower income group. Let us assume, it can be argued, during the next two or three decades that the notion succeeds in raising the standard of living of all citizens to such an extent that all become more or less "middle income" citizens. If that occurs, and even such a skeptical economist as Robert Heilbroner admits this possibility,[47] then it seems reasonable to suppose that an accompaniment of increased incomes will be a substantial increase of middle income life-styles—including those most relevant to effective medical care.

Indeed, certain groups in our population might be raised a number of notches in income without radical changes either in life-styles or in utilization of our system of health care. These groups have long elected to stand a little outside the mainstream of American "middle class" striving for status, increased income, and other conspicuously middle income values. I have in mind, for instance, the large Polish--American and other Slavic groups in cities like Chicago and Cleveland. As various sociologists have noted, these groups remain relatively low in income, produce relatively few "upward mobile" families, and retain a fair degree of older and certainly lower income values. Increased income, and even increased patterns of consumption are not likely to institute or constitute radical changes in their life-styles.

It is, I would contend, simply too optimistic a view that would maintain: "give them another two or three decades and they will efficiently be serviced by our health services." Even if this contention were true, the consequences of the "wait out" period ought critically to be reviewed. Efficiency, let alone compassion, demands such a review. Meanwhile a little tinkering here and there, a few reforms here and there, and even a great deal more money allocated to our health services will hardly give anything like the promised equality of care.

Is the United States Unique?

I wish to add a note about the probable relevance of my argument to conditions in other countries. Of course, there are great differences between the United States and other nations, and between their respective systems of medical organization. Many countries have more universal medical coverage and so perhaps their health personnel have had more experience with lower class patients. Less industrialized countries have less massive organizations for health care than does the United States. The dominant private practitioner control of American hospitals is in marked contrast to state-organized medicine elsewhere. The continental size of the United States, the diversity of its population and complexity of its class structure lead to sharper differences between staffs and patients than may obtain in smaller countries, or in lands with more homogeneous populations and less complex class systems. And many governments in nonindustrialized countries—principally in Asia, Africa and South America—recently much interested in the health of their citizens have focused strongly on bridging the gaps between Western medicine and native beliefs and practices.

Despite such provisos, I suspect many details of my paper are applicable to many other countries. Suppose one thinks of a continuum running from countries (or areas of countries) where modern medicine predominates to countries (or areas) where it is hardly practiced. In nations which fall toward the latter end of the continuum, large portions of their populations are relatively unacquainted with Western medicine and its implementing facilities. The gap between modern medicine and native practice, belief, and styles of living are much like the gap depicted in the foregoing pages. In addition, there may be sharp ethnic and/or class differences between the health personnel and various sectors of the population in these countries. Or the personnel are so Westernized (or in Europe, scientized) that they no longer empathize with, or have patience with, attitudes of their own ethnic groups. Moreover the staffs are likely to have less control over the carrying out of regimens, once patients have the medical facilities, than do personnel in the United States. And if the patient is well motivated and understands the regimen, native or local life-styles are likely to prevent his faithful following of the regimen.

About the more industrialized and urbanized countries, perhaps all that needs to be said here is that—despite the even greater scope of population under medical care than in the United States and greater governmental control of medical organization—much the same model of medical training and medical "treatment" exists. Also, it is probable that the prevailing national organization of health care surely is least effective in those regions which are least urbanized or industrialized. For countries in the middle range, my own observations have suggested that except in the central cities—and there not even with respect to recent immigrants from their hinterlands—the mismatch between organization of medicine and the actual care of patients is great, sometimes greater than in the United States with regard to our lower class patients.

Only comparative studies can tell us how, where, and to what degree such mismatching exists around the globe. Such studies are badly needed. Meanwhile policy cannot stand still. Nevertheless, policy makers in each country might profit from thinking within the framework offered here. Especially I would emphasize that plural systems of medical belief and practice exist in all countries and every class level; hence the conclusion that health officials and personnel everywhere would do well to come more directly—and imaginatively—to grips with the problem of meshing their own systems of medical care with the plural medical observances and life-styles of all segments of their populations.

NOTES

1. Most of the data on which my argument, and critique, is built are readily available. I have used mainly the published research of social scientists about lower income life-styles and utilization of medical services. In addition, I am in heavy debt to Drs. Eliot Freidson, Lee Rainwater and Melvin Sabshin, for extended memos (including recommendations) dealing with aspects of medical care as related to lower income populations, and to Dr. Hylan Lewis for research materials on Negro family life; and to Shizriko Fageshaugh for very useful interviewing. Robb Burlage, of the Institute for Policy Studies, offered many ideas in a careful reading of a first draft of this paper. Of course I drew also on my own experience as a sociologist who has had considerable research experience in medical areas both in the U.K. and abroad.

2. See *New York Times*, January 8, 1965, p. 16.

3. Public Health Service Publication No. 1000—Series 10—No. 9, issued May, 1964. The report is based on data collected in household interviews.

4. Four categories of family income are compared throughout this government report. The two lowest income groups are, respectively, under $2,000 and $2,000–$3,999. The next two classes are, respectively, $4,000–$6,999. The population of all ages for July, 1962–June, 1963 in the United States was approximately for each of the above income categories: 22,590,000; 32,485,000; 61,675,000; and 57,082,000 (9,334,000 were of unknown income). *Thus the two lower income groups constitute a high proportion of the American population.* In percents of the total population (183,146,000), they constitute, respectively about 12 percent and 18 percent (see p. 168).

5. From his abstract of *The Changing Roles of Government in Health Implications for the Future*, delivered on April 30, 1965.

6. Arthur Lesser, *Current Problems of Maternity Care*, U.S. Department of Health, Education and Welfare, speech delivered May 10, 1963.

7. In a more general context, Dr. George Silver has made a similarly strong statement. Summarizing certain findings in his *Family Medical Care: A Report on the Family Health Maintenance Demonstration* (Cambridge: Harvard Univer-

sity Press, 1963), he remarks that *"Nor is utilization based simply on economic access or availability.* In this light, one of the arguments used for (and against) compulsory health insurance loses considerable force. It isn't only economic factors that serve to deprive people of medical care, and equally it isn't true that removal of the economic barrier will inundate the doctor with unnecessary demands for service. *The present organization of medical practice is defective and that is what leads to inadequate service on the doctor's part and improper use on the patient's part. Consideration should be given to restructuring medical practice:* provisions should be made for the added time, family interest and concern, skills in guidance, and perhaps team approach, that would enable the professional people to understand and cope with the complex variables of patient demand and use" (p. 151). Italics not in original quote.

8. As Alonzo Yerby, Commissioner of Hospitals of New York City, summarized in his "The Disadvantaged and Health Care," a paper given at the White House Conference on Health, 1965, "Health care of the disadvantaged is piecemeal, often inadequate, underfinanced, poorly organized and provided without compassion or concern for the dignity of the individual. It remains as a legacy of the Poor Law, little changed in concept or application while discoveries in medicine and other health sciences have advanced with lightning speed. Certain groups of the disadvantaged in America, notably the Negro, get even less than their share of health services even though there is ample evidence that their needs are greatest. We can no longer tolerate a two class system of health care."

9. Furthermore, failure to reorganize efficiently may help to lower quality medical care for higher income patients. Increasing numbers of lower income consumers will be entering the medical market through increased incomes, voluntary insurance and federal financial underpinning. No planning for reorganization, or planning only in terms of delivering in much the same old ways more medical services to previously deprived Americans, almost certainly will lead to some unfortunate consequences for some higher income patients.

10. Daniel Rosenblatt and Edward Suchman, *The Underutilization of Medical-Care Services by Blue-Collarites,* in *Blue-Collar World* edited by Arthur Shostak and William Gomberg. pp. 341–349. Prentice-Hall 1964.

11. Harris Peck, Frank Riessman and Emmanuel Hallowitz (preliminary working draft). *The Neighborhood Service Center: A Proposal to Implement a Community Mental Health Network,* Lincoln Hospital Mental Health Services, Department of Psychiatry, Albert Einstein College of Medicine, pp. 7–8.

12. *Passage Through Crisis,* pp. 56–57. Bobbs-Merrill, Indianapolis, 1963.

13. Eliot Freidson notes, of patients who participated in the Family Health Maintenance Demonstration (Montefiore Hospital), that "high social class was associated with a greater degree of sensitivity to insult, and to feeling like a 'charity case,' and with a critical and manipulative approach to medical care. In contrast, the lower classes were somewhat more insensitive to their status as patients and were rather more passive and uncritical in their approach to medical care . . . lower-class patients were more reluctant to 'bother' the doctor and more eager to accept the substitute services of the . . . nurse." See his "Social Science Research in the Family Health Maintenance Demonstration," in George A. Silver, *Family Medical Care,* Harvard University Press, 1963, especially pp. 233–235.

14. "The Underutilization of Mental Health Services by Workers and Low Income Groups: Causes and Cures," *Am. J. Psychiat.*, 121 (1965).

15. *Ibid.*, p. 799.

16. Bernard Scholz, formerly Chief of the Police Assistance Division of the District of Columbia Department of Public Welfare, writes: "Frequently we ask . . . patients to bring . . . whatever medications they are taking at the present time, and you would be amazed to see the shopping bags they bring in and the pills, tablets, capsules and liquids of all sizes, colors, smells and descriptions they spread out on the table. Frequently we find that they are under treatment in different speciality clinics for different complaints, and that some of the medications prescribed for them and some of the drugs liberally handed to them at the District Pharmacy may either neutralize each other or in combination cause very questionable side effects . . . We professional people in our well-appointed houses, have medicine cabinets cluttered up with an amazing array of save-up medications which we identify, when need arises, and the date when the doctor prescribed it, but here we are dealing with illiterate people, or people with very limited education, who often don't know the name of the doctor who saw . . . and prescribed . . . We give them medications with such white-middle-class instructions as 'one after each meal,' when actually we mean three pills, six hours apart during the day, but this schedule may have nothing to do with the time (when they eat) . . . " From: "Medicine in the Slums." *Clin. Proc. Child. Hosp., Columbia*, 18, 351, 1962.

17. See Arthur J. Lesser, *op. cit.*

18. "And I do think the treatment would have been different if Albert had been white. I mean, if the ambulance had of come in there with a little white boy and he had fell off the third floor perch, they would have had everybody in there working on him. They would have called all the nurses to hold him and everything. And they probably thought I wasn't home or something with the kids, and what was the mother doing (when Albert fell) — why should they rush." Quoted from an interview document with a Negro mother, by permission of Professor Hyland Lewis, Howard University (from his study of child-rearing practices in Washington, D.C.).

19. As John Knowles, General Director of the Massachusetts General Hospital and Lecturer on Medicine at the Harvard Medical School notes, "the goals of the medical school are teaching and research—the teaching of medical students and the conservation and expansion of knowledge, all for *tomorrow's* health wants and needs. The goals of the teaching hospital are first and foremost, the care of the sick and service to the community *today*. In instances where teaching and research . . . have dominated the hospital, the attitude has become set that the patient exists for the teaching program and not that the hospital exists for the patient. Selective admitting policies, shabby patient facilities and deteriorating physical plant, wards full of special 'research' patients, failure (or refusal) to accept alcoholic patients or expand emergency facilities, a two-class system of care with frequent town-gown battles within the walls of the hospital and disregard for the outpatient department all lead to a demoralized and spiritless institution. Such a hospital will never send its roots deep into the community for moral or financial support as a consequence of having served the *Community's* wants and needs rather than just its own." He adds, "Only recently

have some of our medical school research plans included studies of the patient care and community service functions. This type of applied research has a better chance of giving something to the community which will improve the organization and distribution of health services." See his "Medical School, Teaching Hospital and Social Responsibility: Medicine's Clarion Call," delivered at the Second Institute on Medical Center Problems of the Association of American Medical Colleges, Miami, Florida, December 9, 1964 (quotation on pp. 16–17).

20. Arthur Lesser, *op. cit.*, p. 10. See the bibliography for several surveys bearing on underutilization of prenatal care. See also Rosenblatt and Suchman, *op. cit.*

21. Reported in Lesser, *op. cit.*, pp. 10–11.

22. *Op. cit.*, pp. 10–11, quotation from Frank McPhail.

23. Rosenblatt and Suchman, *op. cit.*, p. 349.

24. Quotation from a memo written for this paper.

25. Rosenblatt and Suchman, *op. cit.*, p. 345.

26. In a study done a decade ago, Earl Koos showed how, in one small city, the lower income population expressed in word and deed the gap between themselves and physicians, and how they frequently turned to remedies, osteopaths and druggists. About the pharmacist, Koos remarks "His place in the health team was sharply limited by law, but his place in the community suffered no such limitations." See *The Health of Regionville*, Columbia University, 1954, p. 87.

27. As one researcher, Nora Piore, notes about New York municipal hospitals, "The city tends to get the patient when he is either very sick or wholly unable to afford treatment." "Metropolitan Medical Economics," *Scient. Am.* 212, 19–27, 1965.

28. William R. Rosengren, "Social Class and Becoming Ill," in *Blue-Collar World*, edited by Arthur B. Shostak and William Gomberg. Prentice Hall, pp. 338–339, 1964.

29. Julius Roth, "Institutions for the Unwanted," published paper, presented to the Tufts Colloquium on Social Science and Medicine, April 8, 1965, pp. 13–14; see also his monograph, "Rehabilitation for the Unwanted" (unpublished).

30. *Op. cit.*

31. Robb Burlage has noted in correspondence with me, that New York City is an excellent example: despite the fact that millions of dollars and much regulatory power has been put into upgrading, affiliating and merging the New York City hospital system in the interest of quality care, there has been little organization *distinctively* for delivery of better care to the lower income population, except for a few hospitals like Governeur and Morrisanis.

32. At one community hospital at which we interviewed, the private physicians working at the clinic do not always "behave very well" toward the new patients (coming there on welfare funds) and the young staff physicians openly express adverse attitudes toward these patients, especially when the patients are Negro. More sympathetic staff members acutely feel the gap between themselves and the new type of patient, but do not know how to bridge it.

33. In fact, the whole situation probably will be contributed to further by the federal government's increasingly great financial support of these voluntary

hospitals while it offers only loose, minimum-standard regulation governing care of federally supported patients.

34. One lady whom we interviewed, for instance, phoned around among her professional friends, including doctors, for recommendations and finally decided on one particular clinic physician. She phoned the clinic to find his days on duty, met him, and makes sure she attends clinics only on the days when he is at the clinic. She has obtained from him the names of other clinic-physicians whom he respects just in case she needs to be seen when he is not in attendance.

35. The prominent psychiatrist, Dr. Melvin Sabshin, has in private correspondence remarked that "many psychiatrists are moving into community psychiatry but not thinking about it very hard. They are moving in a practical sense to develop clinics, develop services, but are not conscious of the necessity for a dialogue between themselves and representatives of the lower classes.

36. And perhaps even sometimes harmful—tending to *increase* the gap between lower income health needs and medical organization.

37. At one psychological clinic in New Haven, the practice of going directly to the homes to get the patients (children) has been highly successful. (Personal communication from M. Levine.) S. Sarason, M. Levine, I. Goldenberg, D. Cherlin and E. Bennett, *Psychology in the Community.*, Wiley, 1966.

38. Irving, Zola, "Illness Behavior of the Working Classes: Implications and Recommendations," in Shostak and Gomberg, *op. cit., pp. 350–361.*

39. Anselm Strauss *et al.*, "The Nonaccountability of Terminal Care," *Hospitals*, 38, 73–77, 1964.

40. *Cf.*, Helen Macgregor, *Social Science in Nursing*, Russell Sage Foundation, 1960.

41. Marjorie Newton and Ande L. Knutson, "Nutrition Education of Hospitalized Patients," *J. Am. diet. Ass.* 37, 222–225, 1960; and Marjorie Newton, "Are Administrators and Dietitians Speaking?" *Mod. Hosp.* 99, 108–114, 1962.

42. Apropos of these points, it is worth noting that health care in the armed services depends to a considerably less extent on "voluntary" action than does civilian care. Even here, there is considerable defection away from care: men do not necessarily hold to regimens, do not necessarily revisit the medical facilities "regularly" or "on time," etc. Despite the services' interest in maintaining some minimum level of health, the organization of health care is consequently far from always effective. (I am grateful for this observation to Dr. Egon Bittner).

43. For instance, in New York City, Dr. George Silver's program at Montefiore Hospital and Dr. Howard Brown's program at Gouverneur Hospital.

44. In a revealing exploratory study, Mary Arnold and Douglas Hink of The California Heart Association interviewed officials of various agencies and facilities working with cardiac patients in one county in California. They were all working in relative isolation, each assuming some other agency or institution was taking chief responsibility for cardiacs. No one was. (Personal communication.)

45. *Cf.*, Frank Riesman's account of low-income participation in a mental health program,"Low Income Culture: The Strengths of the Poor." *J. Marriage and the Family*, 26, 420–421, 1964.

46. Robb Burlage, in correspondence with this author: "The basic public policy questions thus become how to provide adequate *public* control at the top

of an increasingly elite-dominated 'corporate' contract system and how to provide quality and appropriate care at the 'bottom,' particularly to difficult cases such as lower socioeconomic groups."

47. "To what extent does that conclusion . . . lead to the prospect of alleviating poverty within the next generation or so? In the short run the outlook is not very hopeful . . . Yet it seems to me that the general dimensions of the problem make it possible to envisage the substantial alleviation—perhaps even the virtual elimination—of massive poverty within the limits of capitalism three or four decades hence, or possibly even sooner." See his, "The Future of Capitalism," *Commentary*, 41, 26, 1966.

48. Gerald Handel and Lee Rainwater, "Persistence and Change in Working Class Life-styles," *Soc. Social Res.*, 43, No. 3, 1964.

Part V

ATTEMPTED SOLUTIONS

Perhaps the most ambitious experiment in the delivery of health services to the poor was the one launched under the auspices of the Office of Economic Opportunity. In all, over fifty neighborhood health centers (NHCs) were established across the country to serve as community-based sources of comprehensive health care for poor populations. The hallmark of these NHCs was an emphasis on community involvement in policy-making and outreach services with maximum employment of indigenous workers.

The evaluation of this extensive undertaking is mixed, both positive and negative. In part this may be attributed to the premises under which NHCs were begun: originally, there was considerable confusion in the minds of the NHC developers about the relationship between health and health care. The initial mission of the NHCs was to improve the health of their targeted communities. Gradually this gave way to other goals, which included the use of health as an issue around which to organize the poor, to increase their access to health care, and finally to provide jobs for a substantial number of people.

Bellin and Geiger focus on attitudinal and situational changes and their influence on utilization patterns in an NHC. Major barriers to use reported by neighborhood residents prior to the establishment of a comprehensive health center were primarily structural: money, time, transportation, babysitting problems, hours of service, and waiting time. The advent of the health center changed the utilization patterns of the population involved, not only because of the improved methods of delivery, but because of changes in attitudes about health care among those who used the center. These changes were reflected in marked increases in use of preventive health measures and less delay in seeking care. The authors suggest that such changes in services and their organization may be an effective means of changing consumers' attitudes.

By way of contrast, the report by Sparer and Anderson describes an attempt to integrate an OEO-eligible poverty population into four middle-class prepaid group practices. The data suggest that such an integration (with the costs borne by a third party, in this case OEO) is quite workable. After an initial catch-up phase during which the health deficiencies of the OEO group were brought under treatment, their utilization pattern came to resemble that of middle-class enrollees. The cost experiences also paralleled those of the regular members with savings resulting from decreased use of hospitals. This suggests that such an approach is feasible on a broad scale.

The reader interested in further information on this subject may refer to the following references listed in the annotated bibliography:

Abrams and Snyder, 1968
Alpert, 1968
Alpert et al., 1970
Arnson and Collins, 1970
Bamberger, 1966
Bates et al., 1970
Beloff and Korper, 1972
Berger and Martin, 1970
Berkowitz et al., 1963
Blum et al., 1968
Bond et al., 1968
Breslow, 1967
Brooks, 1973
Bugbee et al., 1968
Chapman, 1973
Cherkasky, 1969
Coe et al., 1967
Coleman, 1969a, 1969b
Collins, 1968
Columbo et al., 1969
Cons and Leatherwood, 1970
Cowen, 1969, 1970a, 1970b
Cowne, 1969
Curry, 1969
Darsky et al., 1958

Davis and Tranquada, 1969
Deas, 1968
Deasy, 1956
Deschin, 1968
Fabrega and Roberts, 1972(a), 1972(b)
Feldman and Salber, 1969
Foster, 1968
Freidson, 1961
Friedman et al., 1973
Garfield, 1970
Geiger and Cohen, 1971
Gerrie and Ferraro, 1968
Gibson, 1968
Ginzberg, 1969
Goldberg et al., 1969
Goodrich et al., 1963, 1970
Gornick et al., 1969
Gould, 1967
Greeley, 1968
Greene, 1970
Greenlick et al., 1968, 1973
Harmon, 1968
Haughton, 1968
Heagart, 1968
Hochstim, et al., 1968

Hoff, 1966, 1969
Hughes et al., 1972
Hurtado, 1969
Hurtado and Greenlick, 1971
Hurtado et al., 1973
Ingles, 1971
Ingram, 1966
Kaplan et al., 1962
Kegeles, 1969
Kelly, 1969
King and Schwartz, 1968
Kissick, 1968
Kluger, 1970
Lepper, 1967
Lepper et al., 1967, 1968
Leveson, 1972
Light and Brown, 1967
McLaughlin, 1968
McNerny, 1969
Mahoney, 1969
Moore, 1969
Muske, 1968
Penna, 1970
Pope et al., 1969
Robertson et al., 1968
Rosenkrantz, 1969
Salber et al., 1971, 1972

Schroeder, 1973

Schumaker, 1972

Shapiro and Brindle, 1969

Stein, 1972

Stoeckle et al., 1969

Tranquada, 1967

U.S. Department of HEW, 1972(a), 1972(b), 1973

Vaughn, 1968

Wallace et al., 1968

Wallach and Blinick, 1969

White et al., 1967

Whitlock, 1969

Wise et al., 1968a, 1968b

9. The Impact of a Neighborhood Health Center

A Study of a Low-Income Housing Project

SEYMOUR S. BELLIN AND H. JACK GEIGER

On December 11, 1965, the doors of a neighborhood health center were opened at Columbia Point, a low-income, public housing community of about 5,500 people situated in Dorchester, Mass. Sponsored by the Tufts University School of Medicine, and supported by funds from the Office of Economic Opportunity, it was established as part of a comprehensive community health action program (also including the Tufts Delta Health Center) "to intervene both in an urban northern and rural southern population in the cycle of extreme poverty, ill health, unemployment, and illiteracy."[1] This was to be accomplished by providing "comprehensive health services, based in multidisciplinary community health centers, oriented toward maximum community participation of each community in meeting its own health needs and in social and economic changes related to health."

A program of research was designed to evaluate the impact of this demonstration project in terms of its various objectives. Two earlier papers, resulting from this research effort and describing the impact of the health center on ambulatory and hospital bed utilization rates,

Originally appeared as "The Impact of a Neighborhood Health Center on Patients' Behavior and Attitudes Relating to Health Care: A Study of a Low-Income Housing Project," in *Medical Care* 10 (May–June 1972), pp. 224–39. Reprinted by permission of the authors and publisher.

Based on data collected as part of a project funded by the Office of Economic Opportunity, CAP Grant No. C688818.

provide the background for the present study, which focuses on attitudinal and situational changes that accompany the dramatic changes in the target population's health care utilization following the advent of the Health Center. One paper dealt with utilization of the Health Center's services and the extent to which it served as a central or regular source of care,[2] and the second documented a major drop in hospitalization for a representative sample of the Columbia Point population.[3]

A brief recapitulation of some of the findings on ambulatory health-care utilization may be useful. More than three out of four residents made contact with the Health Center at least once during a given twelve-month period. Following the opening of the Health Center, average utilization by this low-income population approximated that reported for more affluent populations. Furthermore, there was a reduction in fragmentation and discontinuity of care. The Health Center was claimed by an estimate of five out of every six residents as their regular source of care. A reduction in noncompliance with medical regimens also was reported.

In addition, a beginning was made in seeking out reasons for the high level of health-care utilization. Residents reported a high level of overall satisfaction with the Health Center and a markedly preferential evaluation of the Health Center (by comparison with two other major alternative sources of ambulatory health care services) on four major dimensions: quality of care, its comprehensiveness, the personal manner in which it was given, and the time typically spent waiting for services.

The present report extends this initial effort to account for success in raising the overall level of utilization of ambulatory health-care services. First, some additional information is presented on aspects of reported utilization, such as promptness in seeking care for health problems, polio immunization, and early case finding. Then we examine attitudes that dispose towards the use of specific types of services, and specific sources of care. Finally, we consider the possible role of such situational variables that could help to explain the changes in utilization of health-care services previously reported, and to draw inference on the extent to which such changes can be attributed to the Health Center and its programs.

COMMUNITY SETTING AND ITS PEOPLE

The Health Center serves a low-income public housing development situated on a peninsula that juts out into Dorchester Bay. It consists of twenty-seven three- and seven-story buildings, housing approximately 1,200 families (or 5,500 persons). The most striking feature of this community is its geographic isolation from the other residential areas, and until recently, from the normal complement of neighborhood-based public and commercial institutions, facilities, and services. This marked isolation from institutional services extends to the health domain. Until the Health Center opened its doors in December 1965, health-care facilities were also inaccessible to the great majority of residents except for a Well Baby Clinic at Columbia Point operated by the City Health Department. The lack of ready access to all kinds of services has been compounded by relatively unsatisfactory public transportation, upon which the great majority of residents depend.

Columbia Point has a distinctive population resulting both from self-selection and from the way formal eligibility criteria are applied by the City Housing Authority.[4] Young people predominate; nearly two-thirds of the population are under twenty years of age, and only 10 percent are sixty-five years of age or over. Since nearly three households in five are husbandless, the adult population is overwhelmingly female. The racial composition of the project has changed over the years. At the time the Health Center opened its doors, in the fall of 1965, about two households in three were white. Two years later, the population of whites had declined to 59 percent.

Family income is very low at Columbia Point. About three households in five have gross weekly incomes which average less than $80.00 or under $4,200 annually. Nearly two households in three depend for their other income solely on sources other than earnings.

TUFTS COLUMBIA POINT
NEIGHBORHOOD HEALTH CENTER

The Tufts Health Center at Columbia Point provides under one roof, comprehensive ambulatory services which span a wide range of preventive and therapeutic services for the total family. These services are provided by three family health-care groups, each consisting of an internist, a pediatrician, several community health nurses, nurses aides, social workers, and indigenous community health aides. The F.H.C.G. draws upon a variety of support services (e.g., laboratory, x-ray, pharmacy, etc.) and incorporates part-time but regular specialty services (e.g., obstetrics, gynecology). In addition, the group takes responsibility for arranging other specialty services or inpatient care at related hospitals. The intent in organizing these services is to provide continuous individual and family-centered care.

At the Health Center, no fees are charged and no means test is used as a barrier to service, since the vast majority of the Columbia Point population have incomes below the poverty guidelines or are eligible for Medicaid or Medicare.

The project also seeks to use the delivery of health services as a point of entry for inducing broader changes in the physical and social milieu that contributes to the cycle of ill health and poverty. An integral feature of this program involved the participation of residents in the design and operation of their health services through a Community Health Association that shares in a wide variety of policy decisions and has independent health-related programs of its own. The goals and programs of the Tufts-Columbia Point Health Center are described more fully elsewhere.[5]

EVALUATION CRITERIA

Ultimately, the justification for health services, whether rendered by the traditional solo practitioner, a hospital outpatient clinic, or a neighborhood health center, rests on demonstrating a reduction in death, disease, and discomfort. Modification of death and disease rates is especially difficult to demonstrate over a short period of time in urban, industrial communities, which have controlled infectious diseases and eliminated hunger and malnutrition for the great majority of their residents. The problem is compounded when the target community is very small as in the case of Columbia Point. Although an effort is being made to measure death and disease rates, we are also conducting descriptive studies of variables such as utilization of health care services which are more easily measurable in the short run.

Since the Tufts Comprehensive Community Health Action Program's objectives are broad, even with respect to health, a variety of criteria must be employed in its evaluation. As has already been noted, the Health Center not only intends to improve the quality of care given to the residents who find their way to the doors, but to reach those who, until now, have not made use of health-care services. Its objective also extends ultimately to a greater emphasis on early detection and primary prevention. The following dimensions of the target population's view of its current health services are reported in this paper, all on the basis of self-reports in response to structured interviews:

1. Promptness in seeking care for health problems.
2. Early case finding; periodic asymptomatic health examinations.
3. Qualities of physicians, e.g., competence, motivation, quality of care rendered.

4. Beliefs about physicians' attitudes towards patients.

5. General evaluation of medical care received.

6. Specific evaluation of the Health Center and a comparative assessment with two other major sources of health care on four dimensions.

In addition, the paper directs attention to such situational factors as money, time, effort—costs and resources—involved in obtaining health care. An examination will be made of the reasons people stated for postponing care, barriers acknowledged in the use of emergency health-care services, times spent in seeking health care, and indebtedness contracted for medical reasons.

SOURCES OF DATA

The data for this evaluation are based on a survey undertaken at two points in time with a representative sample of Columbia Point residents.[6] The initial survey consisted of interviews with 357 household heads and was conducted just prior to the opening of the Health Center in December 1965. It provides a baseline picture of what people at Columbia Point believed, felt, and did about their health problems and the health-care facilities available to them before the Health Center was available. Two years later, the survey was repeated with those families who were still in residence in the community. This before and after study makes it possible to assess any changes that may have occurred which might be attributed to the Health Center.

Of the original sample of 357 households, 253 were still in residence two years later and, of these, 219 (or 86 percent were successfully reinterviewed. At the time of the repeat health survey, this panel sample was supplemented by an additional random sample of 215 households not previously interviewed in the second survey. Thus, a total of 434 households were interviewed in the second survey.

Two major surveys, undertaken two years apart, are treated here as if they were independent random samples. A comparison of these samples on major demographic variables reveals that with the exception of race and income, no statistically significant differences exist (Table 1). Despite the fact that the second survey had a somewhat higher percentage both of black persons and of households with a higher income distribution, the two study populations were similar with respect to key health attitudes and self-reported behaviors.

The health surveys received public endorsement by the Columbia Point Health Association, an elected council of local residents, which

TABLE 1. Selected Social Characteristics of the Columbia Point Survey Samples: Wave I Health Survey (November 1965) and Wave II Health Survey (November 1967).

Social characteristics of respondents	Baseline health survey Nov. 1965 $N = (357)$* % = 100.0 Per cent	Follow-up health survey Nov. 1967 $N = (436)$* % = 100.0 Per cent	χ^2
1. Age of household heads			
Under 25	14	13	
25–44	49	47	
45–64	15	17	n.s.
65 and over	21	23	
2. Race			
White	66	59	
Non-white	34	41	p < .05
3. Family income			
Under $60/week	55	52	
$60–$70	30	18	p < .001
$80 and over	15	30	
4. Marital status			
Married	41	38	
Not married (separated, divorced, widowed, single)	59	62	n.s.
5. Presence of minor children			
Yes	69	67	
No	31	33	n.s.
6. Health insurance			
Yes	29	25	
No	71	75	n.s.

* Percentages exclude "no answers."

speaks for the community in formulating policy and initiating programs on health-related issues. (It also serves as an advisory board to the Health Center on matters affecting policy and practice.) The actual interviewing was carried out by Daniel Yankelovich, Inc., which employed nonresident interviewers. The interviews were conducted in the home and respondents were assured in detail of confidentiality and anonymity. An effort was made to explain to respondents the purpose of the survey: to find out what the community's health needs and desires were, how satisfactory or unsatisfactory health services were, and to find ways of improving them. Evaluations of the Health Center were obtained in a variety of forms—including both open and structured questions. The critical incident technique also was used to encourage respondents to cite specific examples of both good and bad experiences at the Health Center. Such questions minimize the risk of eliciting socially approved responses or "response set" biases.

FINDINGS

Aspects of Reported Use of Health Care Services

Early Detection: Asymptomatic General Health Examinations. Although there is no unanimity of opinion about the value of periodic general physical examinations, a majority of public health authorities favor it. Prior to the Health Center, however, only 28 percent of the respondents reported that they had *ever* had such an examination for preventive purposes.

Two years after the Health Center opened, the proportion of respondents who in the previous twelve months had received a general health examination in the absence of any known or specific health problem increased dramatically from 17 to 59 percent (p = < .001).

Preventive Health Measures: Polio Immunization. Success in primary prevention of illness has tended to be uneven where effectivenss depends on the initiative and cooperation of the individual. Polio immunization campaigns, for example, have usually been least effective in low-income communities. Columbia Point has been no exception. Before the Health Center opened its doors, only 57 percent of the adult respondents and 78 percent of their youngest children had been immunized against poliomyelitis (Table 6). Eighteen months later, the prevalence of reported polio immunization was virtually unchanged among adults (59 percent) but increased to 92 percent among children (p = .01).[7]

Delay in Seeking Care. Twenty-three percent of the people interviewed before the Health Center opened acknowledged that they or someone in their family had put off seeking medical care in the preceding six months. This figure underestimates the actual prevalence of delay in seeking medical attention, since not all persons had medical problems during that period and individuals differ both in their ability to recognize early signs or symptoms of illness and in their definition of those which merit medical attention. Two years later, the proportion of families who reported that they or someone in their family had postponed medical care in the preceding six months declined from 23 percent to 10 percent (p = < .001).

Beliefs and Sentiments Relevant to Health Behavior

Attitudes about illness and sources of health-care services are important to the extent to which they influence actual health behavior and can help to account for the gains in utilization of health-care services previously described. Our attention will be directed initially to beliefs about when medical attention should be sought. Two issues are singled out for consideration: (a) beliefs about the importance of asymptomatic physical examinations, and (b) beliefs about what kinds of signs and symptoms of illness should be brought to a physician.

Subsequently, our attention will turn to attitudes that relate to the choice of health-care sources and the kinds and levels of utilization of health-care services. These attitudes include an overall assessment of one's own medical care, an explicit evaluation of the Health Center, and structured questions evaluating various aspects of the doctor-patient relationship, including patients' beliefs about physicians' attitudes toward patients. Next, respondents' comparative evaluations of and preferences among major alternative sources of health care will be examined. Our aim is to ascertain to what extent there are correlative changes in attitudes that might help to explain the changes in levels of utilization based on Health Center records reported in a previous paper, and in self-reported use of preventive and curative services described earlier here.

Beliefs Regarding When a Physician Should Be Seen. (1) Knowledge of symptoms which merit medical attention. Even prior to the opening of the Health Center, a relatively high degree of sophistication with respect to signs and symptoms of illness which should be brought to the attention of a physician was evident among Columbia Point residents (Table 2). Agreement was highest on the most serious signs of illness—for example, severe shortness of breath (89 percent), a cough that lasts for several weeks (80 percent), or an unexplained loss of ten pounds (73 percent). There was also a high degree of agreement on what appear to be the least serious symptoms: a sore throat (30 percent), foot corns (21 percent), and a slight cold (4 percent).

Two years later, there was a higher proportion of respondents who felt that medical attention should be sought for every item. Even though the percentages were high in 1965, they were even higher in 1967. The gains were greatest for upper respiratory infections, i.e., sore throats (from 30 to 50 percent), and foot corns (from 21 percent to 39 percent), undoubtedly reflecting the attitudes of elderly patients who appreciated the podiatry services made available to them.

The substantial increase in level of utilization of ambulatory health-care services cannot be attributed to gains in knowledge about signs and symptoms of a more serious nature that deserve prompt attention. Even before the advent of the Health Center, there already was considerable sophistication and consensus with respect to such symptoms, and according to information reported by respondents, serious ailments (e.g., chronic nature) were likely to be brought to a physician's attention sooner or later. This opinion suggests, however, an increasing disposition by Columbia Point residents to bring to the attention of physicians symptoms at an *earlier* stage when they were less painful or disruptive to the daily routine, or of a more minor nature. This interpretation is consistent with the findings cited earlier in this paper that a reduction occurred in the proportion of residents who reported that needed medical attention had been put off.

(2) Beliefs in asymptomatic checkups. Perhaps an even more significant index of the disposition of people to seek prompt medical attention (than recognizing the medical significance of particular signs of illness) may be the belief about the value of asymptomatic general health examinations. There was a marked increase in the proportion of people who endorsed the utility of such an examination. At the time of the first survey, 47 percent disagreed with the statement that "there is no need to see a doctor regularly if you are not sick"; in the second survey two years later, the figure was 62 percent (p = < .001).

Attitudes toward Sources of Ambulatory Health Care. Respondents were asked to rate their current medical care, health-care services available to the Columbia Point community, two open-ended questions about the Health Center, structured questions about physicians and their relationships to patients, and for a comparative evaluation of major sources of health care.

(1) General Evaluations of Medical Care and the Health Center. The proportion of respondents who reported that they were "very satisfied" with their own health care, services increased sharply from 56

TABLE 2. Conditions for Which a Doctor Should Be Seen

	Baseline Health survey Nov. 1965 N = (357) % = 100.0 Per cent	Follow-up health survey Nov. 1967 N = (436) % = 100.0 Per cent	Improvement or decline	x^2
Serious				
Severe shortness of breath	89	92	+3	n.s.
Lump or discolored patches of skin	88	92	+4	n.s.
Rash or itch for week or more	84	90	+6	.05
Cough for several weeks	80	87	+7	.05
Feeling of dizziness	73	77	+4	n.s.
Unexplained loss of 10 lb.	73	78	+5	n.s.
Mixed				
Frequent headaches	70	80	+10	.01
Feeling tired all the time	69	80	+11	.001
Backaches fairly often	66	78	+12	.001
Diarrhea or constipation	57	65	+8	.05
Minor conditions				
Sore throat, runny nose	30	50	+20	.001
Foot corns	21	39	+17	.001
Slight cold	4	9	+5	n.s.

to 81 percent, after the Health Center was established. It is conceivable, although highly improbable on the basis of what we know about developments in other ambulatory health-care services for which Columbia Point residents would be eligible, that the gain in satisfaction of this magnitude would be attributable to sources other than the Health Center. To minimize the inferential nature of our conclusion, we examined replies to a question in which respondents were asked to rate on a five-point scale various features of the community including its health-care services. This question provides a more direct assessment of the Health Center as the primary health resource of the community. The proportion of residents who rated health facilities in the community as "very good" or "good" was a strikingly low 24 percent just before the Health Center's doors were opened. Two years later, this figure increased dramatically to 91 percent (Table 3). after the construction of a nearby major shopping center, and schools, after a new school was built, showed comparable increases in favorable assessment. Since only 71 percent of the respondents acknowledged the Health Center as their regular source of care, a majority of those who claim some other source, or no regular source at all, must nonetheless have concurred in the more favorable evaluation of this aspect of Columbia Point.

(2) Specific Evaluation of the Health Center. What people like and dislike about it. Such global evaluations, of course, offer us no insight as to the bases for the favorable assessment. In view of the geographic isolation of this community from major sources of health-care services in the past, sheer convenience may be the decisive consideration in accounting for the shift in overall assessment, assuming that no counterbalancing disadvantages are experienced in other salient aspects of health care delivery, e.g., quality of care, the personal manner in which it is rendered, etc. The Health Center was designed explicitly to do more than simply provide equivalent services at greater convenience; its purpose is to assure good quality, coordinated, continuous, and personal centered care, a new organizational form of health-care delivery and a more comprehensive definition of health, as well as accessibility and relevance. It is, therefore, important for both practical and theoretical reasons to understand the actual bases for patronage by residents of this community.

An examination of responses to two sets of open-minded queries makes clear that while convenience in access (e.g., reduction of travel and waiting time) is a highly salient concern to residents in this community, considerations of quality of care and interpersonal relationships are also important. Respondents were asked to specify what they liked and disliked about the Health Center. Responses to this question, previously reported in more general form, are pre-

TABLE 3. Selected Aspects of the Columbia Point Community Which Are Rated "Very Good" or "Good" in the Baseline and Follow-up Surveys

Aspects of Columbia Point	Baseline health survey Nov. 1965 N = (357) % = 100.0° Per cent	Follow-up health survey Nov. 1967 N = (436) % = 100.0° Per cent	Improvement or decline Per cent	χ^2
Health facilities	24	91	+67	.001
Police protection	14	16	+2	n.s.
Teenager's behavior	6	12	+6	.05
Shopping facilities	24	92	+68	.001
Upkeep of housing	25	16	−9	01
Recreation facilities	33	35	+2	n.s.
School facilities	42	72	+30	.001
Helpful neighbors	42	44	+2	n.s.

° Does not add up to 100 per cent since each aspect of Columbia Point was rated by all respondents.

sented here in greater detail. In addition, they were asked to recall at least one experience that had increased confidence in the Health Center and another which undermined their confidence in it. In order to reduce the possibility that respondents would feel inhibited about reporting personal negative experiences at the Health Center, respondents were asked (for both favorable and unfavorable incidents) to report experiences that happened to them *or* to someone else they knew. Ninety-six percent of the people whom we interviewed mentioned something they liked about the Health Center but only 37 percent mentioned something they disliked. In response to the "critical incident" questions, similarly, 73 percent were able to recall an important favorable experience at the Health Center and only 22 percent an important unfavorable experience.

Three aspects of the Health Center services were favorably mentioned by relatively large numbers of residents. Convenience—that is, proximity of medical services and the reduction of waiting time—received the most frequent mention (60 percent). Since Columbia Point is so inaccessible to the health services previously used by most residents, and a great majority of residents used hospital outpatient clinics and emergency rooms, the salience of convenience is understandable. Not far behind in frequency of mention was interpersonal relationships with the staff—the personal attention and courteous treatment received (47 percent). Quality of care was mentioned by 36 percent and good facilities by 23 percent (Table 4).

Although the great majority of community residents are very satisfied with the Health Center, responses to the two open-ended questions disclose a few focal points of dissatisfaction. Responses to the question, "What do you dislike about the health center?" centered on the same three themes: inconvenience mentioned by 8 percent, or a maximum of 13 percent if we include complaints about "insufficient staff," poor quality of care (10 percent), and unsatisfactory interpersonal relations (8 percent). Hence, the very same aspects of the Health Center which are the focal points of dissatisfaction by some residents are the source of favorable mention by several times as many others. The "negative incident" question resulted in a similar pattern of responses which differed primarily in that it elicited concrete instances of patient dissatisfaction with the Health Center. While it is probably utopian to expect fully to satisfy everyone in a single facility, it is extremely important for those responsible for any service to consider in detail each grievance or complaint. (The Health Center since its inception has had a joint grievance committee with consumers to deal with patient complaints.)

(3) Attitudes about Physicians. In addition to these open-ended questions, several aspects of the health-care delivery system were

TABLE 4. Reasons Given for Liking and Disliking Health Center by Columbia Point Residents, 1967 Survey

A. Reasons for Liking Health Center

Total Respondents	N = (436)	% = 100.0*
1. Convenience	262	60
2. Personal service, attention	205	47
3. Quality care	156	36
4. Good facilities	99	23
5. Any cost reference	55	13
6. Nothing liked	4	1
7. Don't know, never been there	–	–

B. Reasons for Disliking the Health Center

Total Respondents	N = 434	% = 100.0*
1. Inconvenience (excludes "insufficient staff")	33	8
2. Lack of personal attention	32	8
3. Poor quality care	44	10
4. Lack of facilities	18	4
5. Any cost reference	0	0
6. Nothing disliked	261	60
7. Don't know, never been there	14	3

* Does not add to 100 per cent since more than one reason may be given by each individual.

singled out for systematic evaluation and embodied in structured questions. Residents were asked to rate physicians, traditionally the key persons in the health-care delivery system, on a number of qualities, including competence, quality of care rendered, communication, personal interest in the patient, and attitudes toward preventive care and minor patient complaints. While a large majority of people credited most physicians, even before the Health Center was established, with being competent and interested in helping their patients (85 percent and 91 percent, respectively), they were somewhat more critical of the quality of care (20 percent agreed that "doctors don't give you a really good examination"), of the lack of sufficient personal interest in the patient (31 percent), of their failure to give patients a chance to explain what their trouble was (28 percent), and most critical of the failure of the physician to explain what their trouble was (43 percent). In addition, some residents imputed to physicians' attitudes which might be expected to discourage patients from seeking asymptomatic checkups or from seeking prompt medical attention for signs or symptoms of illness at an early stage. Twenty-five percent complained that "doctors only want to see you when you're sick. . ." (i.e., are not interested in preventive care), and a similar percentage maintained that doctors were not interested in hearing about minor complaints (Table 5).

Two years later, Health Center physicians as a group were favorably rated on virtually all qualities by larger proportions of residents. The proportion of residents who attributed competence and dedication in general remained high (89 percent and 92 percent, respectively). The proportions that complained that doctors do not give good examinations dropped from 20 to 11 percent. Doctor-patient communication as a source of dissatisfaction also declined; the proportion who agreed that "doctors don't explain enough to their patients" decreased from 43 percent to 14 percent and that "they don't give patients a chance to tell them exactly what their trouble is" decreased from 20 to 11 percent. Relatively fewer residents complained about the lack of personal interest by the physician. The percentage was reduced from 31 to 12. Finally, the disinterest in preventive health examinations imputed to physicians also declined; the proportion of residents who agreed that "doctors only want to see you if you're sick—they don't want you to come in just for a checkup" declined from 25 percent to 8 percent. The percentage who felt that doctors "are not interested in hearing about minor things" decreased from 26 percent to 14 percent.

(4) Comparative Evaluation of Major Sources of Care. As has been reported elsewhere, respondents were asked to compare the Health Center, hospital outpatient clinics and emergency room services, and

TABLE 5. Evaluation of Physicians

Attitudes toward doctors*	Baseline health survey Nov. 1965 N = (357) % = 100.0	Follow-up health survey Nov. 1967 (436) 100.0	χ^2
	Per cent who agreed		
Competence, Quality Care			
Doctors are competent and know what they are doing	85	89	n.s.
The doctors don't give you a really good examination	20	11	<0.1
Communication			
They don't tell you enough about your condition; they *don't* explain just what the trouble is	43	14	<.001
The doctors *don't* give you a chance to *tell them* exactly what your trouble is	28	11	<.001
Rapport, personal interest			
Most doctors are really interested in helping you	91	92	n.s.
They don't take enough personal interest in you	31	12	<.001
Doctors don't really know your medical history, the illness you have had, your reactions to medicine	26	15	<.001
When to seek medical attention			
Doctors only want to see you if you are sick—they *don't want* you to come in *just for a checkup*	25	8	<.01
Doctors *aren't* interested in hearing about *minor* things	26	14	<.01

* These questions were asked about doctors *in general* in the Wave I Health Survey. In the second survey, they were asked about Columbia Point physicians.

private practitioners on four major dimensions: quality of care, its comprehensiveness, the personal manner in which it is given, and convenience. A majority of respondents chose the Health Center over its nearest rival by a better than 2 to 1 ratio of all four criteria; still others rated the several sources as equivalent on each criterion.[8]

Finally, the residents were asked which source of health care they would prefer if all alternative sources of care were free of charges. Although some who use the Health Center stated they would shift their patronage, the Health Center was preferred over the private practitioner, the next most preferred source of care by more than 3 to 1, even in this hypothetical situation (Table 6). If all other sources of care were just as accessible as the Health Center, undoubtedly, still others would shift. Nonetheless, it is clear that a majority of residents now feel they are able to enjoy the benefits of free, convenient care without sacrificing either quality of care or the personal manner in which it is rendered.

TABLE 6.   Sources of Regular Health Care Which Would Be Chosen if All Sources Were Cost-free

Hypothetical choice of regular source of medical care if all facilities were free	Wave 2 health survey Nov. 1967	
	N	Per cent
Private Doctor	87	20
Columbia Point Health Center	275	63
Hospital Outpatient Department	57	13
Other	17	4
Total	436	100

Situational Determinants

The barriers of time, energy, and cost constitute another important class of determinants of patterns in the utilization of helath-care services.[9] Access to and use of health-care services are affected not only by means tests and fee schedules, location, availability of public transportation, and times when services are available, but also by personal circumstances of the patient. This includes not only his potential resources in money, but also in time, energy, and social credits (e.g., availability of assistance from others), as well as the social claims upon these resources (e.g., responsibility for children, extra-household employment, etc.). The various components of resources and liabilities (or costs) have a limited interchangeability: the time-energy costs of health services which are difficult to reach by public transportation can be reduced by car or taxi. The inflexibility introduced by responsibility for small children can be offset by access to baby-sitters—for hire, in a child-care area at a health center, or through other forms of reciprocity. In accounting for underutilization of health-care services among the poor and for subsequent improvement in utilization attributable to the Health Center, such situational factors constitute a major alternative (although not necessarily a mutually exclusive) explanation to the frequently cited hypothesis that underutilization reflects learned behavior, a social class subculture, a culture of poverty, or the like.

Our findings confirm the expectation that the potential cost barriers to health-care utilization are markedly reduced subsequent to the introduction of the Health Center. This will be documented by an examination of responses to several questions included in the interview schedule: (1) reasons cited by respondents who acknowledged postponing needed health care; (2) reported barriers to the use of emergency health care services; (3) time spent door-to-door, in seeking medical care as estimated by respondents; and (4) reported financial indebtedness for medical reasons.

Reasons for Postponing Needed Medical Care. We noted earlier that 23 percent of the respondents, interviewed before the Health Center opened its doors, acknowledged that they or someone in their family had put off medical attention. When respondents were asked about the reasons for the delay, financial cost, and convenience—i.e., considerations relating to geographic inaccessibility, hours of service, and waiting time—were identified as major impediments. Forty-five percent said they were unable to pay for physicians' services or for medicine. Seventeen percent said they could not afford transportation to the sources of care. Twenty percent complained that it took too long to get there, and 10 percent felt too ill to travel. Female heads of more than one in five households reported that they were unable to find anyone to take care of children or dependent adults while they sought medical care.

Two years later, among the relatively fewer households that still acknowledged putting off needed medical care, the reasons reported were scattered over a wider variety of categories although considerations relating to money cost (e.g., physicians' fees and medicines) and transportation remain numerically the most significant. Such respondents probably are among the minority ineligible for welfare medical benefits, who continue to patronize other sources of health-care services than the Health Center.

Barriers to Use of Emergency Services. Respondents were also asked whether they had actually made use of emergency health services and, if so, whether they had experienced difficulty in using those facilities because of problems in arranging for child care, in reaching emergency room service, or arising from a long wait for treatment. Among persons who had occasion to use a hospital emergency room before the Health Center was established, a maximum of 18 percent had difficulty in arranging for care of younger children,[1]/ 27 percent mentioned trouble with transportation, and 47 percent mentioned the long waiting time at the emergency room. Two years later, fewer respondents experienced such barriers in access to emergency room service—whether at a hospital or at the Health Center, since the Health Center also provided transportation to nearly all emergency services required by its patients. Among households that made use of emergency health-care services subsequent to the inception of the Health Center, the proportions who reported difficulties in arranging for babysitters, obtaining transportation, or with long waiting periods for care dropped substantially: the figures are, respectively, 6 percent, 7 percent, and 12 percent.

Time Spent in Obtaining Services. The time spent, door-to-door, in obtaining needed medical care also decreased markedly after the Health Center opened its doors. Previously, 84 percent of the respondents reported that they spent two hours or more each time they sought care. (Fourteen percent reported spending five hours and longer per visit.) Two years later, the percentage reporting two or more hours declined to 17 percent.

Among residents who used the Health Center, 79 percent reported that they received care within a half hour of their arrival. The proportion who complained about excessive waiting time in the physician's office declined from 56 percent before the inception of the Health Center to about 20 percent afterwards.

Financial Considerations. The significance of financial considerations in affecting access to, and utilization of, health-care services is underestimated by the data presented thus far. The reader will recall that relatively few respondents, in reply to the open-ended question as to what they liked about the Health Center, made any reference to the absence of fees for comprehensive health-care services, including laboratory services and pharmaceutical supplies. Although such considerations are usually prominent among reasons for postponing care, only a fraction of Columbia Point residents are so affected. A major reason for this is that a substantial proportion of Columbia Point residents were eligible for welfare medical benefits. Even before the Health Center opened, residents who were willing to pay a price in inconvenience and accept emergency room and hospital outpatient clinic care were able to obtain some health-care services in Boston. This is reflected in the fact that prior to the Health Center, virtually all chronic medical ailments were reported to have been brought to the attention of a physician at some time during the history of the medical ailment. Only half of these chronic conditions, however, were under continuing medical supervision.

It is also likely that financial considerations may have discouraged residents from seeking medical care at earlier stages of illness or taking advantage of preventive health services. Although half of the families made *no* outlays for medical care or related transportation expenditures prior to the inception of the Health Center, the remaining families spent an average of $8.00 monthly for these purposes. (Much of this, it should be kept in mind, was for emergency room and outpatient clinic care.) Eleven percent of the respondents reported that medical expenses led to financial indebtedness, a figure which was reduced to 3 percent two years later.

Summary

This paper is one of a series reporting the results of a comprehensive evaluation of the impact of a neighborhood health center on its target community two major sources of data are drawn upon for this evaluation: (1) data on *actual* utilization based on medical records, and (2) attitudes toward, and reported use of, health-care services based on a survey of random sample of households interviewed at two points in time—just before the inception of a neighborhood health center and two years later.

A previous report, based on actual utilization, showed high levels of utilization of Health Center services by this low-income community, approximating comparable figures for more affluent populations. We noted further a shift in actual utilization from such major sources of ambulatory health-care services as Boston City Hospital (outpatient department and emergency room), heavily used by Columbia Point residents in the past, to the Health Center. A great majority of residents subsequently acknowledged the Health Center as their central or regular source of care.

The before-and-after studies described in the present report show, for example, marked increases in the reported use of such health services as asymptomatic checkups (from 17 percent, prior to the establishment of the Health Center, to 59 percent two years later), poliomyelitis immunization in children (from 78 percent to 92 percent, reaching two children in three who previously had been without a polio vaccination), and a reduction in families that reported postponing needed medical care (from 23 percent to 10 percent).

Taken together, these and other reported findings demonstrate a major and significant change in behavior relating to medical care and utilization of numerous aspects of the health-care system. One would anticipate that such a major behavioral change would be paralleled by and associated with significant change in attitudes, leaving aside for a moment the question of causality. The present study found that major attitudinal changes had occurred. Recognition of various signs and symptoms of illness as reasons for seeking medical care uniformly increased; this was particularly marked for symptoms of an earlier stage in the disease process, e.g., "sore throats" which increased from 30 to 50 percent. The proportion of respondents who acknowledged the value of an asymptomatic checkup also increased from 47 to 62 percent.

Attitudes toward sources of ambulatory care were also found to have improved markedly after the inception of the Health Center. The proportion of residents who reported that they were "very satisfied" with their (own) medical care increased from 56 to 81 percent, and the proportion who rated health-care services available at Columbia Point as "very good" or "good" increased from 24 to 91 percent. Ninety-six percent of survey respondents mentioned something they liked about the Health Center and only 37 percent mentioned something they disliked.

Respondents were asked to rate physicians in general, on the basis of experience prior to the establishment of the Health Center, with those staffing the Health Center on a number of dimensions: competence, dedication, quality of care given, the personal manner in which care was given, and doctor-patient communication. Attitudes towards physicians at the Columbia Point Health Center were consistently more favorable than those expressed toward physicians prior to the establishment of the Health Center. The proportion of respondents, for example, who complained of poor quality of care declined from 20 to 11 percent, of the lack of personal interest by physicians from 31 to 12 percent, and of the physicians' failure to explain what was the matter with the patient from 43 to 14 percent.

Respondents were also asked systematically to compare the Health Center with two other alternative sources of care—the private practitioner and a hospital outpatient clinic or emergency service—on four major dimensions. A majority of residents preferred the Health Center over its closest rival by a ratio of at least 2 to 1 on each of the four dimensions. In response to a hypothetical situation in which medical care from any source would be free to the patient, the Health Center was favored by a ratio of 3 to 1.

Changes in second set of variables might also be expected to accompany (or help account for) the changes in reported utilization of health-care services—situational variables such as time, convenience, and money. The present study found that such factors did affect reported utilization of services. Almost uniformly, past problems in obtaining medical care were reported to have declined dramatically with the advent of the Health Center. For example, the proportion of residents who reported that they spent a minimum of two hours, door-to-door, in the typical effort to obtain medical care declined dramatically from 84 to 17 percent. The percentage who complained about excessive waiting time in the doctor's office decreased from 53 to 20 percent. Finally, financial indebtedness incurred for medical reasons declines from 11 to 3 percent, a figure which is noteworthy when account is taken of the fact that a high proportion of this community was eligible for welfare or other third-party medical reimbursement.

Discussion

We have already shown that the advent and development of a Health Center which eliminates traditional barriers to comprehensive and community-relevant health services can significantly increase utilization of physicians and use of the health-care system by a low-income, urban population. We now find that advent of the Health Center also significantly changed attitudes, knowledge, and beliefs about health and health care, particularly in the critical areas of early diagnosis and treatment, and asymptomatic checkups, areas which in the past (probably for situational reasons), have received least attention from the poor. Since no systematic effort was made to modify beliefs and attitudes of the community through mass educational campaigns, we suggest that it is experience—the experience of the Health Center—which induced changes in attitudes as well as in actual behavior. In this respect, our inferences are paralleled by evidence from studies of racial integration, that it is not necessary to bring about changes in attitudes before achieving integration; both behavior and attitudes are likely to change in a positive direction as a *consequence* of social integration. The new health experience, however, has to meet the situational needs (time, cost, convenience, etc.) of the health consumers to be meaningful and to facilitate attitudinal and behavioral change. This may be the root issue of the failure of many "health educational" campaigns aimed at the poor in the past—efforts which tried to change the health attitudes and behaviors of the poor without changing the health-care system. For many low-income consumers, this must have seemed to be an attempt to lead them back into a grossly unsatisfactory system—and into a set of experiences which merely reinforced their previous negative attitudes. But if, in contrast, there is a change in the available health-care system, then both attitudes and behavior may change.

If this is so, then something even more important than changes in utilization may have been occurring among the residents of Columbia Point after the advent of the Health Center with its situational advantages. One may at least hope that the changes in health-related attitudes and knowledge described in this study may persist beyond the consumer's length of residence at Columbia Point. A major effect of a Health Center, then, may be to increase the continuing and informed demands by the poor for significant improvement in the health-care system available to them—improvement not only with respect to situational factors but also to meet their new expectations of early diagnosis and treatment, good preventive care, and high quality professional services delivered with concern and respect.

The significance of a new institution like a health center thus may extend beyond its immediate effects on (or advantages to) its target population? it may additionally create informed dissatisfaction with the present system and informed demands for change in the system to meet newly perceived needs for good primary and preventive care. Perhaps, for the health consumers as well, experience is the best teacher.

NOTES

1. Tufts University Comprehensive Community Health Action Program Report to the Office of Economic Opportunity, Department of Preventive Medicine, Tufts University School of Medicine, 1966 (mimeo).

2. S. S. Bellin, H. J. Geiger, and C. D. Gibson, The impact of ambulatory health care services on the demand for hospital beds, *N. Engl. J. Med.* 280:808, 1969.

3. S. S. Bellin, and H. J. Geiger, Actual public acceptance of neighborhood health centers by the urban poor, *JAMA* 214:2147, 1970.

4. Yankelovich, Daniel, Inc., The Columbia Point Housing Project: A Description of a Public Housing Population in the Urban North (575 Madison Ave., New York, N.Y.) April 1966, 68 pp. (mimeo).

5. H. J. Geiger, The Poor and the Professional: Who Takes the Handle off the Broad Street Pump? Paper read at the Special Session on the New Partnerships in Delivery of Health Services, American Public Health Association, Nov. 1, 1966, at San Francisco, Calif. (Tufts University School of Medicine Department of Community Health and Social Medicine, Boston, Mass.); The Neighborhood health center: education of the faculty in preventive medicine, *Arch. Environ. Health* 14:912, 1967; see also C. D. Gibson, The neighborhood health center—the primary unit of health care, *Am. J. Public Health* 58:1188, 1968, Cynthia H. Kelly, Fighting poverty with health care. *Am J. Nursing* 68:1504, 1968,

J. Solon, Changing patterns of obtaining medical care in a public housing community: impact of a service program, *Am. J. Public Health* 57:772, 1967.

6. The original census of all households in residence in the community from which the subsequent household sample was drawn and the two subsequent health surveys were designed by the firm of Daniel Yankelovich, Inc., in collaboration with the Tufts Department of Community Health and Social Medicine. The first is located at 575 Madison Ave., New York, N.Y.

7. A special survey was undertaken of a random sample of households in connection with a Medicaid Sign-up Campaign in which a question was included on poliomyelitis immunization.

A spot check by staff pediatricians, in 1968, revealed that a substantial minority of children had not had their complete series of immunizations, and they pointed up inadequacies in the follow-up procedure in effect at that time.

8. Bellin and Geiger, Actual public acceptance of health centers.

9. Time and effort are costs typically neglected in accounting for human decision behavior.

10. This figure is not adjusted for childless households.

10. Utilization and Cost

Experience of Low-Income Families in Four Prepaid Group-Practice Plans

GERALD SPARER AND ARNE ANDERSON

Since early 1965 the Office of Economic Opportunity (OEO), through its Office of Health Affairs, has assisted in the funding of different types of health-services delivery and financing demonstrations. These demonstrations for providing health services to low-income families have ranged from solo-fee-for-services contract arrangements and newly established freestanding neighborhood health centers, to "buy in" arrangements with established prepaid group-practice plans.

This study reports on four demonstrations in which a comprehensive range of health-care services was purchased from prepaid group-practice plans for a selected number of low-income families. Three plans are located on the West Coast: Kaiser at Fontana, California; Kaiser at Portland, Oregon; Group Health of Puget Sound, Washington; and one on the East Coast, the Health Insurance Plan of New York (HIP) at Suffolk County. All the plans were contracted to enroll approximately 500 families except Kaiser, Portland, which accepted 1,500 families. The major reason for attempting the buy-in arrangements with selected group plans was to provide low-income families with an opportunity to receive health-care services through organizations that provide quality health services, are efficient, with administrative experience in delivering health services, provide health-care services in a manner that can affect the overall cost of health, and provide services to the "new" client group with the same resources as "regular" clients. If the same utilization results could be achieved for low-income families as for regular-plan members, the

From the *New England Journal of Medicine* 289 (July 12, 1973), pp. 67–72, reprinted by permission of the authors and publisher.

arrangements could provide a satisfactory alternative model to deliver and finance health services for the low-income persons.

STUDY OBJECTIVES

This study will present and analyze actual data on use of prepaid health services by low-income families, costs of these services, and utilization of services and costs as compared to regular-plan members. It is our hope that this study may provide information that will aid in the deliberation and development of emerging prepaid group-practice plans and Health Maintenance Organizations, and in the drafting of legislation leading to some form of National Health Insurance.

Findings presented will also show how low-income persons use health services provided by a prepaid group-practice plan and will help in projecting utilization rates, staff needs and the cost of including such persons in prepaid group practices or other delivery mechanisms. The data presented in this study only partially address the policy issue of whether or not prepaid group practices are an effective means of providing health services to the 26 million poor.

METHODS

The data were gathered as part of the management-reporting requirements for Comprehensive Health Services Projects.[1] Only the Kaiser, Portland, project had previously documented and published utilization data on its operation.[2] Each of the participating plans welcomed the study and cooperated with the site visit teams in describing its programs and helping to furnish data.

STUDY DESCRIPTION AND DATA COLLECTION

Visits were made to each of the four participating prepaid group-practice plans. Data were collected on regular-plan members and those enrolled in the project through OEO sponsorship. At three of the four plans, utilization, premium and expenditure data were available from existing reports. In one plan, Group Health of Puget Sound, Washington, it was necessary to draw a 20 percent random sample from medical records to construct the utilization of OEO enrollees and families. Cost data were developed from information that had been used to produce the plans' standard premium rate schedules. Additional information on expenditures for specific services provided only to the OEO group was added to the standard schedule where appropriate. Every attempt was made to identify expenditures for each service provided.

Information on utilization, premium and expenditures was gathered for monthly and quarterly periods for as long as the information was available. Since the start-up period is an important aspect of the demonstration effort, and since very little information exists on utilization in this early period, a special effort was made to collect utilization and cost data on the first one and one-half years of operation as an OEO project.

BACKGROUND OF LOW-INCOME PREPAID PLANS

Three of the plans have been serving the low-income families with OEO assistance for about eighteen months, and the fourth program, Kaiser-Portland, for about four and one-half years. Generally, the capitation formula for estimating the premium for the low-income families was identical to that of the regular-plan member.

In addition to paying the premium for every low-income enrollee, OEO provided additional funds so that supportive-type services usually provided in OEO-assisted Comprehensive Health Service projects[3] — such as social, community and outreach services, patient transportation, staff training, home health and mental health — would also be available to these low-income members of the group-practice plan. Supplementary expenditures were also used to provide full coverage for such services as prescribed drugs and eyeglasses for OEO members. Regular members are usually required to make a copayment for these services. To provide services at a level of intensity not required for regular-plan members, funds were also directed toward providing OEO members additional personnel support in medical, mental and home health services and administrative activities.

An enrollment selection process for OEO members was in effect at each of the four prepaid plans included in the study. The screening process usually included an interview at which basic information on family characteristics was collected. Information gathered included such items as family income, number of members per family, welfare status, location of residence and medical needs. On the basis of this information, those eligible for services were selected for participation in the project.[4]

FINDINGS

Enrolled Population Profiles —
Low-Income and Regular Members

The characteristics of low-income OEO-assisted members differed from those of the regular-plan members, and also from the characteristics of the poor throughout the nation (Table 1). The projects usually placed a priority on the selection of larger, high-risk families with current illness or recent pregnancy. The size of OEO families enrolled ranged from 4.3 to 5.6, and is smaller than the 5.1 average family size of national poor even when the group over 65 years of age is excluded. The OEO-enrolled population is younger than the national poor (Table 1). The differences in age distribution affect utilization rates of physician as well as other services. Since the public policy question is the impact of further use of prepaid groups for the provision of health services to the national poor, utilization rates have been age-adjusted where appropriate for consistency with medical utilization rates for the poor nationally. If we wished to compare utilization rates of OEO members with those of regular members, an age adjustment of the regular-member rates would be appropriate. If, however, universal financial entitlement for health services was to be extended to the national poor, the age distributions of prepaid enrollees among the poor should be similar to the national poor. Therefore, age adjustment of OEO members to national poor is chosen for the main analytical issues of this study.

Benefit Packages

The low-income families were provided with specific services beyond the basic comprehensive physician services usually provided to plan members. To make cost comparisons, the services were grouped into categories so that the same benefits could be compared between plans and groups within plans. The cost differences shown between the plans and groups, therefore, are not due to differences in service benefits, but to management and administrative differences. Regular-plan members usually have restrictions on benefits such as prescribed drugs, outpatient mental-health services, home health services and eyeglasses. For the OEO-supported members, these services were paid for in full. Beyond traditional personal health services, the OEO-assisted families were provided additional benefits. Support staff advised and helped enrolled families with public-assistance questions, employment opportunities and identification of community services that would be useful. Home health services were provided by

Table 1. Characteristics of Enrolled Population According to Group Covered for Each Plan.

Name of Plan & Group Covered	No. of Families	No. of Members	Average Family Size	Percentage Distribution According to Age					
				<5	5-14	15-24	25-44	45-64	65 & over
OEO poor:									
HIP, NY	518	2,278	4.4	20.5	41.4	16.0	16.1	4.8	1.2
Group Health Puget	505	2,148	4.3	12.9	37.2	17.5	22.4	8.3	1.7
Kaiser-Fontana	500	2,805	5.6	12.5	41.6	18.8	19.4	7.1	0.6
Kaiser-Portland	1,497	6,773	4.5	12.2	39.7	26.5	13.6	7.2	0.8
National poor (all ages)*		25,814,000	3.9	11.9	24.6	14.7	16.0	14.6	18.2
National poor (excluding aged)		21,109,000	5.1	14.5	30.1	17.9	19.6	17.8	—
Regular plan:									
HIP, NY	282,000	753,000	2.7	6.2	21.5	14.1	23.0	24.9	10.2
Group Health Puget	—	144,000	—	8.4	20.1	17.8	24.7	21.6	6.9
Kaiser-Fontana	341,000	944,000	2.8	8.2	21.8	17.3	27.9	20.5	4.3
Kaiser-Portland	51,000	145,000	2.8	9.5	22.0	17.4	23.1	19.7	8.3
Total population†		203,212,000	3.5	8.4	20.0	17.5	23.6	20.6	9.9

*Current Population Survey, Mar, 1970, US Bureau of the Census.

†Census reports for 1970, General Population Characteristics.

family-health workers from the community, as well as help in health education, training and nutrition. Transportation services were available to help families get to and from the health center.

Utilization of Services

Comparison of utilization rates for specific services between OEO-assisted families and regular-plan members shows some differences (Table 2). These rates have not been age-adjusted to show the current comparison, and potential impact on existing community premium rates. Physician utilization rates have a major cost implication: only at Fontana did the rate of 4.12 for the OEO group exceed appreciably the 3.72 rate for regular members. If visits by nurses and other nonphysician practitioners are added to the physician utilization rates for the OEO group (only Puget Sound reported providing such services to its regular clients), the total medical visit rates for the OEO group are above the regular-member rates in every case but Puget Sound.

Table 2. Annual Utilization Rates per Member for the Four Plans* (Low-Income and Regular Members).

SERVICES	HIP, NY		GROUP HEALTH OF PUGET SOUND		KAISER-FONTANA		KAISER-PORTLAND	
	LOW INCOME	PLAN MEMBERS	LOW INCOME	PLAN MEMBERS	LOW INCOME	PLAN MEMBERS	LOW INCOME	PLAN MEMBERS
Medical-physician	2.88	4.20	4.00	3.91	4.12	3.72	3.29	3.14
Nonphysician	1.74	NA	0.66	1.0	1.20	NA	0.70	NA
Totals	4.62	4.20	4.66	4.91	5.32	3.72	3.99	3.14
Laboratory	1.77	4.01	2.24	4.33	NA	NA	3.49	4.08
X-ray	0.27	NA	0.50	0.66	NA	NA	0.97	0.97
Prescriptions	NA	NA	NA	6.33	3.78	3.21	NA	4.14
Home health	1.70	—	2.30	—	3.37	—	1.34	—

*Plan-members data relate to 1971; low-income utilization relates to 12 mo ending Mar, 1972, except for Puget Sound (12 mo ending July, 1972). NA indicates data not available, & — not applicable.

The use of nonphysician providers suggests a useful trade between physician and other service providers that may have implications for regular-plan services. Rates for laboratory tests and x-ray procedures comprise both inpatient and outpatient services for each plan except

HIP, which includes ambulatory services only. Estimates at one plan show that up to 22 percent of laboratory and 10 percent of x-ray procedures are used for inpatient care. In each case, except Portland, where the rates are almost the same, the OEO group used laboratory services at almost half the rate of the regular membership. The high proportion of children in the OEO group undoubtedly accounts for much of this difference, but other factors may be influential as well. OEO clients also used 1.4 to 3.4 home health visits per enrollee per year, a service not provided regular plan members.

Physician Utilization Rates Adjusted for Age and Sex

If prepaid group practices included large numbers of the poor in their regular membership, what would be the impact on utilization and premium costs? One way of estimating the impact is to adjust the utilization rates for the OEO enrollees as if they represented the national poor in terms of age and sex, and comparing the adjusted rates to those for the regular-plan membership (Table 3). In every case except Puget Sound, for both OEO and regular groups the utilization rates are lower in the group plans than national average rates (reported by the National Center for Health Statistics) for all ages and also when those over 64 are excluded.

Table 3. Physician Utilization Rates per Enrollee Adjusted for Age and Sex.

| PLAN | OEO LOW-INCOME ENROLLEES | | | REGULAR MEMBERS | |
| | UNADJUSTED RATE | ADJUSTED TO NATIONAL POOR | | | |
	all ages	*all ages*	*excluding 65 +*	*all ages*	*excluding 65 +*
HIP, NY	2.88	4.00	3.15	4.20	3.70
Group Health of Puget Sound	4.00	4.65	3.85	3.91	3.80
Fontana	4.12	NA	NA	3.72	NA
Portland	3.29	4.45	4.00	3.14	3.05
National data*		4.5†	4.1†	4.3‡	4.1‡

*Current Population Survey Mar, 1970, Bureau of the Census. NA indicates not available.

†US National Center for Health Statistics. Vital & Health Statistics. Health Characteristics of Low-Income Persons (Series 10, No. 74), 1969.

‡US National Center for Health Statistics. Vital & Health Statistics. Physician Visits, Volume & Interval since Last Visit. United States (Series 10, No. 75), 1969.

Start-Up Utilization

Prepaid group practices would appropriately be interested in the potential cost of catching up with the unmet medical-care needs of newly enrolled low-income persons. Examination of physician utilization rates for the OEO group (Table 4) shows only a modest, but consistent, downward drift in utilization over time.

Table 4. Utilization Pattern of First Six Quarters of Operation.

PLAN	START-UP DATE	CALENDAR QUARTER (3-MO PERIOD)					
		1	2	3	4	5	6
HIP:							
Physician-encounter rate*	Oct,	3.01	3.20	3.04	2.37	2.73	3.37
New enrollees (%)†	1970		7	22	4	4	19
Group Health of Puget Sound:							
Physician-encounter rate	Feb,	6.47	4.63	4.57	4.06	3.87	3.50
New enrollees (%)	1971		120	9	0	1	1
Kaiser-Fontana:							
Physician-encounter rate	Nov,	3.03	4.62	4.73	3.55	3.92	4.26
New enrollees (%)	1970		112	7	5	4	2
Kaiser-Portland:							
Physician-encounter rate	Oct,	4.43	3.94	2.69	2.68	2.96	2.68
Increase in enrollment (%)‡	1967		21	−6	−1	0	22

*Annualized rates/person/quarter.

†Added enrollees during quarter over total enrollees at end of previous quarter.

‡At Portland additions & terminations are not available; therefore, increase in total enrollment is given.

In three of the four projects the fifth-quarter rates were lower than the first-quarter rates. At Fontana, the fifth quarter was higher. Although each project may have experienced start-up lags, Fontana's first-quarter rates were exceeded in each succeeding quarter, indicating, perhaps, a more than usual start-up lag in utilization. The sixth-quarter rates for Fontana were lower than the second quarter. At Portland, the oldest project, current utilization rates were lower than their first year's rates, but modestly higher than the annual rates for the year's period between six and eighteen months of project operation. If there is an early surge in utilization, it is not apparent after six months. The newly enrolled clients will move toward a stable utilization rate, subject, of course, to seasonal fluctuations.

Hospitalization

A serious concern in developing prepaid capitation rates for low-income persons has been the very high hospitalization rates of the poor in nonorganized medical-care systems. Prepaid group practices organized with strong controls over hospital usage have experienced hospitalization rates far lower than those for the general population. For each of the regular-plan members, the annual inpatient hospital days per 1,000 persons fell under 600 (Table 5). The HIP rate was highest at 549, and the others grouped closely between 440 and 465 days. This compares to the annual 1,150 inpatient days per thousand for the United States population, or 849 days for those under 65 years of age and has been cited as a major advantage of the prepaid groups. The OEO clients used less than 600 days per 1,000 persons per year in the three West Coast plans. Table 5 also presents data on the average length of stay. Because the rates for length of hospitaliza-

Table 5. Hospital Utilization Rate, 1971.

Category	Hospital Admissions*	Inpatient Days	Average Length of Stay
OEO low-income:			
HIP, NY	NA	NA	NA
Puget Sound	88	597	6.8
Kaiser-Fontana	101	562	5.6
Kaiser-Portland	91	410	4.5
US low-income, all ages[†]	114	1580	13.9
<65	102	1136	11.1
Group-practice regular member:			
HIP, NY	73[‡]	549[‡]	7.5[‡]
Puget Sound	92	466	5.1
Kaiser-Fontana	79	468	5.9
Kaiser-Portland	84	443	5.3
US total, all ages[§]:	145	1150	7.9
<65	127	849	6.7

*Rates/1000 persons. NA indicates not available.

[†]United States National Center for Health Statistics. Vital & Health Statistics. Health Characteristics of Low-Income Persons (Series 10, No. 74), 1968.

[‡]1967 data.

[§]Hospitals, Jan 16, 1971.

tion could not be standardized for age and sex, the higher rate for the regular enrollees may be ascribed to their older age as compared to the OEO group, or the national low-income population. Annual admission rates for the OEO group ranged from 88 to 101 per 1,000 persons, which was generally higher than the regular-plan range of 73 to 92. As compared to the 102 admissions per 1,000 persons for the low-income under 65 nationally, hospital admission rates among OEO prepaid-plan members were not high.

The important finding is that a prepaid group practice, exercising a reasonable gatekeeper function over hospitalization, can expect to reduce hospital days consumed by low-income persons to the comparable levels being experienced by regular-plan members.

Cost of Demonstration Groups

An analysis of the cost experience for these demonstrations shows the combination of expenditures for regular-plan benefits, based on a premium structure, and the enriched package of services, budgeted on a line-item basis (Table 6). Regular benefits such as comprehensive physicians' services, prescribed drugs, mental health and hospitalization are covered as part of the basic premium structure.

The range of costs for regular-plan members is about $125 at Portland, Fontana and Puget Sound (with some minor benefit variations) and $154 at HIP. For the OEO low-income group the cost is about $180 at HIP, and ranges from $127 to $141 for the rest, or about 12 percent more than the cost for non-OEO enrollees at each of the plans. At Portland, all OEO premium rates are the same as the community rates for regular members, showing a very strong commitment to providing organized health to the poor. At Puget Sound only the annual comprehensive physician service rates are higher for the OEO group, $86.83 as compared to $72.05 for regular enrollees. At both HIP and Fontana, the comprehensive physician services and hospital rates are higher for the OEO enrollees, with the $27 differential for hospitalization at HIP being attributed to an estimate of about 800 hospital days per year per 1,000 enrollees. This rate is subject to adjustment based on experience.

There are additional basic supplemental services offered, ranging from $8.69 worth of eyeglasses and nurse services at Portland to $19.78 for eyeglasses, nurse services and extended care at Fontana. Each plan has varied these services, for which careful utilization analysis should help document a need-related range. Additional support services, including home health, social and community services and transportation, range from $47 per person per year at Fontana to $65 at Puget Sound. The different outlays for these supporting

Table 6. Annual Cost of Services (in Dollars) per Member According to Type of Services—Comparison of OEO and Regular Plan, 1971.

Benefits	HIP, NY LOW INCOME	HIP, NY PLAN MEMBERS	GROUP HEALTH OF PUGET SOUND LOW INCOME	GROUP HEALTH OF PUGET SOUND PLAN MEMBERS	KAISER-FONTANA LOW INCOME	KAISER-FONTANA PLAN MEMBERS	KAISER-PORTLAND LOW INCOME	KAISER-PORTLAND PLAN MEMBERS
Basic services:								
Comprehensive physician services*	76.98	75.00	86.83	72.05	70.83	64.74	69.58	69.58
Prescribed drugs	12.12	11.16†	13.06	13.06	16.57	16.57	13.71	¶
Mental health	6.96	10.80	4.65	4.65	5.64§	5.64§	3.36	¶
Hospital	84.11‡	57.72	34.51	34.51	44.35	40.32	54.57	54.57
Total premium	180.17	154.68	139.05	124.27	137.39	127.27	141.22	124.15
Supplemental services:								
Nurse services	15.58	—	5.79	—	14.14	—	2.07	—
Extended care	—	—	3.52	—	1.40	1.40	—	—
Eyeglasses	—	—	3.38	—	4.24	4.24	6.62	¶
Total supplemental	15.58	—	12.69	—	19.78	5.64	8.69	—
Supporting services:								
Home health	28.21	—	36.06	—	35.14	—	29.31	—
Social & community	6.94	—	5.79	—	1.10	—	9.34	—
Transportation	21.03	—	23.44	—	11.16	—	10.47	—
Total support	56.18	—	65.22	—	47.40	—	49.12	—
Research & evaluation	25.77	—	14.52	—	15.86	—	15.83	—
Administration	68.10	—	31.64	—	40.96	—	45.21	—
Grand total	$345.80	$154.68	$263.29	$124.27	$261.39	$132.91	$260.07	$124.15

*Includes comprehensive physician & nurse services, laboratory & x-ray services.

†Amount reflects fully prepaid if drugs are obtained by mail order; otherwise, 80% reimbursement from local pharmacies.

‡Hospitalization costs are for an expected utilization rate of 800 days/1000 for the low-income & the 1967 rate of 549 days/1000 for plan members at the prevailing cost of $105 per day.

§Plan members pay $5 for visit after the 20th visit; low-income members have no such limit but pay the same premium.

¶The basic premium includes: a discount on drugs, mental health coverage where the member pays 50% of cost with a $1000/yr limit & $10,000 lifetime limit, & eye examination at $1 to $2 charge & a discount on glasses. The premium paid for the low-income members eliminates these charges.

health-service items suggest an opportunity to document the importance of these services to the clients, in terms of appropriate utilization and efficiency in delivering health care. In addition, research, evaluation and administrative expenses ranged from $93.87 per person per year at HIP to $46.16 at Puget Sound.

DISCUSSION AND POLICY ISSUES

This analysis of the utilization and cost data from the four OEO-assisted demonstrations that served 500 to 1,500 families provides information on how low-income families use services of prepaid group practices. Low-income families enrolling in a prepaid group-practice plan are generally larger than the regularly enrolled families, and the premium structures of prepaid plans based on a family size of three may need to be considered for revision if large numbers of low-income families become enrolled in these plans. The newly enrolled OEO group initially used physician services at a higher rate than regular-plan members. After about six months, the physician utilization rate among OEO members leveled off to approximately that of regular members. The most important finding that may affect policy planning is that the OEO low-income group used hospital days at a rate more like that of regular-plan members, which was some 50 percent lower than the low-income rate under 65 years of age nationally. Although admission rates were about equal to the national rates, the length of stay was lower.

In the area of costs, the differences between the OEO members and the regular-plan members for the basic benefits package ranged from no difference in costs to 15 percent more for the low-income person. With the inclusion of other benefits such as laboratory, x-ray, pharmacy, hospital, eyeglasses and mental-health services along with necessary research, evaluation and administrative expenses, the package could be purchased for under $170 per person per year. If supporting-type health services consistent with OEO's concept of a broader health-services delivery system were to be added, the annual cost per enrollee would add another $47 to $65 to the amount. Early assessment of the usefulness of these supporting outlays would be desirable. Research and administrative expenses ranging from $46 to $94 appear high, and reviews of these costs should be initiated.

The policy implications of these demonstrations are that modest numbers of the poor can effectively be integrated into existing prepaid group practices at current community rates. Savings in hospitalization can be assumed for prepaid plans offering effective gatekeeper functions regarding hospital use. If large numbers of the poor were to be covered, consideration would have to be given either to an increase in the average community premium rate or to the establishment of a rate for the low-income subscribers that would be about 12 percent more than the rate charged for regular-plan members. Better documentation of each component of supporting health services must be undertaken to assess the effect of outreach and transportation on appropriate utilization and enriched social services on family functioning. Now, only few anecdotal data suggest that not even minimal utilization would occur without the support services. If this hypothesis is true, the question still remains of how support services relate to what changes in utilization and for how much and how long.

NOTES

1. *Reporting Requirements of Comprehensive Health Services Projects* (OEO Manual 6128-2). Washington, D.C.: Office of Economic Opportunity, November, 1972. Collection of the data presented in this paper was supported partially through OEO contract B1C-5291 with System Sciences, Inc. Data-collection efforts were subcontracted to Geomet, Inc., which carried out on-site collection for information not already available from existing data. On-site assistance and staff support from Raymond Fink, HIP, New York, Joel Kovner, Kaiser-Fontana, Theodore Colombo, Kaiser-Portland, and David Chivers and Dorothy Mitchell at Group Health in Puget Sound are appreciated.

2. Colombo, T.J., Saward, E.W. and Greenlick, M.R. The integration of an OEO Health Program into a prepaid comprehensive group practice plan, *Am. J. Public Health* 59:641-650, 1969.

3. Sparer, G., Anderson, A. Cost of services at neighborhood health centers: a comparative analysis. *N. Engl. J. Med.* 286:1241-1245, 1972.

4. *Guideline for Service through Comprehensive Health Services Program* (OEO Guidance 6128-1). Washington, D.C.: Office of Economic Opportunity, March, 1970; *OEO Income Guidelines revised* (OEO Instruction 6004 1c). Washington, D.C.: Office of Economic Opportunity, November 10, 1971.

Part VI

LOOKING AHEAD–
IMPLICATIONS FOR
FUTURE PLANNING

The accomplishments of American medicine have been partially obscured by the growing recognition that there are major deficiencies in the delivery of health care.[1] Academic observers have verified the real nature of the health crisis; *Time, Fortune, Business Week*, CBS, and NBC, recently reporting on the medical scene, find it "chaotic," "archaic," "unmanageable." One of the main criticisms is that a large segment of the American public is not now receiving adequate medical care and that a sizeable proportion of those who do are dissatisfied with some aspects of it.[2] Although the United States spends more on medical care than any other country in the world, it ranks low with respect to health. In 1974 alone, when the nation's health bill totaled $100 billion, or approximately 8 percent of the gross national income, the United States ranked below twenty other countries in male life expectancy. The women of seven other nations outlive American women. Even more significant is the fact that the United States ranks fourteenth in infant mortality, the figure generally accepted as the most accurate indicator of a nation's health.[3]

Although somewhat slow in responding, the medical profession is now moving more vigorously to take the lead in resolving this critical national problem. This response has been motivated by the pronouncements and activities of the federal government and other non-medical organizations. American medicine is in a state of transition, marked by an acceleration of studies and critical appraisals of the delivery system, accompanied by a proliferation of medical innovations and modifications in the existing system.

215

PLANNING AND THE FEDERAL GOVERNMENT

Planning and accountability are key words today. Federal policies have shifted toward more deliberate, preset goals: funding agencies are awarding contracts rather than grants, which allows them to specify the results expected — though many in the academic community have criticized this practice as frustrating creativity and scientific freedom. The government also tends to use funds to encourage particular outcomes, such as preferential funding for training primary-care providers and decreased funding for research specialists. Health planning activities have been stimulated by the establishment of comprehensive health planning agencies, which have the potential to become regional health authorities. These activities have been increasingly well funded.

A related development has been the notable shift of federal funding sources from basic to applied research. Here again, the emphasis is on finding ways in which health care can be more effectively delivered and practical information disseminated. For behavioral scientists, this means an opportunity to collaborate in determining pragmatic predictors and other factors that affect health-care utilization behavior.

SHIFT FROM CHARITY TO WELFARE

Underlying much of these new developments, particularly as they relate to the delivery of medical care to the poor and minority groups, is a transition dating back to the Depression, in the way we think about health—from "charity" to "welfare." Certain services are now considered a right rather than a gift bestowed by a bountiful upper class. With increased militancy the poor and minority groups are demanding more representation and more services. This stance will mean a much larger role for the federal government and a decreasing role for private charities. This balance will continue to adjust if current federal policies to restrict welfare expenditures continue while large foundations sponsor major research activities; yet it seems clear that the government will continue to be the dominant source of support for undertakings involving the poor. Also evident is a shift toward more federal input (and therefore more control) in state and local programs, which should result eventually in a greater standardization of programs. This changing orientation will encourage the development of additional programs targeted at minorities and the aged, as these people represent the bulk of the poverty group.

INSURING THE NATION'S HEALTH

A major force for a more unified medical service in the near future will be the passage of a national health insurance program. The United States is ready for such a program. People are concerned as never before with skyrocketing medical costs, realizing that they can be financially destroyed by a serious medical problem. Labor unions and civic organizations, congressmen and senators are openly advocating passage of a national health insurance plan. A variety of proposals has been put forth. The major question is whether it will be government run, government financed, or merely government required. Also to be established are whether the program is to be voluntary or compulsory, how extensive the coverage is to be, and how much is to be paid by insurance and how much by the individual.[4]

The effect of such a program on utilization of medical services by the poor is unclear. One would hope that passage of such a bill would be accompanied by a determined effort to improve and expand the medical care delivery system, particularly for those who are the predominant nonutilizers. And, one could easily argue, that good medical care is a right of all Americans, and poor people especially would come to view good medical care for themselves and their families as normal and expected, therefore cooperating in treatment programs more frequently than in the past.

However, this increase in utilization might bring about a new set of problems. An increased demand for services in the face of limited supply would create a new set of market pressures. If the price is controlled by a single payer, i.e., the government, then other factors will also determine supply. It is not inconceivable that the poor might suffer even more, owing to social discriminations on the part of providers who would prefer to treat persons more like themselves. If economic rewards are equalized, the differences in achievable results, patient gratification, and provider satisfaction may become key issues in the allocation of services. In an even more pessimistic projection, a program of national health insurance could produce a single class of care on a level with that previously offered to the poor.[5] This new single level of quality would offer no increase in benefits to the poor and no hope of social mobility.

We must retain some skepticism about the likelihood that any form of health insurance will provide significant assistance to the poor. The experience with Medicaid provides some evidence that a new source of payment may not result in improved or in increased services. Olendzki suggests that Medicaid has benefited primarily the young and the less sick.[6] Reviewing the experience in New York City, Bellin and Kavaler report significant overutilization and fraud.[7]

The data from Medicare is no more encouraging. In a study conducted during 1966–70, Coe and Andrews found "(1) there was virtually no coordination of health care facilities in any of the communities studied. (2) Typically, Medicare was used as a justification for expanding acute care capabilities of general hospitals. (3) Medicare had little effect on the way doctors went about their business although (4) Medicare did broaden the doctor's role in the whole health care scheme. (5) Medicare did provide an impetus for needed service–home health care."[8]

Results like these must be considered in our projections for the impact of social programming on health issues. Although we desperately want to believe that large investments to develop such programs will be effective in alleviating the health plight of the poor, there is more than adequate reason for caution and controlled enthusiasm.

HEALTH MANPOWER—FUTURE EXPECTATIONS

Maldistribution and Shortages of Primary Care Providers

There is general agreement in the health field that much of the health care crisis in this nation is caused by a critical shortage or a maldistribution of health manpower, or both.[9] The lack of manpower has a direct effect on the quality of medical care received by poor people. Some view the situation as one of too many specialists (particularly surgeons) and too few primary care providers. Naegele details many factors that contribute to the expansion of medical specialties.[10] While there is some debate as to whether the number of physicians available is adequate, maldistribution is recognized as a major problem. Hepner and Hepner emphasize the manpower dimension in proposing major components for improved health care delivery: "(1) more and better qualified health manpower; (2) better planning for health manpower utilization; (3) reorganization of the health care delivery system; and (4) better financing arrangements for the population."[11] A recent White Paper report spelling out the Administration's plans with respect to health priorities specified some of these manpower problems as "poor distribution of physicians, both in geographical location and type of practice, poor utilization of our manpower resources, and financial difficulties of our professional schools."[12] The Carnegie Commission (1970), studying the same problem, concluded that "The most serious shortages of professional personnel in any major occupational group in the United States are in the health services."[13] The reasons for the manpower shortage are many, but it is primarily due to three related causes: "increased demand for care, inadequate expansion in the supply of health care personnel, and problems within the health care team."[14]

Several factors are behind the increased demand for care. While the population of this country increased 28 percent from 1950 to 1965, the number of physicians increased only 14.3 percent. Moreover, a growing proportion of this nation's population, both in terms of percentages and sheer numbers, are moving into the older age groups. This increased number of older people, who use medical services more frequently than others, will create greater need for medical and hospital resources.[15]

The rising affluence of the American public has played an important role in increasing the demands for medical services. As people become economically secure, they become more concerned about improving and maintaining their health; many Americans are now seeking medical care at times when they did not do so in the past. Also, as the American public has become better educated, they have sought better medical care, particularly preventive care. The long series of medical breakthroughs, such as the organ transplant program, have led the public both to appreciate and want to take advantage of these spectacular medical advances.

As noted earlier, Americans are coming to accept the belief that medical care is a right, and minorities and the poor have moved aggressively to demand these rights. The resultant federal, state, and local government health programs have brought about a need for additional health manpower.

Instead, the supply of manpower has been falling steadily behind for several years. Contributing to this lag is the fact that many medical schools are using student admission formulas based on population growth projections developed several years ago.[16] Faculties and physical plants at most schools grew with the aim of upgrading and accelerating basic research. In such an atmosphere it is not surprising that medical students entered the specialties rather than going into general practice. Thus, even fewer physicians were available for providing primary care, particularly in rural areas, since specialists locate principally in urban areas. Similar problems were experienced in other health manpower fields. Medical personnel generally locate in middle-class suburban areas. As a result, rural areas, ghettos, and other undesirable urban neighborhoods receive limited medical care services.

Still another facet of the health manpower problem stems from confusion and overlapping of roles within the field itself. While various national and state statutes and license laws clearly prescribe who may function as physician, nurse, or allied health personnel, the specific functions of each remain, in many respects, undefined. Thus one finds duplication and conflict within the physician role, as, for example, who should practice surgery, and between role functions— between, for example, the nurse anesthetist and the medical anesthesiologist. Role ambiguity extends even to the case of who should give immunizations—the physician, the nurse, or the medical aide. Many nurses and physicians are reluctant to delegate tasks to the least trained person capable of performing them. These multiple role conflicts result in an inefficient utilization of available and potential manpower, increased expense, and, indirectly, a poorer quality of medical care.

Fortunately, many changes are bringing about a more effective use of existing medical manpower. Both the number of medical schools and the enrollments of existing schools are increasing, largely as a result of federal programs, augmented by funds appropriated by the various states. Additionally, medical schools have of late been more inclined to select students likely to enter practice in rural areas, ghettos, and other areas that lack physicians and related medical personnel.

The development of medical departments of family medicine and the upgrading of the family practitioner's status, through the establishment of family practice as a specialty comparable to internal medicine or pediatrics, have improved the supply of primary care physicians. Reversing the trend of several years, students are electing to enter this new specialty. Complementing this situation, an increasing number of general practitioners are returning to obtain their specialty in family medicine; this should upgrade the general quality of medical care throughout the nation.

Another major source of physicians has been the foreign doctors who immigrate to the United States. Although this practice does not set well with countries who need their skilled people at home, it has helped somewhat to alleviate the physician shortage here. But not without some problems: there is some concern that the large influx of foreign medical graduates will have an adverse effect on standards of care. Many in the medical profession feel that doctors trained abroad do not in the long run represent a satisfactory solution to the manpower shortage.[18]

The Emergency Health Personnel Act of 1970 established a National Health Service Corps wherein young doctors could elect to serve as physicians in needy communities, many of which had never before had such services, as an alternative to serving in the armed forces. The incentive for joining the Corps has largely been lost, however, by the discontinuance of the Selective Service draft.

The Physician Assistant Program

Because of the shortage of physicians, large numbers and new types of supporting personnel are entering the medical field. One of the newest, and perhaps most significant, medical manpower innovations is the physician assistant (PA) concept. Though new to this country, such programs have been practiced in other countries for several years. Perhaps the oldest example is the feldsher program of the U.S.S.R.; originating with the Czar's armies during the seventeenth century, the program has grown to 400,000 persons, or one feldsher for every 600 people in Russia.[19]

Similarly, the physician assistant program in the United States originated in the armed forces' medical service. For several years, particularly during World War II, medical aides and corpsmen were trained to perform many of the tasks normally handled by physicians. These corpsmen administered first aid, treated minor complaints, made routine dressing changes, gave immunizations and intravenous transfusions, took temperatures, administered medicines, sutured wounds, and maintained records. The range of functions carried out by the corpsmen was remarkably large, particularly in situations such as those on submarines, where no medical doctor was available except through radio communication. In the main, corpsmen worked under the supervision of one or more physicians, carrying out many routine medical tasks and freeing the medical doctors to give attention to more difficult problems. The program worked surprisingly well and is still used in all branches of the armed forces.

The physician assistant training program adapts this concept to the civilian sector. While program specifics vary, there are some common principles. Most programs are located in medical schools. Students selected for admission are at least high school graduates, and a large percentage have attended college for one or more years. Many are ex-medics or medical corpsmen who have had previous medical training and experience in the armed forces. Training usually includes some rudimentary theoretical material with a heavy emphasis on clinical work, including clinical rotations in outpatient clinics and hospital wards. In most training programs, the students are placed in preceptorships with practicing physicians in the community for additional practical experience prior to graduation.[20]

The physician assistant concept has been well accepted by both patients and physicians in most settings where the plan has been put into operation. Evaluation studies indicate that a large majority of patients accept the PAs once their role has been explained by the practicing physician. A survey of physicians' attitudes toward the program in Wisconsin disclosed that, while 70 percent of the physicians were in favor of the program, only 40 percent felt ready to use the services of physician assistants in their own practices.[21] This suggests that although this program is gradually being accepted, the concept still needs to be sold to many doctors.

If many physician assistants come from disadvantaged populations themselves, and if they give physicians more time for patients with greater and more complex needs, they could help solve some parts of the complicated problem of providing medical care to the poor. Physician assistants represent a way to provide the much needed personal involvement with patients and their families that often makes the difference in patient compliance.

Allied Medical Personnel and the Team Concept

Accompanying the concern with the supply of physicians and primary specialists has been a growing acceptance of the proposition that many different kinds of personnel are needed to deliver adequate medical care to the American public. There has also come the gradual recognition that other medical personnel can effectively carry out many functions that were formerly the physician's. One result has been a more extensive use of the medical team in which several kinds of personnel work together with the physician as team captain. This has in turn produced a dramatic increase in the need for allied health personnel and a corresponding broadening of their training to prepare them to perform new functions — part of a general tendency for all health personnel to expand their functions. Nurses, for example, are going into private practice where they deliver limited primary medical care to patients, or in other instances take over technological functions customarily reserved for physicians or other medical specialists. Pharmacists are becoming members of the medical team in outpatient clinics and provide regular input about drugs and other medications.

The passage, during the early 70s, of federal legislation to fund such training has helped raise the number of available personnel, yet manpower is still not sufficient to meet the ever-growing demands for medical care. We can therefore expect to see the allocation of even more funds for such programs in the future.

To view any of these manpower developments as a panacea to the health-care dilemmas of the poor is very dangerous. It seems likely that the major benefits will continue to be reaped by those more socially and economically able to utilize them: yet some spillover of benefits to the poor seems inevitable.

The situation in some other cases is less clear. At present, we have very little data on the suitability of family practice for poor patients. Given the frequently unstable family structure of the indigent, this modality of care may be quite inappropriate. Its emphasis on the behavioral sciences, however laudatory, may simply be unsuited to a population whose environmental realities leave them unable to cope with such factors as compliance or reaction to social stress.

Similarly, the physician assistant may not have any significant impact on the poor communities. Experience suggests that acceptance of these physician surrogates is better in middle-class communities than in ghetto neighborhoods, where they are viewed as indicating second-class medical care. Because health care is so heavily imbued with social values, we frequently find ourselves faced with a paradox. Those most in need of a fresh approach may be the least accepting of it because it seems some form of experimentation or exploitation. Ironically, in their pursuit of a middle-class ideal the poor may be less willing to try new ways of doing things than are the middle class they seek to emulate. Thus, we see the ghetto neighborhood that wants nothing to do with a medical school or that closes its clinic to physician assistants and insists on "real doctors" it may never get.

EFFORTS TO DISTRIBUTE
HEALTH CARE MORE EQUITABLY

Prepaid Group Practice Plans

One of the most promising developments with respect to the health delivery problem has been the introduction of the prepaid group practice plan. The first such plan of any significance was started by the Kaiser Industrial Organization for the workers in Kaiser's shipyards and steel mills in World War II. It is now a program involving 60,000 employees, working in 242 major plants and facilities located in 35 states and 23 foreign countries.[22] Nonprofit and self-sustaining, the plan offers comprehensive medical care services for persons enrolled.[23] The aim is to keep patients healthy so that they do not require medical care, an objective pursued by means of preventive screening techniques, comprehensive services, and rewards to doctors for keeping their patients well. The spread of medical programs similar to the Kaiser model has been held back by laws in many states prohibiting prepaid health plans. However, attitudes are changing.

One sign of these changes is the growth of health maintenance organizations, or, as they are commonly called, HMOs. Similar to the Kaiser plan, HMOs have been fostered by federal legislation and by both labor and management. The HMOs attract many people by their promise of providing comprehensive medical care for a reasonable cost, considerably below the national per capita cost of total medical care services.[24]

One caution frequently expressed about such programs is that they may become insensitive to consumer needs. Moreover, as they become competitive, HMOs could repeat the practice of private insurance carriers in the days before Medicare, when certain carriers avoided high-risk people such as the elderly and minorities.

Clearly, more and more medical care in the future will be delivered in one form of group practice or another; it is less clear whether this will be prepaid, as in health maintenance organizations, or a fee-for-service practice, in which groups of physician specialists share the costs for equipment and facilities used. Group practice, in any case, has finally become an accepted modality of care, and an increasing portion of graduating medical students are interested in it. In all likelihood this trend will be accelerated by the institution of national health insurance bills.

The growth of HMOs can play a primary role in improving medical care to the poor, especially in the area of preventive medicine for children. This potential is emphasized by those medical professionals who maintain that the long-term solution to this nation's health problem must be based on prevention and health maintenance.

Neighborhood Health Centers

One of the more successful innovations in providing health care to the poor has been the neighborhood health centers (NHCs), a program originally sponsored by the Office of Economic Opportunity. These centers, which are located in communities and rural areas throughout the United States, are an outgrowth of the War on Poverty Program inaugurated by the late presidents Kennedy and Johnson. Persons responsible for directing Community Action Programs on both the local and national level realized that in order to help the poor adjust to the problems of living in modern society, it would be necessary to provide them with good health care and related services. This required either extensive changes in existing medical services or the development of new ones. Three neighborhood health centers were organized in 1965; by the summer of 1966, eight demonstration neighborhood centers had been approved. Four years later, the program was well established with fifty-eight projects in operation, six more approved, and fifteen planning projects underway.[25]

Most centers are located close to the target population, often with several smaller satellite health stations situated even closer to the poor neighborhoods. Neighborhood health centers emphasize comprehensive medical care, including health maintenance, the treatment of physical and emotional problems, and the personalized service with emotional and educational support necessary for persons within the center's catchment area. Consumers play an important role in deciding policy and in carrying out the functions of the neighborhood health center. Poor people serve on the board of directors as well as work at every type of job in the center for which they can be prepaid. Centers are typically organized for the convenience of the consumer and designed to fit the life style of their constituents.

Future federal support for neighborhood health centers is uncertain: the program could be eliminated completely, reduced with respect to function and expenditures, retained as is, or markedly expanded in terms of both numbers and types of services offered. This uncertainty is due to several factors. The centers appeal to only a small proportion of the population within their catchment areas; treatment has been very expensive, with no conclusive evidence that the centers deliver quality medical care to hard-to-reach persons any more economically than do other medical centers. Probably outpatient clinics of community hospitals and neighborhood health centers will be more closely combined in the future than they are today. Yet much remains to be done if an adequate system of ambulatory care is to evolve from such a merger. Many aspects of the neighborhood health center should be preserved, particularly its emphasis on quality of care and consumer participation.

Quality of care, how to measure it, and how to improve it have become a national concern. Recent amendments to the Social Security Act (PL92-603) call for the formation of Professional Standards Review Organizations (PSROs) in each section of the country.[26] Physicians are charged with the responsibility to devise ways satisfactory to the government to monitor the standards of care in their areas. Thus far, our techniques for measuring quality are relatively primitive, with the emphasis on hospital care rather than ambulatory care. Patient satisfaction is one dimension of this concern, but it has not been evident in most of the PSRO activities to date. An awareness of the ways in which the delivery of medical care fits into the patient's total social and cultural milieu would be an added sophistication in PSROs that has not yet been shown. It is not clear at this point whether quality of care through PSRO-type activities will ever reach the stage of looking at outcomes of care rather than the process of care itself.

Consumers, of course, have unique information about how the health-care system fits in with the rest of their total life style; this information should not be lost, particularly if we are trying to increase utilization among minorities and the poor. Thus far consumer participation has been minimal, almost to the point of tokenism. Much depends upon the future organization of the health-care delivery system; if this is modeled after the group health cooperative, then the consumer may have much greater input. At present, we lack a good system for merging consumer and provider interests.

Community Mental Health Centers

In 1961, the Joint Commission on Mental Illness and Health published its report *Action for Mental Health*, recommending the establishment of community mental health centers for every 50,000 persons.[27] This figure was later changed to serve geographically limited population groups of 75,000 to 200,000 people. A program of comprehensive community mental health care was to be carried out through the construction of centers where services would be made available to all persons, regardless of their ability to pay.[28] Long-range plans call for the development of enough mental health centers to serve every area of the United States. Emphasis is to be given to keeping people mentally healthy — preventive mental health — and treating those in the community with problems. This objective is to be accomplished by providing outpatient treatment at a nearby community health center, with other supplementary services such as marital counseling and employment offered through cooperation with other agencies. Only the more seriously impaired patients would receive inpatient treatment on a limited basis at the community health center closest to their home or, when necessary, at a mental hospital. In the latter case, the staff of the mental hospitals would work closely with the staff of the mental health centers, resulting in a marked reduction in resident patient population.[29]

As mental health centers have grown in number, they have also taken on additional services and developed new programs to meet the many needs and problems encountered. For example, centers now offer family therapy programs, inpatient services, drug treatment programs, and consultation services to schools, churches, juvenile courts, and welfare agencies.

Although they have experienced many problems, community mental health centers have been generally accepted by both professionals and the public as one means of dealing with the mental health problem. Notwithstanding this general acceptance, there are growing doubts about their present and future programs.[30] For example, a recent critical appraisal of community health centers found the system to be "irrational, expensive, and grossly wasteful of manpower."[31] Another serious criticism, reported in the same appraisal, was that the centers suffered from severe conflicts of interest, as they were frequently dominated by medical schools or community agencies more interested in building their own empires than in developing community mental health centers. At a minimum there is clearly a need to improve both their functioning and public image.

Nevertheless, we foresee that community mental health centers will eventually serve the entire United States, continuing to improve and expand their services to the point of reaching far more people than they now do. Our admittedly optimistic forecast is based on the expectation that community mental health services will receive adequate "expenditures of time and money, community understanding and support, and the presence of trained medical health professionals."[32] This will involve providing services to the poor, who have more than their share of mental health problems.

Regional Systems

Since the early 1920s, writers have been describing the inefficiencies of health care and the need for more organized approaches. Over and over again, they have articulated models that begin with small field clinics, which relate to satellite clinics such as neighborhood health centers, which in turn relate to local hospitals, which are similarly related to specialty or regional medical centers, or both. Various efforts have been used to encourage such a system. The Regional Medical Program originally began with the idea of establishing such regional centers for heart, stroke, and cancer. But it is difficult to see how this will come about in an entrepreneurial system such as ours unless there is strong legislation to prevent duplication of services. Some states have already passed certificate-of-need legislation requiring approval of new construction.

The growth and mounting costs of medical technology contribute to the need for consolidation in the interests of efficiency.[33] The danger is that our fascination with technology may make us increasingly less person-oriented. White and his associates comment: "People's needs, not availability of technology, should determine policies and priorities for its application in health services. Technology can improve efficiency and assist in solution of problems, but cannot 'drive the system' or cure all ills."[34] Nonetheless technology, properly utilized, can provide the opportunity to expand accessibility of medical care by substituting machines for people.

We have not yet begun to tap the potential for health education using new technology. Most assuredly, medicine will become regionalized as this new technology, together with other promising developments, is introduced into the medical field. In the meantime, our supposition is that neighborhood health centers, community health centers, HMOs, and similar programs will all become tied into large medical centers. These centers will, in turn, tie in with regional centers, all of which will be joined together through the use of computers, television, and other technological devices.[35] Through this arrangement, all the medical resources in the nation will be instantly available to all persons needing medical or psychiatric help, including the suburban housewife, the isolated farmer, or the black living in the ghetto.

Such a situation should increase the availability of quality medical care for all Americans, rich or poor, but its actual implementation in the foreseeable future depends on a change in social attitudes. As Ginzberg warns, we cannot be overly optimistic about such developments, because of the close ties between the nation's health system and its value system and institutions.[36] Health care must first be universally recognized as a common social commodity, the availability and accessibility of which should take precedence over other traditional values such as profit, autonomy, and ambition. As a society, we have generally been reluctant to give up our personal liberties for a greater good except in times of crisis. It is not yet clear whether the crisis of the poor is perceived as such at this time.

Waitzkin and Modell conclude from their study of the contemporary Chilean situation several precepts that have relevance for the United States:

1. Health care is inextricably linked to a nation's political and economic systems.

2. Conflicts within the health system reflect the inherent conflicts of a stratified society.

3. Incremental reforms in health care have little meaning without basic change in the social order.[37]

NEW PERSPECTIVES ON THE POOR

It is no longer enough to attribute the nonutilization of health services by the poor to such limited factors as a lack of motivation, education, or other personal characteristics. This change in perspective, which emphasizes a much more comprehensive view of man, can be attributed to three factors: (1) a growing recognition that the customary way of perceiving and responding to poor people has contributed to their poor utilization rates; (2) indications in an increasing number of studies that lack of education and motivation are only two of many factors influencing their behavior,[38] and (3) a growing emphasis on the conflict between the life styles of the poor and modern scientific medicine.[39] Thus, rather than viewing the poor as lacking some personal characteristic — education, intelligence, or motivation — many health personnel and social scientists now see the incongruity between the life style of the poor and the rationale underlying modern health delivery systems as central to the problem of utilization. This view accepts the fact that although the poor are not particularly knowledgeable or motivated with respect to scientific medicine, they are motivated with respect to a whole host of phenomena that make sense to them personally and that are congruent with their society's values. Those who hold this view — among them, Anselm Strauss — argue that if delivery is to be increased, medical services to these people must fit their life style and be consistent with their value system as well.

There is also evidence that differences in the medical behavior of the poor frequently disappear or diminish when certain contributing factors are held constant. For example, several studies disclose that many significant differences between the poor and middle- and upper-class persons with respect to preventive behavior, such as receiving immunizations, diminish when marital status is held constant.[41] Similar findings have been reported with respect to other contributing factors, such as alienation, low self-image, and high mobility[42] Collectively, these studies suggest that poor people make less extensive use of medical services because they more frequently experience these negative factors. Yet these explanations are not totally adequate, for other studies indicate that some poor people utilize existing medical services less extensively than other persons even when contributing factors are held constant.[43] Thus, there are contradictory findings, with the consensus indicating that both positions are tenable, depending upon the particular situation and the individuals involved. A growing proportion of health personnel are working to develop programs that deal not only with personal characteristics, but also take into account such factors as education, security, values, and personal needs.[44]

The increased involvement of the poor in the decision-making process has also made for broader perspective.[45] Agencies, hospitals, and other community institutions are including them as consumers in the planning and employment areas of health activities. This trend has been accelerated by poor people themselves, who have organized into pressure groups to demand a much more important role in decision-making about medical care delivery and other important community functions.

Emphasis is now given to the idea that maintaining a workable patient-practitioner relationship is almost impossible when the practitioner is ignorant about the patient's way of life. Traditionally, it was held that the patient seeks out medical services and complies with medical instructions if he is educated and motivated. Now, however, spokesmen for the poor are forcefully pointing out instances in which medical transactions are undermined by medical personnel whose behavior conveys to the patient a feeling that he is considered an inferior. To combat these problems, several efforts are already underway — from recruiting minorities and humanistically oriented medical students to emphasizing behavioral science in postgraduate education.[46]

In essence, instead of being perceived and responded to as inferior persons, the poor and other disadvantaged people are now more frequently considered as individuals whose experiences, life styles, and motivations are to a degree incongruent with medical delivery systems and other community services. Lack of education and motivation are still important factors affecting utilization and related behavior. But a growing number of observers insist that the development of a medical delivery system capable of delivering quality medical care to all Americans will depend upon the acceptance of a more comprehensive and meaningful perspective of the poor than is afforded by models used in the past.

To summarize: the problem is not whether we have a national health problem or whether we should attempt to deliver health care to the poor and disadvantaged, but rather *how to get the job done.* As John Norman puts it:

> Good health is universally recognized as a basic right of all citizens. In practice, however, millions of Americans are denied the full benefits of medical science because they are poor and because they are confined by social, economic, and cultural forces to isolation in the ghettos of our large urban centers. Their health needs can no longer be ignored. Conscience, stimulated by a rising crescendo of voices from the ghetto itself, is forcing a substantial change in the attitudes of health professionals, government, and indeed all Americans who recognize that the evils of inequality, prejudice, and discrimination must be eliminated from the national scene.
>
> The question is not *whether* to respond to the health needs of the ghetto, but *how* to do so effectively.[47]

Given the complete incongruence of current services with the life styles of the poor and disadvantaged, many authorities argue that we will never be able to deliver them quality medical care until we totally reorganize or replace existing medical services in this country. Others maintain that this goal can be achieved by a change in orientation and a modification of existing medical services. We prefer the latter view — emphasizing the major revisions necessary to accomplish this objective — and expect to see an acceleration of this change of orientation and the consequent reorganization of *existing* medical services.

A GROWING ROLE FOR SOCIAL SCIENTISTS

Social scientists, particularly medical sociologists, are being employed more frequently as consultants and evaluators on health projects — a sign of growing recognition that the organization and distribution of services is a sociological problem, involving people in social transactions.[48] Anselm Strauss, supporting this view, has argued that an effective national health delivery system will, in all likelihood, depend on major reforms in existing medical delivery systems designed to make them more compatible with the life style of those not now receiving medical care. Irving Leveson similarly comments: "The health levels of the poor are depressed not only because of inadequate health services but also because of problems associated with poverty. Although health services often do not deal with the causes of illness, they can make an important contribution. Many changes are required to restructure the service delivery systems which do not respond to the needs of the poor and the ill."[49]

Increasingly, those responsible for training medical personnel and improving the medical care distribution system are citing such observations, and in all likelihood social scientists will play a major role in resolving these problems. An attempt to predict their future role, however, must also consider the attitudes of other medical professionals. Medical students, for example, frequently change their interests and attitudes. In the early sixties, we saw the emergence of the Student Health Organization, with its concerns about the political implications of health and a strong emphasis on social activism. The much more conservative students who followed were concerned with providing for their own futures, minimizing their work and maximizing their income. At the present time many students are interested in delivering personal health care services and attracted to primary care. Here there is a very strong potential role for the behavioral sciences.[50]

If social scientists are to enter the medical world successfully, they must be able to relate their theories to practical concerns. If they remain pure theorists, their entrance into medicine will be slow and short-lived. But if they are able both to contribute to social theory and develop dependable and workable answers to practical medical problems, their integration into the medical field will be rapid and permanent.[51]

NOTES

1. See R. Fein, *The Doctor Shortage: An Economic Diagnosis* (Washington, D.C.: Brookings Institute, 1967); E. Ginzberg and M. Ostow, *Men, Money and Medicine* (New York: Columbia University Press, 1969); and U.S. Department of Health, Education and Welfare, *Towards a Comprehensive Health Policy for the 1970s, A White Paper* (Washington, D.C.: U.S. Government Printing Office, 1971).

2. J. Ehrenreich and B. Ehrenreich, *The American Health Empire: Power, Profits and Politics* (New York: Vintage, 1971), p. 3; A. L. Strauss, Medical organization, medical care and lower income groups, in this volume, and M. Gorman, The impact of national health insurance on delivery of health care, *American Journal of Public Health* 61 (1971), pp. 962–63.

3. Insuring the national health, *Newsweek*, June 3, 1974, pp. 73–74.

4. E. M Burns, A critical review of national health insurance proposals, *HSMHA Health Reports* 86 (1971), p. 112.

5. E. Freidson, *Professional Dominance: The Social Structure of Medical Care* (New York: Atherton, 1970).

6. M. C. Olendzki, Medicaid benefits mainly the younger and less sick, *Medical Care* 12 (1974), pp. 163–72.

7. L. Bellin and F. Kavaler, Policing publicly funded health care for poor quality, overutilization and fraud — The New York City Medicaid experience, *American Journal of Public Health* 60 (1970), p. 811.

8. R. M. Coe and K. R. Andrews, Effects of Medicare on the provision of community health resources, *American Journal of Public Health* 62 (1972), pp. 854–56.

9. See D. D. Rutstein, *Blueprint for Medical Care* (Cambridge: M.I.T. Press, 1974), pp. 52–53; and A. J. Zweifler and L. Corey, Physician manpower and the health care team in *Medicine in a Changing Society*, ed. L. Corey, S. E. Saltman, and M. F. Epstein (St. Louis: C. V. Mosby, 1972).

10. K. Naegele, *Health and Healing* (San Francisco: Jossey-Bass, 1970).

11. J. O. Hepner, and D. M. Hepner, *The Health Strategy Game* St. Louis: C. V. Mosby, 1973), pp. 184–87.

12. HEW, *Toward a Comprehensive Health Policy . . .*, p. 38.

13. Carnegie Commission on Higher Education, *Higher Education and the Nation's Health: Policies for Medical and Dental Education* (New York: McGraw-Hill, 1970).

14. Zweifler and Corey, Physician manpower and the health care team, p. 117.

15. O. W. Anderson and R. M. Andersen, Patterns of use of health services, in *Handbook of Medical Sociology*, ed. H. E. Freeman, S. Levine, and L. G. Reeder (Englewood Cliffs, N.J.: Prentice-Hall, 1972), pp. 386–403.

16. Zweifler and Corey, Physician manpower and the health care team, p. 118.

17. See R. Coe, Processes in the development of established professions, *Journal of Health and Social Behavior* 11 (1970), pp. 59–67; and L. H. Powers, The community hospital and ambulatory care, in *Functional Elements of Outpatient Care* ed. C. G. Oakes, (Spartanburg, S.C.: Converse College, 1971), p. 26; and D. D. Rutstein, *Blueprint for Medical Care* (Note 9).

18. C. C. Sprague, The foreign medical graduate — A time for action, *New England Journal of Medicine* 290 (1974), pp. 1482–83.

19. Zweifler and Corey, Physician manpower and the health care team, p. 120.

20. A. M. Sadler, Jr., B. L. Sadler, and A. A. Bliss, *The Physician's Assistant — Today and Tomorrow* (New Haven: Yale University School of Medicine, 1972); and V. W. Lippard and E. F. Purcell, eds., *Intermediate-Level Health Practitioners* (Baltimore: Port City Press, 1973).

21. Zweifler and Corey, Physician manpower and the health care team, p. 123.

22. C. H. Keene, Kaiser industries and the Kaiser-Permanente health care partnership, in *The Kaiser-Permanente Medical Care Program*, ed. A. R. Somers (New York: Commonwealth Fund, 1971), p. 13.

23. E. Saward, The relevance of prepaid group practice to the effective delivery of health services, *Office of Group Practice Development: U.S. Department of Health Education and Welfare*, 1969.

24. M. R. Greenlick, Medical services to poverty groups, *The Kaiser-Permanente Medical Care Program*, ed. A. R. Somers (New York: Commonwealth Fund, 1971). p. 146.

25. L. B. Schorr, The neighborhood health center — background and current issues, in *Medicine in a Changing Society*, ed. L. Corey, S. E. Saltman, and M. F. Epstein (St. Louis: C. W. Mosby, 1972), p. 141.

26. C. E. Welch, PSROs — pros and cons, *New England Journal of Medicine* 290 (1974), pp. 1319–22.

27. D. Mechanic, *Mental Health and Social Policy* (Englewood Cliffs, N.J.: Prentice-Hall, 1969), p. 59.

28. D. J. Scherl, The community mental health center and mental health services for the poor, in *The Practice of Community Mental Health*, ed. H. Grunebaum (Boston: Little, Brown, 1970), p. 171.

29. S. Yolles, The community mental health center in national perspective, in *The Practice of Community Mental Health*, ed. H. Grunebaum (Boston: Little, Brown, 1970), pp. 787–88.

30. Mechanic, *Mental Health and Social Policy*, pp. 148–49.

31. Ehrenreich, and Ehrenreich, *The American Health Empire*, pp. 77–94.

32. M. E. Chafetz and M. J. Hill, The alcoholic in society, in *The Practice of Community Mental Health*, ed. H. Grunebaum (Boston: Little, Brown, 1970), p. 158.

33. J. O. Hepner and D. M. Hepner, *The Health Strategy Game — A Challenge for Reorganization and Management*, (St. Louis: C. V. Mosby, 1973), pp. 252–60.

34. K. L. White, J. H. Murnaghan, and C. R. Gaus, Technology and health

care, *New England Journal of Medicine* 287 (1972), p. 1223.

35. D. D. Rutstein, *Blueprint for Medical Care*, (Cambridge: M.I.T. Press, 1974), pp. 15–26.

36. E. Ginzberg, and M. Ostow, *Men, Money and Medicine* (New York: Columbia University Press, 1969), pp. 261–62.

37. H. Waitzkin and H. Modell, Medicine, socialism and totalitarianism: Lessons from Chile, *New England Journal of Medicine* 291 (1974), p. 175.

38. D. Mechanic, *Medical Sociology: A Selective View* (New York: Free Press, 1968), pp. 259–70; see also Andersen and Andersen, Patterns of use of health services (note 15).

39. E. A. Suchman, Sociomedical variations among ethnic groups, *American Journal of Sociology* 70 (1964), pp. 319–31; L. Saunders, *Cultural Differences and Medical Care* (New York: Russell Sage, 1954); see also Anselm Strauss' essay in this volume.

40. E. A. Suchman, Social patterns of illness and medical care, *Journal of Health and Human Behavior* 6 (1965), pp. 2–12.

41. R. M. Gray, J. Kesler, and P. Moody, Alienation and immunization participation, *The Rocky Mountain Social Science Journal*, 4 (1967), pp. 161–68.

42. R. M. Gray, P. Moody, and J. R. Ward, The use of oral polio vaccine as related to some possible determinants, *Inquiry* 6 (1969), pp. 52–56; and R. M. Gray and R. Geertsen, Familistic orientation and inclination toward adopting the sick role, *Journal of Marriage and the Family* 32 (1970), pp. 638–46.

43. R. Andersen and O. W. Anderson, *A Decade of Health Services: Social Survey Trends in Use and Expenditures* (Chicago: University of Chicago Press, 1967); and M. Lerner and O. W. Anderson. *Health Progress in the United States, 1900–1960* (Chicago: University of Chicago Press, 1963), p. 91.

44. B. M. Gross, The State of the Nation: Social Systems Accounting, in *Social Indicators*, ed. R. A. Bauer (Cambridge: M.I.T. Press, 1966), p. 224.

45. C. G. Oakes, *The Walking Patient* (Columbia: University of South Carolina Press, 1973), pp. 22–28; and R. E. Tranquada, Participation of the poverty community in health care planning, *Social Science and Medicine* 7 (1973), pp. 719–28.

46. D. Mechanic, Problems in the future organization of medical practice, *Law and Contemporary Problems* 35 (1970), pp. 233–52.

47. J. C. Norman and B. Bennett, Foreword, *Medicine in the Ghetto*, ed. J. C. Norman (New York: Appleton-Century-Crofts, 1969), p. xxi.

48. H. E. Freeman, S. Levine, and L. G. Reeder, Present status of medical sociology, in *Handbook of Medical Sociology*, ed. H. Freeman, S. Levine, and L. G. Reeder (Englewood Cliffs, N.J.: Prentice-Hall, 1972), pp. 501—21.

49. I. Leveson, The challenge of health services for the poor, *The Annals of the American Academy of Political and Social Science* 399 (1972), p. 22.

50. See R. M. Coe, *Sociology of Medicine*, (New York: McGraw-Hill, 1970); S. Bloom, *The Doctor and His Patient* (New York: Free Press, 1965); R. S. Duff and A. B. Hollingshead, *Sickness and Society* (New York: Harper & Row, 1968); G. E. Jaco, ed., *Patients, Physicians and Illness* (New York: Free Press, 1972); and G. Reader and M. Goss, eds., *Comprehensive Care and Teaching* (New York: Cornell University Press, 1957).

51. A. B. Hollingshead and F. C. Redlich, *Social Class and Mental Illness* (New York: Wiley, 1958); A. H. Stanton and M. S. Schwartz, *The Mental Hospital* (New York: Basic Books, 1954); and H. S. Becker, B. Geer, E. C. Hughes, and A. L. Strauss, *Boys in White: Student Culture in Medical School* (Chicago: University of Chicago Press, 1961).

Part VII

ANNOTATED
BIBLIOGRAPHY

The bibliography is the result of an extensive review of the literature through July 1974. The works cited were chosen for one or more reasons. Most represent information, expressed in terms of either data or opinions, about one or more aspects of the utilization of health-care services by the poor. Some authors suggest solutions to this problem.

The article abstracts are presented alphabetically by the last name of the first author. For each article abstracted, information is keyed to the identification of problems and proposed solutions. Each citation is organized into five headings for rapid review:

 I. Reasons given for inadequate utilization of health-care services by the poor
 II. Data provided to support these reasons
 III. Solutions proposed
 IV. Data provided to support these solutions
 V. Specific comments on other aspects of the utilization problem

Missing numbers in the annotations indicate that those headings were not applicable to that reference.

This bibliography has been compiled from a number of sources. We have used computerized indexing systems, such as MEDLARS and MEDLINE, as well as specific searches of the following journals:

American Anthropologist
American Journal of Diseases of Children
American Journal of Medical Science
American Journal of Nursing
American Journal of Obstetrics and Gynecology

American Journal of Orthopsychiatry
American Journal of Psychiatry
American Journal of Psychotherapy
American Journal of Public Health
American Sociological Review
Annals of Internal Medicine
Annals of the American Academy of Political and Social Science
Archives of Environmental Health
Archives of Otolaryngology
British Journal of Preventive Social Medicine
British Medical Journal
Bulletin of the New York Academy of Medicine
California Medicine
Canadian Journal of Public Health
Cancer
Clinical Pediatrics
Clinical Research
Geriatrics
Health Education Monographs
Health Services Research
Hospital and Community Psychiatry
Hospital Management
Hospital Progress
Hospitals
Human Needs
Human Organization
Industrial Medicine and Surgery
Inquiry
International Journal of Health Services
Johns Hopkins Medical Journal
Journal of Chronic Diseases
Journal of Clinical Psychology
Journal of Health and Social Behavior
Journal of Medical Education
Journal of Nervous and Mental Disease
Journal of Pediatrics
Journal of School Health
Journal of Social Issues
Journal of the American College of Dentistry
Journal of the American Dental Association
Journal of the American Geriatric Society
Journal of the American Hospital Association
Journal of the American Medical Association
Journal of the American Pharmaceutical Association
Journal of the American Podiatry Association
Journal of the Kansas Medical Society
Journal of the Kentucky Medical Association
Journal of the National Medical Association

Journal of the South Carolina Medical Association
Lancet
Marriage and Family Living
Maryland Medical Journal
Medical Care
Medical Times
Mental Hygiene
Milbank Memorial Fund Quarterly
Modern Hospital
New England Journal of Medicine
Nursing Outlook
Nursing Research
Pacific Sociological Review
Patient Care
Patient Education
Pediatrics
Pennsylvania Medical Journal
Phylon
Postgraduate Medicine
Psychiatric Quarterly
Psychiatric Research Reports
Public Health Reports
Public Welfare
Rehabilitation and Health
Rocky Mountain Social Science Journal
Rural Sociology
Scientific American
Social Forces
Social Problems
Social Science and Medicine
Social Security Bulletin
Social Service Review
South African Medical Journal
Southern Medical Journal
Transaction
Transcultural Psychiatric Research
West Virginia Medical Journal

Abrams, H. K., and R. A. Snyder. Health center seeks to bridge the gap between hospital and neighborhood. *Modern Hospital* 111 (May 1968): 96–101. I. Negroes claim white doctors are impolite and discriminatory; long waits for service, excessive charges, and ignorance of health matters are also contributory. II. Primary: information collected at North Lawndale Neighborhood Health Center. III. Allow local people to participate in health programs; train the poor in medical skills. IV. One year after start of program many jobs in NHC were filled by local people; the health team approach was working well.

Aday, Lu Ann, and Robert Eichhorn. *The Utilization of Health Services: Indices and Correlates — A Research Bibliography.* U. S. DHEW Publication No. (HSM) 73 (December 1972): 3003. I. Some of the findings of the authors: (1) When the price of medical services to the consumer is reduced through charity care, insurance, or government financing programs, more services will be purchased; (2) distance influences the choice of the site for the visit, but not the volume of services consumed; (3) the consumption of physicians' services increases as educational level increases, owing primarily to the greater use of preventive services by the better educated; (4) hospital admissions increase when the supply of physicians is low or the supply of hospital beds high. II. An excellent review and correlation of some 207 publications.

Adler, Leta McKinney, et al. Failed psychiatric clinic appointments — relationship to social class. *California Medicine* 99 (December 1963): 388–92. I. Lower class tend to blame problems on environment rather than self. Lower class are more "present oriented" ("don't plan for future"). Unskilled and unemployed had highest appointment-breaking record. II. Primary: study of 199 consecutive new applicants to psychiatric outpatient clinic of Los Angeles County General Hospital. V. Applicants who were supported by family and friends or family physician were most likely to keep appointments.

Aitken-Swan, Jean, and Ralston Paterson. The cancer patient: Delay in seeking advice. *British Medical Journal* 1 (March 12, 1955): 623–27. I. Factors in underutilization: fear of terminal illness, ignorance of the significance of the symptoms, fear of doctors and hospitals, fear of operations and treatment, and domestic difficulties. II. Primary: interviews with 75 men and 239 women patients and their relatives, at Christie Hospital, Manchester, England. III. Public needs better education on symptoms of cancer; more confidence in treatment programs is needed on the part of the public.

Aledort, Stewart, and Henry Grunebaum. Group psychotherapy on alien turf. *Psychiatric Quarterly* 43 (July 1969): 512–24. I. Factors: resentment of disadvantaged by professionals, language and cultural barriers. II. Primary: an account of a group therapy situation with Negro adolescents in Roxbury, Massachusetts, ghetto. IV. A meaningful group experience *can* be provided by a white middle-class psychiatrist to Negro ghetto residents. Group members showed definite signs of change and growth over the course of a year. Utilization increased as therapist and adolescents increasingly accepted each other on equal terms.

Alexander, Benjamin. Chronic illness — fact of life for the rural poor. *Hospitals* 43 (July 1, 1969): 71-74. I. Value system of rural poor accepts chronic illness as a way of life. Major health barriers include transportation, lack of physicians, lack of health education, discrimination, lack of money, and legal problems. II. More research is needed to get facts, then correct these barriers.

Alexander, C. A. The effects of change in method of paying physicians: The Baltimore experience. *American Journal of Public Health* 57 (August 1967): 1278-89. I. Method of payment to physicians affects utilization. II. Secondary: analysis of utilization data in Baltimore's Medical Care Program for the indigent. III. Replace capitation with fee-for-service. IV. Utilization rates before and after show utilization of physician services and prescriptions increased. Utilization of inpatient care and clinic services did not.

Alpert, J. J. Effective use of comprehensive pediatric care. *American Journal of Diseases of Children* 116 (November 1968): 529-33. I. Medical care for low-income families is episodic, fragmented, crisis oriented, and anonymous. II. Primary: 489 low-income families were divided into control and experimental groups and their characteristics were compared. III. Comprehensive, family-focused pediatric care by a health team (physician, PH nurse, and social worker) was offered to experimental group. IV. Results: fewer operations, hospitalizations, and physician visits for illness, and more physician visits for health care. V. The study tests the hypothesis that large-scale comprehensive medical care programs for low-income families result in measurable differences in cost, morbidity, utilization, attitudes, and knowledge toward health. A plea is made for additional and continued experimental efforts in the delivery of medical care.

Alpert, J. J., et al.(a) Medical help and maternal nursing care in the life of low-income families.*Pediatrics* 39 (May 1967): 749-55. I. The attitude of mother toward health determines utilization patterns. She is the family member who takes action in response to symptoms. II. Primary: repeated interviews with families who were users of the Emergency Clinic at Children's Hospital Center in Boston. V. The mother is the primary agent in the family for defining and organizing response to symptoms of illness; she analyzes the type of action taken and the type of medical help sought for various symptoms of illness.

Alpert, J. J., et al.(b) A month of illness and health care among low-income families. *Public Health Reports* 82 (August 1967): 705-13. I. Low-income families are less likely to use existing health facilities; they used medical services when symptom in-

dicated need for attention only 14.3 percent of the time. Up-
setting events caused mothers to seek medical advice only 8.4
percent of the time. Telephone calls to physicians were underutilized compared to middle-class populations. II. Primary: data
collected in diary form from families using Children's Hospital in
Boston. III. Increase regular visits and improve relationships with a
family physician, who should have a more complete family history.

Alpert, J. J., et al. The types of families that use an emergency clinic.
Medical Care 7 (January-February 1969): 55–61. I. Lack of stable
source of care by either physician or hospital causes health-care
pattern which is episodic and fragmented. Disadvantaged tended
to use clinic more often for nonemergency visits and less often had
any stable relationship with a hospital. II. Primary: data collected
at Medical Emergency Clinic of Children's Hospital, Boston —
4,320 families were surveyed over a six-month period. V. A typology was developed to screen patients upon entry at an emergency
clinic to learn if they had stable relationships with the physicians
designated as "own doctor."

Alpert, J. J., et al. Attitudes and satisfaction of low-income families
receiving comprehensive pediatric care. *American Journal of
Public Health* 60 (March 1970): 499–506. I. Low-income families
have attitudes of dissatisfaction because of long waits and inadequate contact with doctor in Boston Children's Hospital Emergency Clinic. II. Primary: 750 low-income families were grouped
into experimental and control groups. III. Comprehensive care was
provided to experimental group. IV. Where care was actually delivered, there was increased satisfaction and increased preference
for a primary physician.

Ambuel, J. P., et al. Urgency as a factor in clinic attendance.
American Journal of Diseases of Children 108 (October 1964):
394–98. I. Unstable relationships with doctors cause underutilization. II. Primary: study of 174 patients at Children's Hospital,
Columbus, Ohio. III. Stress the importance of keeping appointments and strive for better communications between doctors and
patients. IV. Good results were obtained when doctors cooperated
and stressed the urgency of return visits.

American Public Health Association Conference Report. Health services for the poor. *Public Health Reports* 84 (March 1968):
192–98. III. Better ways are needed to disseminate information
about health services. Consumer participation is important.

American Public Health Association. *Abstracts of Contributed
Papers, U. S. Department of Health, Education, and Welfare.*
Washington, D.C.: U. S. Government Printing Office, 1972. V.

This government publication has a section on "Utilization." It is an excellent resource for current research on this subject.

Andersen, R., and O. W. Anderson. *A Decade of Health Services.* Chicago: University of Chicago Press, 1967. II. Primary: describes health-care utilization and expenditure patterns for the decade 1953–63. V. Comprehensive data show that the level of use of personal health services has been rising for low-income groups relative to high-income groups, although the level of use has increased for high-income groups as well. For general hospital care, the lowest income groups now use more hospital services than the high-income groups.

Andersen, R., and L. Benham. Factors affecting the relationship between family income and medical care consumption. In *Empirical Studies in Health Economics,* ed. H. E. Klarman. Baltimore: Johns Hopkins Press, 1970. II. Secondary: interviews obtained in a national survey, 1964, by Center for Health Administration and NORC. V. The study assessed factors that may influence the relationship between family medical care consumption and family income in general; families with lower permanent incomes had more illness but spent less per illness episode than those with higher permanent incomes; however, utilization was not highly associated with expenditures.

Andersen, R., et al. *Medical Care Use in Sweden and the U.S. — A Comparative Analysis of Systems and Behavior.* Center for Health Administration Studies, Research Series No. 27. Chicago: University of Chicago Press, 1970. II. Secondary: data are based on comparable social surveys conducted in Sweden and the United States in early 1964. V. The stated purpose of this book is to consider the reasons underlying the differences in the use of services in Sweden and the United States.

Anderson, J. G. Demographic factors affecting health services utilization: A causal model. *Medical Care* 11 (March–April 1973): 104–20. I. Supply of hospital beds is a major determinant of utilization. II. Secondary: demographic information from 1960 U.S. Census and August 1, 1969 Guide Issue of *Hospitals.* III. Use of the model proposed here permits predictions as to future demands on the health-care system. V. A demographic model correlating hospital bed-population ratio; percentage unemployed; median education; median age; net emigration; and percentage nonwhite, Spanish-American, and agriculturally with utilization.

Anderson, O. W. The utilization of health services. In *Handbook of Medical Sociology*, 1st ed., ed. H. E. Freeman et al., pp. 349–67. Englewood Cliffs, N.J.: Prentice-Hall, 1963. II. Secondary: author uses data from national surveys and other studies regarding health care and its utilization. V. An introduction to O. W. Anderson's classification of utilization variables and indices regarding utilization from national surveys and other studies. The relationship of sociodemographic and social-psychological characteristics to utilization is explored.

Anderson, O. W., and R. M. Andersen. Patterns of use of health services. In *Handbook of Medical Sociology*, 2nd ed., ed. Howard E. Freeman et al, pp. 386–406. Englewood Cliffs, N.J.: Prentice Hall, 1972. II. Primary: data presented by authors in their book, *A Decade of Health Services*, and secondary data from other studies on health-care use. V. O. W. Anderson's typology of usage and updated major national trends in health-care utilization.

Antonovsky, A. A model to explain visits to the doctor. *Journal of Health and Social Behavior* 13 (December 1972): 446–54. II. Secondary: following Suchman's model (1967) of agent, host, and environment, the author concludes that these factors conjointly operate in the direction of encouraging visiting in the state of Israel, which differs radically from other countries in the extraordinary high usage of outpatient medical services. V. Some significant data: 90 percent of Israeli population are covered by health insurance schemes; the people have a strong belief that "nothing is worse than illness" (from Zborowski and Herzog, 1952).

Apostle, Donald and Frederick Oder. Factors that influence the public's view of medical care. *Journal of the American Medical Association* 202 (November 1967): 592–98. I. Nonuse is primarily related to socioeconomic factors, unfavorable attitudes toward doctors and the medical profession. II. Primary: personal interviews with 438 households in Monroe County, New York. V. Attitudes of households in a large metropolitan community toward medical care and the medical profession are correlated with the frequency of use of various medical facilities, age, sex, and socioeconomic status. The study demonstrates the value of factor analysis as a tool for identifying important variables in utilization.

Apple, Dorrian. How laymen define illness. *Journal of Health and Human Behavior* 1 (Fall 1960): 219–25. I. Until the patient himself thinks he is ill, he will not see a doctor. II. Primary: data collected by Boston University School of Nursing. III. Patient education in recognizing health problems is needed. IV. Patients were asked what action they would advise when certain symptoms were present. For illness of long duration or illness symptoms they did not understand, 80 percent advised seeing a physician.

Arnson, A. N., and R. Collins. Treating low-income patients in a neighborhood center. *Hospital and Community Psychiatry* 21 (April 1970): 111–13. III. Center should offer and utilize flexibility of time in the length of contacts and hours of service. It should use neighborhood resources and avoid lengthy intake sessions.

Baca, Josephine E. Some health beliefs of the Spanish speaking. *American Journal of Nursing* 69 (October 1969): 2172–76. I. Folk beliefs about the nature and treatment of illness contradict modern medical knowledge and practice. The culture and social organization of the Spanish-speaking support activities of folk healers and reject many actions of PH personnel. Anglo doctors usually lack ability to communicate in Spanish and regard folk-medical beliefs with incredulity. Folk healers communicate well, contribute to an atmosphere conducive to successful treatment, and tend to have a sincere interest in their patients. II. Data from author's personal experience, with several examples of folk beliefs about illness and the usual course of treatment.

Badgley, Robin F., and Robert W. Hetherington. Medical care and social class in Wheatville. *Canadian Journal of Public Health* 53 (October 1962): 425–31. I. Upper social class respondents reported fewer illnesses per household, subscribed more frequently to voluntary health insurance programs. II. Primary: patterns of medical care utilization described for small Canadian prairie town. V. No reported difference in general physician utilization.

Bamberger, L. Opportunities for official health agencies in CAP. *American Journal of Public Health* 56 (April 1966): 595–99. II. Author's subjective viewpoints. III. Need to adapt services and programs to the way of life of the poor, render care in circumstances acceptable to recipients, and involve the poor in planning.

Banks, F. R., and M. D. Keller. Symptom experience and health action. *Medical Care* 9 (November-December 1971): 498–502. I. Low-income groups are more "symptom-insensitive." II. Primary: 445 respondents in four samples were asked questions regarding twenty-nine disease symptoms. V. Study found that persons with previous symptom experience expressed less health concern than those without previous experience.

Bashur, R. L., et al. Some ecological differentials in the use of medical services. *Health Services Research* 6 (Spring 1971): 61–75. I. Distance and sociocultural factors influence choice of medical facilities. II. Primary: socioeconomic background, race and reasons for choice of a particular facility were examined for each of several travel patterns. III. For satisfaction and a workable system of health care, one must examine ecological and social factors involved in the distribution of health care.

Bates, J. E., et al. Provision for health care in the ghetto: The family health team. *American Journal of Public Health* 60 (July 1970):

1222–24. I. Programs are not designed to meet the life styles of the poor. II. Opinions and observations of authors. III. Create family health teams, acculturate staff by working with patients and community, and educate the poor to be receptive to new procedures and attitudes.

Baum, O., and S. Felzer. Activity in initial interviews with lower social class patients. *Archives of General Psychiatry* 10 (1964): 345–53. I. Lower-class patients do not respond to the usual approach; they have difficulty verbalizing problems and understanding the problems and procedures of psychotherapy. II. Primary: a two-year study of lower-class patients at Temple University Medical Center. III. The study proved the need for early, flexible, and meaningful activity in the initial interview; this is essential to establishing a therapeutic relationship. the patient's expectations should be discussed openly at the outset. Study also showed that fantasy production was considered taboo, a sign of weakness by lower-class patients. V. Over one-third of the patients had an I.Q. below 90, which contributed to their inability to verbalize and understand psychotherapy.

Baumgartner, Leona. Medical care of children in public programs. *American Journal of Public Health* 51 (October 1961): 1491–99. I. Lack of efficiency in public programs, chaos in health administration, and lack of coordination in specific programs compound problems for the poor in obtaining health care. II. Primary: survey of 200 low-income families and case studies obtained by welfare adminstrator. III. A reorganization of health services is needed. Coordinate services into a more efficient plan, and apply more funds for needed facilities.

Beck, R. G. Economic class and access to physician services under public medical care insurance. *International Journal of Health Services* 3 (Summer 1973): 341–55. I. There are financial barriers for the poor: other factors were implied but not determined in this study. II. Secondary: from records of Saskatchewan Medical Care Insurance Plan correlated with tax return stated incomes. V. There was considerable disparity in access to physician services (as measured by inverse ratio of zero-utilizers) by income class prior to introduction of public insurance. Rates of accessibility of low-income groups increased more rapidly than that of high-income groups; however, disparity by income class still remains after six years' experience with medical care insurance.

Becker, Marshall H., et al. Motivations as predictors of health behavior. *Health Services Reports* 87 (November 1972): 852–62. I. Inadequate compliance results from a low value being placed on the outcome of compliance and a low expectancy that proper compliance will result in an unproved situation. II. Primary: compliance records of 125 mostly black females bringing children to a comprehensive child care clinic were related to various motivating factors. V. The study examined the value of employing the health motivations and perceptions of mothers as predictors of their compliance with regimens prescribed for their children.

Beloff, Jerome S., and Meiko Korper. The health team model and medical care utilization: Effect on patient behavior of providing comprehensive family health services. *Journal of the American Medical Association* 219 (January 1972): 359–66. I. Traditional private practice and prepaid group-practice programs provide only "illness" care; poverty patients' greatest problems may be social and emotional, the solutions of which may be an important factor in improving health behavior. II. Primary: utilization patterns of thirty-one multiproblem families were studied for thirty continuous months of comprehensive care provided by health-care team. III. and IV. Care provided by health-care team (physician, nurse, health aide, and social worker) with continuity, coordination, and constant availability of care, resulted in illness-response pattern changing to health-orientation response pattern. Increased use of nurse counseling, psychosocial guidance, employment assistance, health education, marriage counseling, and rehabilitation; and decreased use of physician services for illness care resulted.

Berger, E. J., and H. R. Martin. Study and analysis of utilization and cost data concerning provision of home health service and extended care service. St. Louis Labor Health Institute Report No. PB 190 (1970): 793. II. Primary: case evaluations and cost studies provided the documentary evidence. V. This brief study demonstrates the savings brought about by the addition of home care and extended services to a prepaid medical plan. It does not provide statistical evidence for the conclusions.

Berkanovic, Emil and Leo G. Reeder. Can money buy the appropriate use of services? Some notes on the meaning of utilization data. *Journal of Health and Social Behavior* 15 (June 1974): 93–99. I. Authors list four factors that complicate the Financial Access Model: (1) "Serious" diseases requiring medical attention are defined differently by various cultures. (2) Available data suggest that the elimination of economic barriers might equalize the utilization of treatment services, but those with the higher levels of morbidity would not necessarily seek higher rates of treatment. (3) If early detection and the use of preventive services are important areas of concern to the health professions, then we need to understand the determinants of their utilization. (4) Recent data suggest that equality in the use of physician services among different income groups is not the result of more frequent visits by the poor, but of less frequent visits by the more affluent. Cultural differences may act as barriers to professional-client encounters because there are apt to be several sets of misfitting expectations; different ordering of problems and priorities; and different vulnerabilities to ego assault in the professional-client encounter. And these barriers are aggravated by the prejudices of health professionals. II. An overview of the problem; good list of references.

Berkowitz, N. H., et al. Patient follow-through in the outpatient department. *Nursing Research* 12 (Winter 1963): 16–22. II. Primary: physicians in fifty-five clinics completed questionnaire about their patients over a period of five clinic visits. III. Patients followed through more consistently when illness was serious and hence motivation for care was high. Educating patient is primary step.

Berle, Beatrice B. *Eighty Puerto Rican Families in New York City.* New York: Columbia University Press, 1958. I. High incidence of tuberculosis related to fear of prolonged hospitalization. Insured individuals have little or no understanding of the services available to them through group policies. The "Welfare Doctor" is held in low esteem. II. Primary: study of ethnic group in New York City. III. Home treatment of tuberculosis will diminish the need to deny the existence of the disease. Establishment of a family service center within the community will study and treat the family as a unit, utilizing visiting nurses. V. Physicians in the community are older or foreign trained, and they are not on the staff of any hospital. Of nineteen Spanish-speaking physicians, eleven did not belong to the County or State medical societies; ten who were registered in the State Medical Directory were graduates of foreign medical schools. Fear associated with illness and a desire for active treatment led this population to use the emergency rooms of local hospitals frequently.

Bice, T. W., and K. L. White. Factors related to the use of health services: an international comparative study. *Medical Care* 7 (March-April 1969): 124–33. II. Primary: studies in Chester, England, Chittenden County, Vermont, and Smederevo, Yugoslavia. V. Although the proportions of persons who visited a physician within a two-week period differed among the areas, the internal patterns of use showed remarkable similarity; the levels of perceived morbidity were closely related to use of services in all areas.

Bice, T. W., and K. L. White. Cross-national comparative research on utilization of medical services. *Medical Care* 9 (May-June 1971):

253–71. II. Authors' opinions, observations, and suggestions. V. This article is mainly concerned with comparing the various methods developed for measuring utilization of health services. It suggests that comparative research on utilization is in the infancy stage and more complex methods and techniques for measuring utilization will develop.

Bice, Thomas W., et al. Economic class and use of physician services. *Medical Care* 11 (July-August 1973): 287–96. I. Medicaid and other assistance programs have diminished the effects of low income and poverty on overall use of health services, but beliefs, life styles, and other noneconomic factors continue to affect the use of preventive services. Among poor adults who have regular sources of care, those least likely to use physician services are nonwhites who have no recognized chronic health problems and who must pay at least a portion of the charges for services. II. Primary: a household survey in the Baltimore Metropolitan Standard Statistical Area, 1968–69. III. Reducing financial barriers to the use of medical services appears to encourage utilization among previous low utilizers. However, authors caution that their data cannot demonstrate conclusively that other factors do not account for the Net Price-Use relationships; there could be a set of variables related to both utilization and eligibility for benefits from social insurance schemes. V. Authors cite P. H. Rossi and D. Blum ("Class, Status, and Poverty," in *On Understanding Poverty*, ed. D. P. Moynihan, 36–63, New York, Basic Books, 1968), who state that lack of education may affect behavior in two different ways. (1) It may produce such direct effects as being unable to cope with complex and abstract ideas or situations such as not understanding the need for preventive medical care. (2) Indirectly, other effects intervene; for example, health professionals may find it difficult to respond to those who have little education and who do not exhibit "proper" behavior; the result may be that clients are denied the opportunity to learn more middle-class behavior patterns.

Blum, Henrik L. et al. The multipurpose worker and the neighborhood multiservice center: initial experiences and implications of the Rodeo Community Service Center. *American Journal of Public Health* 58 (March 1968): 458–62. I. The fragmentation of health, welfare, and probation services leads to counselors being unconcerned about areas of wellbeing outside their individual spheres of interest; this fragmentation also leads to uncoordinated service efforts on the part of community workers. II. Primary: the development of a project to provide comprehensive well-being services in a small, working-class community. III. Primary counselors were

trained to provide multiphase services to families from neighborhood multiservice center. Specialist services were made available
through the primary counselors when needed.

Bond, L. W., et al. Contract health services for rural counties —
success and failure. *American Journal of Public Health* 58 (March
1968): 469–72. I. Limited tax bases, funds, personnel and health
resources cause PH services to be inadequate in rural counties. II.
An historical review of the development of contract health services
for rural counties in California. V. Counties with population less
than 40,000 in California contract with the State Department of
Public Health for the provision of public health services. In 1963,
for the first time, all counties in the State of California were
covered by organized local public health services, 16 of 58 through
the contract mechanism.

Booth, A., and N. Babchuk. Seeking health care from new resources.
Journal of Health and Social Behavior 13 (March 1972): 90–100.
I. Except under emergency conditions, people are likely to seek
advice from a layman before contacting a physician. The most
isolated in society, the poor and the aged, have greatest need for
information, but are least likely to have such services available. II.
Primary: 800 adults, age 45 and over, were asked specific
questions related to the selection of health services. V. The study
focuses on events that occur after an individual initially considers
using an unfamiliar health service, what laymen he consults, the
time lapse involved, and other related decisions.

Breslow, L. New partnerships in the delivery of services — a public
view of the need. *American Journal of Public Health* 57 (July
1967): 1094–1099. I. Factors: poor settings in which care is rendered, limited hours, travel inconvenience, and negative attitudes
of health professionals toward poor patients. II. Secondary:
author's opinions and observations. III. Create partnerships between traditional and new health agencies to respond directly to
community needs.

Breslow, L. The urgency of social action for health. *American
Journal of Public Health* 60 (January 1970): 10–16. I. Health
crisis exists in America in delivery of health services, especially to
the poor. Specific examples cited. II. Secondary: author's opinions
and suggestions. III. Develop overall strategy for health care based
on human needs to replace independent hit-or-miss programs.

Brinton, D. M. Value differences between nurses and low-income
families. *Nursing Research* 21 (January-February 1972): 46–52. I.
Value differences between nurses and low-income families were in
some areas less sharp than nurses thought they were; if nurses
approach low-income families with the assumption that the

families do not care about health, many important cues will be missed. II. Study of twenty low-income families and twenty-three young, white nurses. V. Study showed that 82 percent of mothers who kept appointments thought it important to take a child to the doctor when he was sick; only 44 percent of those who failed to keep appointments thought it was important. More mothers who kept appointments scored high on fatalism and low on reflectiveness. Thus one wonders if, for families with an urban background, fatalism no longer denotes rejection of scientific medicine, such as Suchman (1963) found in respondents with rural backgrounds. Once drawn into a health care system, these people may think very little about it, and continue returning out of force of habit. One interesting result: nurses, the nurses' perceptions, and mothers were all low in future orientation; this may reflect the present life style.

Brooks, C. H. Associations among distance, patient satisfaction, and utilization of two types of inner-city clinics. *Medical Care* 11 (September-October 1973): 373–83. I. Utilization will increase with distance for large, bureaucratically structured clinics, and will tend to decrease for small-neighborhood clinics. Larger, older clinics tend to be more separated from populations served, have initiated "outreach" programs to attract users living miles away, and rely on formal referral system for patients. Small-neighborhood health clinics are designed to serve population contiguous to clinic location, and recruit patients through informal channels such as fliers, door-to-door canvassing, meetings with neighborhood organizations, and word of mouth. II. Primary: from analysis of data on client attitudes and behavior in four clinics in Detroit, Michigan. V. Also examines the relationship of patterns of patient satisfaction according to large versus small clinics.

Brown, H. J. Delivery of personal health services and medical services for the poor: concessions or prerogatives. *Milbank Memorial Fund Quarterly* 46 (January 1968): 203–23. I. Services to poor are inadequate, impersonalized, hurried, and social problems of the poor often interfere with seeking care for health problems. II. Secondary: data from several health surveys. III. More money should be provided for services to the poor. Incentives for doctors to serve low-income patients should be established. Medical schools should train their students in community health problems. Existing facilities should be improved and their efficiency upgraded. Social welfare and health services to the poor should be unified under one comprehensive service, and, lastly, the poor themselves should demand better care.

Brown, R. D. Poverty and health in the United States. *Clinical*

Pediatrics 8 (August 1969): 495–98. I. Factors: lack of knowledge of how to obtain care, orientation to medical care instead of health care, lack of money, and insufficient knowledge of disease. II. Secondary: author's opinions, observations, and suggestions. III. Dedicate resources of country to solving problems of poverty.

Bugbee, G. Medical care for low-income families: an introduction. Proceedings of the Tenth Annual Symposium on Hospital Affairs, Center for Health Administration Studies, University of Chicago. *Inquiry* 5 (March 1968): 5–7. I. The poor are unable to use middle-class systems of medical care. Service is of substandard quality, and the price of medical care has increased drastically so that they cannot afford it. II. Secondary: author's opinions, observations, and suggestions. III. Find new funds to care for poor and create new organizations to use money more effectively and efficiently. V. Care for the poor is most pressing need in the medical field.

Bugbee, G., et al. Organizing the hospital for care of the poor: panel discussion. *Inquiry* 5 (March 1968): 49–64. I. Service for the poor is not geared to the poor, is not long-term or preventive, but isolates and dehumanizes patients. II. Secondary: discussion between several eminent professionals in the health care field. III. Reorganize hospitals to meet the needs of the poor. Provide high-quality care. Provide incentives for doctors to care for the poor. Allow the poor representation on boards that decide what their care will be. Gear hospitals to the communities they serve and to the needs of the local people.

Bullough, B. Poverty, ethnic identity and preventive health care. *Journal of Health and Social Behavior* 13 (December 1972): 347–59. I. Lack of income and education is a significant factor in predicting preventive health care, excluding a new baby's checkup and the mother's postpartum visit. A broken-down car, no money for a baby sitter, no bus fare, or the threat of the loss of a day's work can be real barriers to seeking care. In addition, the culture of poverty includes feelings of powerlessness, hopelessness, and social isolation, and these affect the level of utilization of preventive care. II. Primary: a sample study of 806 women from three Los Angeles poverty neighborhoods.

Cauffman, J. G., et al.(a) Medical care of school children: factors influencing outcome of referral from a school health program. *American Journal of Public Health* 57 (January 1967): 60–73. I. Children were less likely to receive attention if they were from a low social rank, members of large families, Negroes, or Spanish American. II. Primary: school health records and interviews with parents of 495 children who had 641 medical defects. III. and IV.

Assess the impact of socioeconomic, attitudinal, and notification factors upon the outcome of referral from school health clinic examinations.

Cauffman, J. G., et al.(b) The impact of health coverage on health care of school children. *Public Health Reports* 82 (April 1967): 323–28. I. Children with insurance received more care. II. Primary: 458 Los Angeles school children with health defects were examined. III. School and community leaders should encourage noninsured families to obtain health insurance coverage; this will lead to higher rates of utilization.

Cervantes, Robert A. The failure of comprehensive health services to serve the urban Chicano. *Health Services Reports* 87 (December 1972): 932–40. I. Anglo staffs lack empathy for Chicanos. The structure of health services is at variance with Chicano social organization; "comprehensive" health is defined from a non-Chicano perspective. II. Secondary: author's observations with quotations from various research on Chicano cultural and social structures. III. Recruit and train Chicano health and mental health professionals; redesign health curriculums and programs to recognize and incorporate the diverse cultural, linguistic, and ethnic elements appropriate to all clients. V. An excellent review of Chicano stereotypes and realities, and a description of the Chicano health care system, which includes the influence of religion, folk medicines, and chiropractors.

Chapman, L. S. The neighborhood health center foundation for health care: a portent for the future or a necessity for survival? *American Journal of Public Health* 63 (October 1973): 841–45. I. Changes in federal health service funding policies and lack of empirical evidence supporting the neighborhood health center type of health-care delivery system have necessitated a reevaluation of sources of future support for neighborhood health centers. II. Secondary: author's own opinions, observations, and suggestions. III. Neighborhood Health Centers may do well to bank together to form Neighborhood Health Center Foundations; such a system would promote better general and financial management practices and reduce staff turnover, thus bringing about a more stable provider relationship. In addition, they should formalize a quality review process based on recognized standards of primary health-care services; organize patient advocacy programs; simplify administrative procedures; and lower overhead costs by means of shared services. V. Tells of approach under consideration to modify corporate structure of Massachusetts League of Neighborhood Health Centers to form a Neighborhood Health Center Foundation for health care.

Cherkasky, M. Medical manpower needs in deprived areas. *Journal of Medical Education* 44 (February 1969): 126–31. I. Factor: not enough services available to ghetto populations. II. Secondary: author's observations. III. Health professionals working with poor require special preparations. In addition to training students in scientific technology, medical schools must prepare doctors to deal with social problems and to work in the community . The story of a demonstration project in which health workers were successfully trained and incorporated into health teams.

Clark, M. *Health in the Mexican-American Culture.* Berkeley: University of California Press, 1959. I. Folk beliefs about health and illness inhibit use of modern, scientific cures. Mexican-Americans have feelings of alienation from Anglo culture and health workers. Also, there is discrimination on the part of Anglos. II. Secondary: author's observations. III. Health workers should be able to speak Spanish, to overcome the language barrier. Find a method to make prepayment of medical care acceptable to the community. Health workers should be used to teach scientific concepts of disease etiology. In general, health professionals need to be sensitive to Mexican-American culture. V. The book tells of the social and cultural life patterns of members in the Colonia, a San Jose Mexican-American community.

Clausen, J. A. Social factors in disease. *Annals of the American Academy of Political and Social Science* 346 (March 1963): 138–48. II. Secondary: author's observations. V. Differences in life styles, diet, physical activity, family patterns, and self-attitudes all tend to make the poor more likely to have poor health. Article reviews Mechanic and Volkhart, and is primarily concerned with social factors and etiology of disease. There are some comments on perception of illness (Koos) and readiness to seek care.

Clifford, M. C. Health and the urban poor. *Nursing Outlook* 17 (December 1969): 62–3. I. Medical programs fail to meet emotional needs of blacks and other poverty groups who are outsiders on the American scene. Society is unwilling to provide a decent standard of living for the poor. II. Secondary: author's observations and opinions. III. Middle-class health professionals must learn to appreciate the values and expectations of the poor.

Cobb, B., et al. Patient-responsible delay of treatment in cancer: social psychological study. *Cancer* 7 (September 1954): 920–26. I. Significant differences in age and life style distinguished the delayers from the prompt seekers of health services. II. Primary: interviews with one hundred patients with cancer: fifty who presented themselves promptly for treatment, and fifty who delayed more than three months. III. Cancer information should be disseminated through agencies that reach lower-income people. Education should be presented in terms that are meaningful to people with different styles of life and only an elementary school education. V. Meaningful information concerning cancer, its symptoms and treatment is probably the most potent weapon with which to combat patient-responsible delay in seeking medical care.

Coburn, D., and C. R. Pope. Socioeconomic status and preventive health behavior. *Journal of Health and Social Behavior* 15 (June 1974): 67–8. I. Education, age, income, and social participation provided the most cogent set of variables for predicting general preventive health behavior. II. Survey of 1,143 male workers in Victoria, British Columbia in 1970; data taken from 1,037 respondents who were working twenty-five hours a week or more. V. The possibility that variables generally used to explain or predict social participation may also be determinants of certain types of preventive health behavior, merits further investigation.

Coe, R. M., et al. The impact of Medicare on the utilization and provision of health care facilities: a sociological interpretation. *Inquiry* 4 (December 1967): 42–6. I. The perception of illness and definition of symptoms as illness affect utilization. II. Secondary: author's own opinions. III. Medicare will increase seeking of medical care for symptoms previously not defined as illness. Also, Medicare will encourage development of sick role that is "non-deviant," and will therefore encourage utilization of services.

Coleman, A. H.(a) A social system to improve health care delivery to the poor. *Journal of the National Medical Association* 61 (March 1969): 192–94 and 204. I. Factors: insufficient involvement of the poor in planning health services and bureaucracy in services. II. Secondary: author's own observations. III. Provide financial support for private care; furnish health teams that provide total health care. V. Describes plan to implement a neighborhood health center in the Hunter's Point area of San Francisco, a typically hard-core metropolitan area. Cites goals for proposed center.

Coleman, A. H.(b) The Hunter's Point-Bayview Community Health Service. *California Medicine* 110 (March 1969): 253–55. I. Factors: crisis orientation, ignorance, and transportation problems of poor. II. Primary: records of the Hunter's Point-Bayview community health service. III. Proposal: radical reorganization of health-care delivery to the poor by (1) providing freedom to choose physicians in health facilities as much as possible; (2) making maximum use of existing facilities, preferably private; (3) altering life styles of the poor as they relate to health; (4) utilizing local people as "social health technicians" in health teams.

Collins, Beverly. Denver builds citywide health network. *Modern Hospital* 110 (May 1968): 102–6. I. Long waits and overcrowded conditions at Denver General Hospital discouraged patients from coming except for extreme emergencies. II. Primary: from records of Denver Neighborhood Health Center. III. Locate centers close to patients' homes: furnish center according to patients' tastes; integrate programs of family centered care, enabling families to receive medical attention at one centralized location. IV. The above measures were successful. There was extensive participation by indigenous personnel.

Collver, A., et al. Factors influencing the use of maternal health services. *Social Science and Medicine* (September 1967) 293–308. I. Rates of attendance at prenatal, postpartum, and family planning clinics are associated with patient background and characteristics such as age, number of living children, and years of school completed. Distance of clinics from patients' homes had substantial effect on attendance. II. Primary: 774 low-income obstetric patients in two hospitals were interviewed to determine extent of prenatal care, and were followed up to determine extent of participation in postpartum and family planning clinics. III. Place branch maternal care clinics in strategic locations, no more than ten miles apart, or use mobile clinics. V. Expressed intentions of patients contribute nothing to prediction of attendance once objective characteristics, including number of children, age, marital status, and education, have been taken into account.

Colombo, T. J. et al. The integration of an OEO health program into a prepaid comprehensive group practice plan. *American Journal of Public Health* 59 (April 1969): 641–50. I. Financial means for building Kaiser Foundation Medical Care facilities were not available until Economic Opportunity Act of 1964. II. Primary: data from Kaiser Foundation Medical Care Center. III. Kaiser Foundation Medical Care facilities made available to indigent in Oregon region. Tells of use of neighborhood health coordinators. IV. A large population of medically indigent persons was integrated into an ongoing medical care system, and medical care services were provided for this group without serious problems.

Cons, N. C., and E. C. Leatherwood. Dental services in community child care programs. *American Journal of Public Health* 60 (July 1970): 1245–49. I. Financing, lack of manpower, transportation, professional prejudice, and consumer ignorance contribute to low utilization. II. Secondary: author's own opinions. III. Suggests providing NHC's with better transportation, health aides, non-tax supported auxiliary services.

Cornely, P. B., et al. Acquaintance with municipal government health services *American Journal of Public Health* 52 (November 1962): 1877–86. I. Factors: lack of knowledge of resources and of the functions of the health department. II. Primary: data from 310 black and 98 white low-income families in Washington, D. C.

Cowen, D. L. Denver's neighborhood health program. *Public Health Reports* 84 (December 1969): 1027–31. I. Low-income families are crisis-oriented toward health care and have little previous experience. II. Secondary: description of Denver Neighborhood Health Center. III. Provide NHC and employ local residents. IV. A combination of good planning, adequate funds, and personnel from the poverty community, a nearby medical school, and the health department, resulted in a successful health center in Denver.

Cowen, D. L.(a) Denver's preventive health program for school-age children. *American Journal of Public Health* 60 (March 1970): 515–18. I. Public health personnel in schools experience almost insurmountable difficulties in working with poor, because of their hostility toward the establishment, broken homes, inadequate housing, poor nutrition, and the lack of any relationships with physicians. II. Secondary: author's own opinions. III. System of NHC's and health stations, family health counselors. Education programs that involve neighborhood people. Cooperation with schools. IV. Description of Denver's successful health program.

Cowen, D. L.(b) Denver. *Hospitals* 44 (July 1970): 61–4. I. Traditional operations of the health department and the Denver General Hospital were insufficient to provide health care for the total population. II. Secondary: statistical surveys. III. Proposals: small clinics to be established in the city's low-income areas; a new General Hospital; upgrading of staff and equipment; and the use of sub-professionals from the target area. IV. Facilities were successfully able to handle 120,000 patients who make 700,000 visits each year. V. Denver's Neighborhood Health Program is demonstrating that a city hospital and a city health department can provide adequate care for lower-income families if enough effort is exerted.

Cowles, W., and S. Poigar et al. Health and communication in a Negro census tract. *Social Problems* 10 (Winter 1963): 228–36. I. Factor: lack of communication; although there was no overall "resistance" to medicine in this area, the poor relied on medical advice from friends. II. Primary: 10 percent systematic random sample of households in Berkeley that had the highest proportion of blacks. III. Improve the use of communication networks: personal contacts with families, the use of mass media, and communications from schools to parents. Use roving practical health educators from the same environment as population being served.

Cowne, L. J. Approaches to the mental health manpower problem: a review of the literature. *Mental Hygiene* 53 (April 1969): 176–87. I. Nondelivery rather that nonutilization is the immediate problem because of the manpower shortage in mental health. II. Secondary: personal observations of author. III. Proposals: downward transfer of functions and increased use of subprofessional personnel. IV. Several programs are cited which were successful in utilizing nonprofessional personnel.

Curry, W. Small health group builds big success in the Southwest. *Hospitals* 43 (July 1, 1969): 95–100. I. Factors: extreme poverty, disorganized programs, and lack of transportation facilities. Cultural differences between Indians, Spanish-Americans, and Anglos add to the problems. II. Study of Presbyterian Medical Services of the Southwest. Secondary: observations by the author of four health centers. III. Four comprehensive health centers have been established in this region, each with a fleet of vehicles to bring patients in for treatment. IV. Based on the success of the present project, plans are being made to develop a comprehensive health care project for entire Rio Grande valley. V. A good example of health care delivery in remote areas.

Darsky, B. J., et al. *Comprehensive Medical Services under Voluntary Health Insurance: A Study of Windsor Medical Services.* Cambridge: Harvard University Press, 1958. I. Patients were not able to afford medical care when needed. II. Primary: interviews with 1,345 people in metropolitan Windsor in 1954. III. A program of prepaid physician services was arranged. IV. Number of residents utilizing medical services *and* number of physician settling in area covered by prepaid physician services increased. V. A useful reference where cost of medical services is a barrier. People without insurance use the hospital more sparingly than others, but once they require a hospital stay, they receive a more extended sequence of home and office care.

Davidson, K. R. Conceptions of illness and health practices in a Nova Scotia community. *Canadian Journal of Public Health* 61 (May-June 1970): 232–42. I. Factors: skepticism toward modern medical care, lack of health consciousness, practice of folk medicine, and self-reliant attitude. II. Primary: based on one year of field work using ethnographic and survey research techniques. III. More attention will have to be focused on reducing cultural chasm between economically deprived and modern medical services.

Davis, M. S. Variations in patients' compliance with doctors' orders: Analysis of congruence between survey responses and results of empirical investigations. *Journal of Medical Education* 41

(November 1966): 1037–48. I. Expectations between doctor and patient for mutual role fulfillment are rarely congruent. Little recognition by doctors that certain types of patients are more compliant than others. II. Primary and Secondary: questionnaires mailed to 132 physicians (with 63 percent return) and 86 medical students (61 percent return). Study compares results obtained from a review of compliance literature with doctors' perceptions of general patient compliance. Income, social class, and education were the most significant predictors of compliance. III. Doctors must develop good rapport, including ability to analyze the significance of social, psychological, and cultural factors affecting the lives of patients.

Davis, M. S. Predicting noncompliant behavior. *Journal of Health and Social Behavior* 8 (December 1967): 265–71. I. Incongruence between norms and values of patient and doctor's advice results in decreased compliance. II. Primary: a sample of 435 men from a five-county area in central Indiana was interviewed in 1955 and again in 1960. III. The doctor must diagnose the social, psychological, and cultural facets of the patient's problem in order to reduce dissonance between medical regimens and patient's norms and values.

Davis, M. S. Variations in patient's compliance with doctors' advice: An empirical analysis of communication. *American Journal of Public Health* 58 (February 1968): 274–88. I Articles are on compliance rather than utilization. Revisits between an authoritative patient and a physician who passively accepts such patient participation may promote patient noncompliance. Unreleased tension in doctor-patient participation may promote patient noncompliance. Unreleased tension in doctor-patient relationships impedes communication and compliance. When doctors seek information from patients without giving them any feedback, the patient is unlikely to follow the doctor's orders once they are formulated. II. Primary: 223 taped doctor-patient interactions were coded into twelve responses and then data collected on what each patient did in complying with doctor's orders. III. The doctor must rely on his ability to establish good rapport in order to inculcate in his patient a positive orientation and commitment to the relationship so that ultimately the patient will follow his advice. In order to do this, the doctor must continually explore and diagnose the social and psychological facets of his interaction with his patients as well as the manifest medical problems.

Davis, M. S., and R. L. Eichhorn. Compliance with medical regimens: a panel study. *Journal of Health and Human Behavior* 4 (Winter 1963), 240–49. I. Social and psychological factors affect compliance with medical regimens. II. Primary: a sample of male farmers with cardiovascular impairment interviewed in 1955 and again in 1960. III. It is naive of a physician to assume his job is completed after he gives a prescription. V. Many compliers in 1956 had stopped complying by 1960; even more who did not comply started to do so in the interim. Those with low work orientation were more likely to continue to comply or begin to comply than high work-oriented cardiacs.

Davis, M. S., and R. E. Tranquada. A sociological evaluation of the Watts Neighborhood Health Center. *Medical Care* 7 (March-April 1969): 105–17. II. Primary: taken from the South Central Multi-purpose Health Services Center in Watts, California. III. Recommended that lay community groups should act as advisers, not necessarily decision-makers. IV. Black community revolted because they were not involved in decision-making. V. An evaluation of the conflict between OEO, USC, and a lay community health council.

Deas, B. W., Jr. A view of health services. *Journal of the South Carolina Medical Association* 64 (November 1968): 453–56. I. Factors: lack of education, poor communications with medical personnel, transportation problems, and long waits before medical help is given. II. Primary: study of 150 indigent Negro families. III. Improve communications with medical personnel, educate the poor, provide transportation, and improve efficiency of health services.

Deasy, L. C. Socioeconomic status and participation in the poliomyelitis vaccine trial. *American Sociological Review* 21 (April 1956): 185–91. I. Members of low socioeconomic groups are less aware of services and their consequences and lack motivation to participate in programs. Mothers in the lowest status group were less likely to allow their children to participate in the vaccine trial. They knew less about the trial and demonstrated a lower level of awareness of the disease. II. Primary: interviews with random samples of mothers of second graders in five public schools near Washington, D. C. III. New orientations are needed to help poverty groups improve use of medical services.

Deschin, C. S. The need to extend medical services beyond the hospital if maternal and infant care is to become comprehensive. *American Journal of Public Health* 58 (July 1968): 1230–36. I. Anomie, alienation, poor self-image, and expectations of friends affected utilization. II. Primary: study of records of Maternity Home Care Program in New York City. III. Social work students asked mothers to come to the hospital to give feedback on home care program. IV. Most mothers said they were in favor of preventive medicine, but did not come to the hospital because of problems at home. V. Program tells of attempt to give follow-up care to postpartum mothers and children.

de Vise, P. The problem isn't how little we spend on the poor, but how badly we spend it. *Modern Hospital* 114 (May 1970): 84–6. I. Irrational and wasteful organization of public payments and health delivery systems gives some of the population a great advantage over others, especially those who are young, black, female, or living outside certain areas. II. Secondary: author's own opinions. III. Better medical care could be provided at a fraction of the current cost with a dual health system of private and public components working together to provide equitable services for all. V. Article details the failure to deliver health services in Chicago.

Dodge, W. F., and E. F. West. Consumers' motivation and acceptance of urinary screening of school children. *Public Health Reports* 85 (September 1970): 828–34. I. Medical and school communities made little effort to motivate parents. Low socioeconomic groups had not been screened for kidney impairment before and thus did not realize the importance of the screening. Follow-through on referrals followed class lines. II. Primary: 10,000 children, with parental permission, were checked for compliance over a three-year period. III. Incorporate preventive health programs in schools. The portion of referred children who do not receive subsequent care could not be explained by availability of care.

Dodge, W. F., et al. Patterns of maternal desires for child health care. *American Journal of Public Health* 60 (August 1970): 1421–29. I. Current maternal opinion and desires with regard to health care are matched by current performance in utilization of care. II. Primary: based on interviews with mothers from a 12 percent sample of all children enrolled in first, second, and third grades of public schools in Galveston County, Texas. V. Differences in use patterns between mothers of different ethnic groups and income levels were not significant.

Donabedian, A., and L. S. Rosenfeld. Some factors affecting prenatal care. *New England Journal of Medicine* 265 (July 1961): 1–6. I. Probable variables associated with inadequate prenatal care are knowledge of hygienic principles, cultural values, feelings of responsibility toward family, availability of time, geographic accessibility, and patient understanding of physician's recommendations. Women in lower income and educational categories were less likely to believe prenatal care was necessary and less likely to seek such care. II. Primary: all women in selected hospitals questioned on second and third postpartum day over period of one month. III. Provide more adequate education to the public on the need for prenatal care. Research further into reasons for neglect, especially by mothers in low education and income brackets who have two or more children. IV. 82 percent of private patients received adequate care compared with 41 percent of clinic patients.

Dummett, C. O. Understanding the underprivileged patient. *Journal of the American Medical Association* 79 (December 1969): 1363–67. I. Factors: discomfort over the cleanliness of the medical world, communication difficulties, lack of finances, long waiting periods, ignorance about health problems, failure to realize importance of keeping appointments, fear of treatments, and over-reactions to grievances. II. Primary: observations of doctors and case studies. III. Warm, amiable attitudes on the part of doctors are valued by the underprivileged more than competence. Patients should be involved in planning medical care programs.

Durbin, R. L., and G. Antelman. A study of the effects of selected variables on hospital utilization. *Hospital Management* 98 (August 1964): 57–60. II. Secondary: a study of selected medical resource variables on hospital utilization — number of beds per 1,000 and the number of doctors per 100,000 persons. Sources: World Almanac, Research Division of AMA, etc. V. Admission rates decreased with increased patient income and the number of physicians, and increased very rapidly as the number of beds increased. The effect of increased health insurance was slight.

Elling, R., et al. Patient participation in a pediatric program. *Journal of Health and Human Behavior* 1 (Fall 1960): 183–91. I. Low identification with clinic; i.e., poor participators had little understanding of problems, felt personnel evaluated them negatively. II. Primary: eighty randomly selected families with children under 12 years of age were studied on utilization in rheumatic fever clinic. III. Increase physician's awareness of his own value judgments and their effect on patient's feelings; develop an index to predict low participators and give them special attention. V. Income was not significantly related to participation in clinic.

English, J. T. New challenges for physicians in the war on poverty. *Journal of the National Medical Association* 60 (January 1968): 38–41. I. Clinics for poor are crowded, uncomfortable, and lacking in concern for human dignity. "Specialty clinics" make it necessary for those with several illnesses to be seen in different clinics on different days. II. Secondary: address by assistant director of OEO with quotes from observations of M.D.s. III. Provide Neighborhood Health Centers to bring family medicine to poor; increase interpersonal involvement with community members; coordinate all types of medical care. Reach rural poor as well as urban poor.

English, J. T. OEO health programs. *Inquiry* 5 (March 1968): 43–48. I. Ill health and poverty reinforce each other. The poor live in conditions that undermine health, and illness prevents utilization of services. Inadequate transportation to facilities is also a barrier to utilization. II. Secondary: author's opinion and description. III. With the aid of federal funds, hospitals should reorganize outpatient clinics to deliver high quality care and to provide transportation for the poor. IV. Describes OEO health program established in Watts area of Los Angeles. The results of organizing services for poor were encouraging.

English, J. T. The dimensions of poverty. *American Journal of Nursing* 69 (November 1969): 2424–28. I. The culture of poverty: inadequate, inaccessible, impersonal fragmented and discontinuous health care all contribute to poor utilization of health services by the poor. II. Secondary: author's own opinions and suggestions. III. Establish more neighborhood health centers, train young physicians to deal with health needs of poor, educate various kinds of health aides. Increased experimentation is necessary to discover effective ways to improve health services.

Fabrega, H. J., and R. E. Roberts.(a) Social–psychological correlates of physician use by economically disadvantaged Negro urban residents. *Medical Care* 10 (May-June 1972): 215–23. II. Primary: survey of low income Negro-Americans in Houston, Texas. Groups differing in degree of physician contact were compared on a variety of social-psychological and demographic variables. V. Initial results showed significant effect of social-psychological variables; controlling for age–sex diminished relationship. Demographic variables seem more significant in determining patterns of utilization than social-psychological variables.

Fabrega, H. Jr., and R. E. Roberts.(b) Ethnic differences in the outpatient use of a public-charity hospital. *American Journal of Public Health* 62 (July 1972): 936–41. II. Primary: records of users of a large public-charity hospital of a metropolitan area in Southwestern U.S. V. Differences in utilization patterns between ethnic groups is mediated by the availability of alternative sources of care. Anglos were the lowest users of hospital facilities and had the highest number of doctors available. Blacks were the highest users of hospital facilities and had the lowest number of doctors available.

Fagin, C. Pharmacists' role expands in the neighborhood health center. *Hospitals* 42 (December 16,1968): 70–72. II. Secondary: author's description of delivery of pharmaceutical supplies in a neighborhood health center. III. Pharmacists in low-income areas could cooperate in providing a group practice in a health facility instead of operating privately. Pharmacists should never ignore patients' questions or hesitate to trace medication problem back to physicians. IV. Tells of success of pharmacy in Montefiore Hospital NHC. Community sentiment was strongly favorable.

Fay, T. H. et al. Audiological and otologic screening of disadvantaged children. *Archives of Otolaryngology* 91 (April 1970): 366–70. I. The disadvantaged give low priority to preventive health measures, such as hearing tests. II. Primary: study of hearing impairment incidence among disadvantaged children taken from Children's Shelter in New York City; 461 disadvantaged children were given hearing tests. III. A very high rate of hearing impairment was found among disadvantaged children (20 percent had problems), possibly due to inadequate medical attention. The study suggests providing services in greater proportion to disadvantaged children.

Feldman, J. J. *The Dissemination of Health Information: A Case Study in Adult Learning.* Chicago: Aldine Publishing Company, 1966. I. With lack of education or intelligence, some people do not understand the message even when they read it; others will forget it, and still others will reject it. II. Primary: NORC Survey, N = 367 households. III. Better educated people are better able to learn from the health materials in the mass media; more use of TV is suggested in order to reach the less literate. IV. Various examples of failures with educational programs through the mass media are cited. V. Some doctors are critical of mass media for unnecessarily arousing popular fears, anxieties, neuroses or phobic concern with illness.

Feldman, J. J., and E. J. Salber. The use of a household survey in neighborhood health centers. *American Journal of Public Health* 59 (August 1969): 1291–92. I. The effectiveness of a health center is greatly enhanced by the involvement of the potential clientele in both planning and operations. Residents of poverty areas have generally not been consulted concerning the health facilities they desire; they are not cohesive enough to exert a major influence. They wait until center is built and then do not use it. II. Secondary: authors' opinions, editorial. III. Use household survey to provide necessary denominator data to make possible the analysis of utilization patterns and to suggest changes in the health facility that will make the services more congenial to the population.

Feldstein, P. J. Research on the demand for health services. *Milbank Memorial Fund Quarterly* 44 (July 1966): 128–62. I. Incidence of illness and cultural, demographic, and economic factors affect utilization. II. Secondary: theoretical article. V. A proposed model of demand for health care, based on patient characteristics and physician choice of particular components of care. Need, cultural-demographic, and economic factors (net price to patient, normal income) affect patients' demands for treatment.

Feldstein, P. J., and J. W. Carr. The effect of income on medical care spending. *Proceedings of the Social Statistics Section, American Statistical Association*, 1964, 93–105. I. A family's level of consumption of medical care is determined primarily by its expected permanent income rather than by transitory income. II. Secondary: data from several national statistical reports on Labor and Health Insurance. V. The purpose of the study was to determine the average net effect of income on private spending for personal health care.

Ferguson, L. A. The medical needs of the ghetto and inner city in Chicago. *Proceedings of the Institute of Medicine of Chicago* 28 (January 1970): 10–18. II. Editorial: a review of health services for ghetto patients in Chicago. III. Allow ghetto residents to have some decision-making power. Prevent unscrupulous physicians from being parasites on the persons they purport to serve.

Fink, R., et al. The reluctant participant in a breast cancer screening program. *Public Health Reports* 83 (June 1968): 479–90. I. Non-participants were older, had less education, included fewer Jews and more Catholics; had less favorable attitudes toward screening examinations; differed in beliefs as to whether cancer can be cured in the early stages and as to whether or not a woman can detect breast cancer before seeing a physician; were less concerned about the possibility of having cancer and had fewer specific symptoms associated with breast cancer. Reluctant participants had characteristics similar to those of the minimum-effort participants. II. Primary: a mail and telephone survey of 11,500 women; 63 percent response. III. Response was increased by use of second mailing and then a follow-up phone call.

Fishman, J. R. Poverty, race, and violence. *American Journal of Psychotherapy* 23 (October 1969): 599–607. I. We promise far more than we give, leading to frustration; we are not responsive to the poor on their terms, and we perpetuate dependency by the structure of our programs. II. Secondary: author speaks from his experience in the ghetto. III. Allow communities to decide what services need to be provided, determine priorities, and establish policies. V. The article describes the overall relationship between our society and its poor and the failure of various programs designed to help the poor.

Flora, R. E., et al. Health facility utilization by people living in West Virginia Hollows. *West Virginia Medical Journal* 63 (September

1966): 316–19. I. Rural people lack knowledge about existing medical facilities, are reluctant to try something new, and have fatalistic attitude toward life and health. II. Primary: 50 percent of survey population had seen a physician in the preceding year; few had utilized services of dentists or public health nurses.

Foster, J. T. Neighborhood health centers: A new way to extend care. *Modern Hospital* (May 1968): 110–95. II. Editorial. V. A one-page introduction to neighborhood health centers. Gives background on development and status of neighborhood health centers.

Freeman, H. E., and C. Lambert, Jr. Preventive dental behavior of urban mothers. *Journal of Health and Human Behavior* 6 (Fall 1965): 141–47. I. Assesses the impact of preventive dental behavior of low-income mothers and related socioeconomic and attitudinal variables on children's preventive dental care. Individual family behavior is often splintered and various behavioral segments only partially overlap. II. Primary: a statistically significant positive relationship was exhibited between family income and preventive dental behavior. The study was drawn from school records of children in first through fourth grades in Brooklyn school.

Freidson, E. *Patients' Views of Medical Practice.* New York: Russell Sage Foundation, 1961. I. Patients seemed to use two interlocking criteria to evaluate health services. First, good medical care requires technical competence; second, it means taking an interest in the patient so that he not only obtains emotional satisfaction from the practitioner, but also the impression that competence is exercised in a more than routine way. II. Primary: surveys of families in various health maintenance and insurance plans, which give the data a basically middle-class orientation that does not relate directly to the problems of the disadvantaged. V. This book reports on a study that explored the attitudes and behavior of patients who have had experience with more than one way of organizing medical practice. Patients experienced the Family Health Maintenance Demonstration, the Montefiore Medical Group, and the conventional fee-for-service practice. The patients came from a culture of strong middle-class virtues of independence, thrift, and cleanliness; they were fearful of being "pushed around" or "taken advantage of," all of which influenced the data in this study.

Friedman, B., et al. The influence of Medicaid and private health insurance on the early diagnosis of breast cancer. *Medical Care* 11 (November–December 1973): 485–90. I. Although Medicaid and private health insurance may eliminate direct expense to consumers of medical care, they have not proved a meaningful stimulus to bringing people in for early diagnosis of serious illness. II. Primary: data collected from nearly all women with breast cancers in a large Massachusetts population base in 1970. III. The importance of noneconomic limits to the effectiveness of consumer incentives in promoting early diagnosis and treatment of serious illness should be more strongly emphasized.

Gales, H. The community health education project: Bridging the gap. *American Journal of Public Health* 60 (February 1970): 322–27. I. The poor do not value health agencies and are handicapped by much "red tape." II. Secondary: author's observations. III. Health aides were hired to encourage poor people in their own neighborhoods to participate in system. Establish teamwork between aides and agency. IV. Five thousand visits were made to those who may not otherwise have had information on health and services.

Gallagher, E. B. Prenatal and infant health care in a medium-sized community. *American Journal of Public Health* 57 (December 1967): 2127–37. I. Mothers were too busy, had no money for health care, had responsibilities with other children, were frightened by doctors, and did not feel preventive care was essential. II. Primary: interviews in homes, 10 percent of all infants born during ten-month period in three midwestern counties. Household survey covered special class, family health behavior, and infant development. Lower-class families were lowest utilizers. III. Clues to more comprehensive health coverage of mothers and infants in lower classes can be found by exploring subgroup and subcultural values concerning health, by determining situational barriers facing mothers wishing to obtain adequate health care, and by PH workers developing more convenient, acceptable ways of organizing health services for target populations.

Gans, H. J. *The Urban Villagers: Group and Class in the Life of Italian-Americans.* New York: The Free Press, 1962. I. Modern folk medicine replaces the Italian equivalent. Doctors are considered "outsiders," but hospitals are held in high esteem. Deepseated fatalism reinforces skepticism. II. Primary: study of an ethnic group in Boston. V. Middle-class doctors are unable to cope with the working-class subculture.

Garfield, S. R. The delivery of medical care. *Scientific American* 222 (April 1970): 15–23. I. Medical care in the U. S. is expensive and poorly distributed, and national health insurance will make things worse. II. Secondary: author's own opinions and observations. III. Reorganize the medical care system by eliminating present paid fee-for-service and facilitate the delivery of preventive and ameliorative health services.

Geiger, H. J. The endlessly revolving door. *American Journal of Nursing* 69 (November 1969); 2436–45. I. Health services for the poor fail to deal with the cycle of poverty and other social ills.

Health as an isolated entity rather than health in its social context prevents involvement in the larger problems that affect health. II. Secondary: from author's experience and opinions as general director of Tufts-Delta Health Center, Mound Bayou, Mississippi. III. Identify real problems, reorder priorities, create new social institutions appropriate to the problems, and have a commitment to change. *Social engineering* is the health professions' responsibility. IV. Author tells of a community health action department within a health center that utilized indigenous personnel and established its own priorities. Food, water, transportation, and housing problems must be worked out *before* health needs can be totally met.

Geiger, H. J., and R. D. Cohen. Trends in health care delivery systems. *Inquiry* 1 (March 1971): 32–36. II. Secondary: general discussion of where health delivery has been and where it is going. III. Future developments in the health field will include: a shift in emphasis from molecular research and concentration on technical aspects of serious illness to the concern over health-care delivery system; change hospital role to an institution devoted to critical, acute and intensive care; shift urban ambulatory care from hospitals to neighborhood health centers; increase community control over health-care systems; increase involvement and responsibility of health professionals for the social issues that underlie health problems; create new funding mechanisms. V. Traces past trends in health-care delivery systems, and points to probable future changes.

Gerrie, N. F., and R. H. Ferraro. Organizing a program for dental care in a neighborhood health center. *Public Health Reports* 83 (August 1968): 633–38. I. Cost, fear, ignorance, indifference, inaccessibility, and lack of effective referral and recall systems contributed to low utilization. II. Secondary: author's plans and criteria for establishing neighborhood dental program. III. To improve utilization, emphasis ought to be on changing dental behavior pattern from crisis orientation to behavior orientation (education programs). V. The operational dental program of Tufts-Columbia Point Medical Service Program is presented.

Gibbs, C. E., et al. Patterns of reproductive health care among the poor of San Antonio, Texas. *American Journal of Public Health* 64 (January 1974): 37–40. I. Situational factors include lack of transportation; problems providing care for children while seeing doctor; cost of services; and inconveniences imposed by clinics; i.e., long distances, poorly scheduled clinic hours, long waits, etc. Attitudinal factors include indifference or apathy, desire to conceal pregnancy (among young patients), and a local cultural tradition that pregnancy is a natural condition which should not require medical or other special attention. II. Primary: study of poor in San Antonio, Texas. III. Patients attending clinics now see the same doctor on each visit, nursing staff is upgraded in skills and interest, patients are informed of the state of pregnancy and the results of examination and tests, and information sharing was personal.

Gibson, C. D. The neighborhood health center: The primary unit of health care. *American Journal of Public Health* 58 (July 1968): 1188–91. I. Existing programs are badly fragmented; there are few physicians in low income areas. II. and III. A good background is given on need for NHC; to improve health care, health center must be in the community, community must participate in operation of NHC, and care must be oriented to entire family unit. IV. Author tells of the success of Tufts-Columbia Point Health Center, but offers no statistical proof.

Ginzberg, E. Facts and fancies about medical care. *American Journal of Public Health* 59 (May 1969): 785–94. I. Poor utilization of medical services is the result of "perverse" ways in which medical services are produced and distributed. III. Better and more comprehensive planning is needed; base future programs on facts instead of fancies.

Glasser, M. A. A study of the public's acceptance of the Salk vaccine program. *American Journal of Public Health* 48 (February 1958): 141–46. I. People lacked definite, positive influence which might direct them to a clinic or doctor's office for inoculation; felt they were not susceptible to disease; lacked specific knowledge about vaccination; and their friends tended not to have been vaccinated. Non-utilizers tended to be of lower social class. II. Primary: from a nationwide survey conducted in 1957.

Glogow, E. Effects of health education methods on appointment breaking. *Public Health Reports* 85 (May 1970): 441–50. I. Because of the lack of symptoms in glaucoma, patients are not convinced of the importance of remaining under treatment. II. Primary: study of 186 patients with suspected glaucoma interviewed on their reactions to differing information. V. The "manner" in which educational materials are presented (warmth, gentleness, and ability to communicate) is more important than educational material itself for reducing broken appointment rates. Positive suggestions are offered for improving utilization of preventive health-care services.

Gochman, D. S. The organizing role of motivation in health beliefs and intentions. *Journal of Health and Social Behavior* 13 (September 1972): 285–93. I. Perceived vulnerability to health problems, perceived benefits attributed to visiting the dentist, and experiences of dental trauma comprise a set of generally significant predictors of intention to visit a dentist. Among children for whom health is more important than appearance, the degree of prediction is greater than among children for whom health is not as important. II. Primary: a study of 774 children, ages 8 to 17, from schools in a large city area. V. Further analyses are required to examine the effects of socioeconomic factors and to determine the relative importance of specific predictors.

Goldberg, G. A., et al. Issues in the development of neighborhood health centers. *Inquiry* 6 (March 1969): 37–47. I. Low priority is given to health by ghetto people. Health-care services are often inaccessible. II. Secondary: descriptive article. III. Establish a neighborhood health center with maximum community participation in planning. IV. Article discusses problems and issues involved in developing a neighborhood health center with high community involvement.

Goldsen, R. Some factors related to patient delay in seeking diagnosis for cancer symptoms. *Cancer* 10 (1957): 1–7. I. Delay in seeking treatment may relate to symptom and worry over possibility of having cancer; the predominant factor is patient's general, customary medical orientation. II. Primary and secondary: analysis of data on 727 patients at hospitals and tumor clinics. III. It is suggested that good orientation to medical services will reduce delay in seeking diagnosis. V. Socioeconomic factors are not discussed.

Goldsen, R. Patient delay in seeking cancer diagnosis: Behavioral aspects. *Journal of Chronic Disease* 16 (1963): 427–36. I. People of little education and low socioeconomic status have little knowledge of cancer symptoms, poor medical habits in general, and less exposure to information regarding cancer. II. Secondary: data from many studies on the factors involved in seeking cancer diagnosis. III. Create an extensive outreach program for those who do not normally have checkups for cancer and a concentrated campaign of direct personal appeal to potential victims of cancer.

Goodrich, C. H., et al. The New York Hospital—Cornell Medical Center Project: An experiment in welfare medical care. *American Journal of Public Health* 53 (August 1963):1252–59. I. Lack of coordination in administering medical services to welfare recipients creates duplication, wastes time, energy, and money, and makes it difficult to control or evaluate effectiveness and quality of care. II. Primary: care was offered to 1,000 newly accepted public assistance cases in New York Hospital Project. III. Break down barriers between public and voluntary agencies. IV. Patients responded well to the invitation offered by the hospitals and did not inundate the hospital facilities. V. Report on organization, origin, research goals, and problems of New York Hospital Project on basis of two-year operation.

Goodrich, C. H., et al. *Welfare Medical Care.* Cambridge: Harvard University Press, 1970. I. The medical care system for the poor in New York state project was fragmented and often interfered with the utilization of patient care. II. Primary: the experimental group receiving medical care through city hospital outpatient clinic increased utilization. One thousand cases selected from newly registered welfare recipients were divided into control and experimental groups and followed for two years. IV. A full range of services was offered under the auspices of one institution to the experimental group. V. Report of New York Hospital—Cornell Project, 1960–1965.

Gornick, M. E., et al. Use of medical services as demanded by the urban poor. *American Journal of Public Health* 59 (August 1969): 1302-11. II. Primary: a sample of 1,000 households was drawn from deprived areas in Baltimore, Maryland. Of the households drawn, 52 percent had some or all members eligible for the Medical Assistance Program. III. Suggestions: more efficient use of resources, support of physicians in area, recruitment of young physicians, and provision of incentives to practice medicine in understaffed areas. V. This study was undertaken to assess the effects of a change in the medical care program for needy persons after the introduction of the Medical Care Program, a publicly financed program.

Gould, R. E. Dr. Strangeclass: Or how I stopped worrying about the theory and began treating the blue-collar worker. *American Journal of Orthopsychiatry* 37 (January 1967): 78-82. I. Writer considers many of the difficulties of middle-class psychiatrists and physicians in reaching lower-class patients to be rationalizations; the difficulties are often biases and limitations within professional groups. II. Primary: twenty-three interviews with union members who sought psychotherapy under a union contract with a psychoanalytic institute. III. Services were offered in a simple, direct, and open manner; they were immediately available, voluntary, and supported by trusted union leaders. Overtures came from the psychiatrists to reduce any fear of rejection. IV. The writer felt that the program was highly successful.

Graham, S. Socioeconomic status, illness, and the use of medical services. *Milbank Memorial Fund Quarterly* 36 (January 1957): 58-66. II. Primary: 35 personal interviews in Butler County, Pennsylvania, in 1954. There was no significant difference between low-income persons and upper-level income groups in their frequency of acute and chronic illness and their use of medical services. III. Study suggests that relationship between socioeconomic status, illness, and use of services should be reexamined.

Gray, R. M., et al. The effects of social class and friends' expectations on oral polio vaccination participation. *American Journal of Public Health* 56 (December 1966): 2028-32. I. Expectations of friends accounted for differences in utilization patterns between upper, middle, and lower-income groups. II. Primary: study of mothers who were provided the opportunity of having their children under 5 years of age immunized against poliomyelitis. V. No significant differences were found to exist between lower and upper-class mothers with respect to immunization rates when the mothers with similar views concerning their friends' expectations were compared separately.

Gray, R. M., et al. Alienation and immunization participation. *The Rocky Mountain Social Science Journal* 4 (April 1967): 161-68. I. Highly alienated people tend to make less use of available immunization clinics, regardless of socioeconomic status, age, education, or social participation. II. Primary: interviews with a sample of mothers from eight rural and urban Utah communities. III. To increase participation: decrease the individual's degree of alienation from society; make the person feel a part of the community health program.

Greeley, D. M. The health department and comprehensive health planning. *Industrial Medicine and Surgery* 37: (1968): 276-78. I. The poor do not know the values of preventive medicine and cannot cope with the present medical care system. II. Secondary: Dr. Greeley was the Director of Medical Care of the Chicago Board of Health. III. & IV. Article tells success of two neighborhood health centers in Chicago. Problems are discussed with suggestions for improving utilization. Three echelons of care are utilized: (1) Public Health nurses and aides, (2) the PHC facilities and personnel, and (3) the patient's hospital. A local advisory council of fifty residents (laymen) was established to assist in determining policy, recruiting, and gaining feedback from the community.

Greene, C. R. Medical care for underprivileged populations. *New England Journal of Medicine* 282 (May 1970): 1187-93. I., III., & IV. A critical review of OEO, Medicare and model cities. Suggestions to improve utilization rates: more (adequate) federal funding, attractive facilities, more compassion, and personalized care. II. Secondary: national statistic—the poor risk dying under the age of 25 at a rate four times that of the national average.

Greenlick, M. R., et al. Determinants of medical care utilization.

Health Services Research 3 (Winter 1968): 296-315. II. Primary: data from a sample of the Oregon Region of the Kaiser Foundation Health Plan. Of those sampled, 87 percent were employed; 81 percent were married. V. The study posits the effect of the intervening variable of disease characteristics on the relationship between background characteristics and medical care utilization.

Greenlick, M. R., et al. Determinants of medical care utilization: The role of the telephone in total medical care. *Medical Care* 11 (March-April 1973): 121-34. II. Primary: a study of telephone use in a prepaid group practice. Telephone calls represented a significant proportion of the total medical care of study population. V. Relative probability of a patient being told to come to the clinic after discussing a symptom varied inversely with certainty of the physician in his diagnosis and directly with the seriousness of the disease as perceived by the physician. Great variation was noted among individual physicians as to disposition of calls.

Gursslin, O. R., et al. Social class, mental hygiene, and psychiatric practice. *Social Service Review* 33 (September 1959): 237-45. I. The mental hygiene orientation of public psychiatric agencies is based on middle-class values; the lower-class population is less likely to find psychiatric practice palatable; because of class value differences, mental illness is less often diagnosed in lower classes. II. Secondary: data taken from the Hollingshead-Redlich study in a New Haven community. III. Use more staff from the lower classes and give more individualized service, taking into account cultural differences.

Hardy, M. C. Parent resistance to need for remedial and preventive services. *Journal of Pediatrics* 48 (January 1956): 104-14. I. The lower the socioeconomic status of a family, the less chance for a child to be referred for care. II. Primary: data taken from hearing and vision records in 128 Chicago public elementary schools. III. Improve parents' understanding and awareness of how healthy vision and hearing affect a child's well-being and a child's chances for a better education.

Harmon, E. L. Third-party payment increases utilization of home care services. *Hospitals* 42 (September 1, 1968): 68-72. I. Home care services have been limited by the lack of eligibility for third-party payment. II. Secondary: administrative records of enrollees in various third-party programs. III. & IV. Third-party payors, such as welfare agencies, Medicare, commercial insurance carriers and Blue Cross, should encourage individuals to use home-care facilities, which are less expensive than hospital and rest home facilities.

Harper, G. L. A comprehensive care program for migrant farmworkers. *Public Health Reports* 84 (August 1969): 690-96. I. Factors: financial, administrative, and cultural barriers, and difficulties with transportation to health-care facilities. II. Primary: development and problems with the San Luis Obispo County (California) Health Project. III. Develop programs geared to specific needs of the people needing care; face the problems of cultural differences. Respond flexibly to specific demands. Recruit aides from the community being served.

Haughton, J. G. Can the poor use the present health care system? *Inquiry* 5 (March 1968): 31-36. I. Welfare medical program excludes important services and gives only a few services to few people. We do not have a system of "care," defined as such, and the present system does not lend itself to proper utilization. II. Secondary; author's observations and opinions. III. Create a health system with the capacity and sophistication to deliver "care" to all persons, and in so doing reduce illness. The system should be soundly financed, efficiently organized, and free of discrimination. The government must take the initiative in leading such a system. IV. Describes a successful health care program developed in New York City.

Haynes, M. A. Some medical and sociological problems of the urban community. *Maryland State Medical Journal* 18 (September 1969): 80-82. I. There is a lack of understanding between health professionals and the poor and a shortage of physicians willing to serve the poor. II. Secondary: author's opinions and observations. III. Provide care with respect and dignity; reorganize and integrate services.

Heagart, M. C., et al. Use of the telephone by low-income families. *Journal of Pediatrics* 73 (November 1968): 740-44. I. There is a lack of true communication between the person calling and the person receiving the call. II. Primary: a random sample of medically indigent families were offered a program of pediatric care that resembled a private group practice. III. With continuous participation in a supportive medical care program, the poor increased their ability to communicate and adopted the telephone patterns of higher income groups. IV. While the study proved that the sample adopted the telephone patterns of higher income groups, difficulties did arise in doctor-patient relationships. Doctors used the phone less than the patients.

Herman, M. W. The poor: Their medical needs and the health services available to them. *Annals of the American Academy of Political and Social Science* 399 (January 1972): 12-21. I. Factors: unavailability of services, lack of personal physician, folk orientation (vs. scientific orientation to medical care), social distance from health professionals, and bureaucratic procedures. II. Secondary: general discussion, supported with factual documentation. III. Provide more financial support, increase personal attention in clinics, and offer more convenient and easy-to-use services.

Hochbaum, G. M. Public participation in medical screening programs: A socio-psychological study. *Public Health Service Bulletin* No. 572, U. S. Department of Health, Education, and Welfare, Washington, D. C.: U. S. Government Printing Office, 1958. I. No single or simple answer exists as to why some people use free public health services and others do not. II. Primary: personal interviews in Boston (451), Cleveland (445), and Detroit (305). V. The study found that three sets of factors were responsible for motivating people to seek a chest X-ray: the psychological state of readiness; situational influences; and environmental conditions.

Hochstim, J. R., et al. Poverty area under the microscope. *American Journal of Public Health* 58 (October 1968): 1815-27. II. Primary: poverty and non-poverty groups in Oakland, California were compared on health and certain economic and social items. V. Residents of poverty areas and those with incomes below the poverty level were more likely to report illnesses at rates above the national average.

Hoff, W. Why health programs are not reaching the unresponsive in our communities. *Public Health Reports* 81 (July 1966): 654-58. I. Preventive health care has low priority among those who struggle to satisfy their needs for food, shelter, and safety. Health agencies and professionals have negative attitudes toward stereotyped poor and minority groups. Inflexible programs and poor communications are also factors. II. Secondary: author's observations as assistant chief, Bureau of Health Education, California State Department of Public Health, Berkeley. III. Give health agency personnel special training in diverse cultural backgrounds of lower socioeconomic groups; involve local personnel as auxiliary workers in the health profession; and use local facilities for health education.

Hoff, W. Role of the community health aide in public health programs. *Public Health Reports* 84 (November 1969): 998-1002. II. Secondary: author's observations and opinions. V. The cultural gap between middle-class professionals and lower-class clients has been successfully bridged by the use of auxiliary personnel from the local community. Article gives a good bibliography of successful project reports on the use of paramedical personnel.

Hollingshead, A. B., and F. C. Redlich. *Social Class and Mental Illness.* New York: John Wiley and Sons, Inc., 1958. I. Lower-class patients who have an insoluble reality situation often have little desire to get better; they have a less favorable attitude toward psychiatrists than do upper-class patients. Techniques providing "insight" do not meet the needs of people seeking "outside" therapy. II. Primary: a community study in New Haven, Connecticut, of patients under the care of psychiatrists. III. More and better mental hospitals are needed, along with a new profession of workers to help the lower classes. Low-cost methods are needed to reach all mental patients. V. Social and cultural conditions do influence the development of the various types of psychiatric disorders at different class levels.

Holloman, J. L. S., Jr. Health care in the inner city. *Journal of the Kansas Medical Society* 70 (August 1969): 349-55. I. Clinics for the poor are dirty, confusing, and impersonal. II. Secondary: author's views. III. Clinics need fewer specialists and more doctors of various races and backgrounds; more NHCs are needed, and these should develop comprehensive health-care programs. V. A good article on general health-care problems, particularly those pertaining to poor blacks.

Hughes, J. S., et al. Patterns of patient utilization in a volunteer medical clinic. *North Carolina Medical Journal* 33 (May 1972): 430-35. I. Medical schools have had only a limited involvement with local communities; students are not community-oriented. II. Primary: the development and patterns of utilization of the Edgemont Community Clinic, Durham, North Carolina, which was staffed by medical students. III. A primary health-care program initiated by students and controlled by the community is a significant stopgap solution to many problems that the poor face in obtaining medical care. IV. This clinic served 860 patients, mostly aged 16-50, for routine physical examinations and for problems requiring continued care.

Hulka, B. S., et al. Scale for the measurement of attitudes toward physicians and primary medical care. *Medical Care* 8 (September-October 1970): 429-35. II. Secondary: author's own comments. III. Both consumers and providers of medical care should be consulted as to their attitudes, concerns, and satisfaction with the medical care provided. V. The methodological development and description of a scale to measure people's attitudes toward physicians and primary medical care is presented.

Hulka, B. S., et al. Determinants of physical utilization: Approach to a service-oriented classification of symptoms. *Medical Care* 10 (July-August 1972): 300-09. I. Perceived seriousness of symptoms, bed-loss days, perception of the physician's ability to relieve symptoms, and race were the significant variables in determining non-utilizers. II. Primary: 160 households in low-income urban area were interviewed; a discrimination function analysis was used on the data.

Hurtado, A. V. The organization and utilization of home-care and extended-care facility services in a prepaid comprehensive group practice plan. *Medical Care* 7 (January-February 1969): 30-40. II. Primary: data from the Kaiser Foundation Health Plan serving 15 percent of urban Portland, Oregon. III. For an efficient use of health facilities, use a screening facility to separate cases requiring hospital care or home care. IV. Description of a successful health program. V. This article describes the preliminary results of a public health service-funded project developed to provide extended care and home-care facilities of Medicare to a population of 100,000 receiving care under a prepaid health plan.

Hurtado, A. V., and M. P. Greenlick. A disease classification system for analysis of medical care utilization, with a note on symptom classification. *Health Services Research* 6 (Fall 1971): 235-50. II. Secondary: author's description of the development of a disease classification system. V. This article describes a new disease classification system developed for the Kaiser Foundation Health Plan. The diseases were classified into three major categories: chronic ailments, pregnancies, and emotional disorders; this helped achieve greater efficiency in the delivery of health care to Kaiser Foundation members.

Hurtado, A. V., et al. Determinants of Medical care utilization: Failure to keep appointments. *Medical Care* 11 (May-June 1973): 189-98. II. Primary: a study of subscribers to the Kaiser Foundation Health Plan in Oregon. V. Of all scheduled appointments, 16.3 percent were not kept. Those most likely to miss appointments were the high medical care utilizers. Demographic and psychosocial characteristics, as well as physician characteristics, were of much less significance in determining patient failures to keep appointments. The medically indigent had a significantly higher rate of appointment failures.

Ingles, T. Where do nurses fit in the delivery of health care? *Annals of Internal Medicine* 127 (January 1971): 73-75. I. Role-confusion exists among health professionals. II. Secondary: from author's background. III. Train nurse practitioners to fill the gaps in patient care.

Ingram, N. R. Planning for healthful communities: The neighborhood health center. *American Journal of Public Health* 56 (December 1966): 1987-89. II. Secondary: editorial. III. Health services should be only one part of multi-purpose community center having intimacy and personal appeal. Administrative planning needs to become more responsive to community needs and desires.

Irelan, L. Health practices of the poor. *Welfare in Review* 3 (October 1965): 1-9. I. Differing beliefs and attitudes of lower classes; less knowledge of resources; discrimination by doctors; social isolation. Public assistance programs have attacked symptoms rather than causes. III. Greater understanding by health professionals of differing values and social relationships. Better coordination between public health, welfare and outreach programs; health care should become a "right" instead of "charity." Health problems of the poor are directly related to the social structures of poverty.

Irvine, J. On not being upper class. *New England Journal of Medicine* 282 (February 1970): 453. I. The American public does not recognize the fact that the American Indian is not receiving his fair share of health services. II. Secondary: infant mortality statistics, TB rates for reservation Indians, income statistics, and Public Health Service Resource Budget. V. This letter to the editor comments that the American Indian represents the poorest of the poor in health services.

James, G. Poverty and public health—new outlooks. *American Journal of Public Health* 55 (November 1965): 1757-71. I. Factors: lack of money to buy services, long waiting lines, and language/cultural differences. Many poor are trapped in the vicious circle of poor health and unemployment. II. Secondary. III. Six suggestions to make medical care more appealing and comprehensive for the poor: (1) improved packaging of treatment, (2) research—to discover better ways of solving medical and social problems, (3) more personnel, new kinds of personnel, (4) more care of families and old people in their homes, (5) less reliance on symptoms and more concern for preventive measures, (6) more concern for the total person; more comprehensive care.

Kaplan, R. S., et al. The efficacy of a comprehensive health care project: An empirical analysis. *American Journal of Public Health* 62 (July 1962): 924-30. I. The "cycle of poverty" (the poor are poor because they are ill and ill because they are poor) is influenced by many complex underlying factors. II. Primary: school attendances in two similar housing projects, one with and one without a comprehensive pediatric care clinic, are compared to determine effect of health clinic on general life style. Improvement in school attendance was noted in housing project with health clinic, but the effect was small compared to other variables.

Kasl, S. V., and S. Cobb. Health behavior, illness behavior, and sick role behavior. *Archives of Environmental Health* 12 (April 1966): 531-41. I. Factors influencing health action: past utilization of medical services, perceived possibility that action produces results, cost of action, perceived value of action, factual information, and demographic variables. II. Secondary: observations gathered by authors. V. A good health behavior model for explaining factors related to the seeking of health care.

Kassebaum, G. G., and B. B. Bauman. Dimensions of the sick role in chronic illness. In *Patients, Physicians, and Illness*, 2nd ed., ed. E. Gartly Jaco, pp. 141-54. New York: The Free Press, 1972. I. Denial of sickness was more often emphasized by male, older, and less educated patients. II. Primary: study of 201 persons with one or more chronic diseases; women in sample outnumbered men three to one; slightly more than half were native-born Americans. III. Implication for further research: specify what dimensions of the sick role are perceived in different social settings.

Kasteler, J. M. Variations in compliance with medical regimens and utilization of medical services among patients with rheumatoid arthritis. *Dissertation Abstracts* 31 (1970): 2512-A. I. Factors: low self-esteem, feelings of alienation, lack of family integration, unhappy family life, little knowledge of disease, and unfavorable attitudes toward the medical profession. II. Primary: interviews with 126 patients with rheumatoid arthritis; half were private patients and half welfare patients in a large teaching hospital. III. Assist low-income families to improve family relationships; educate the public to increase knowledge of disease and symptoms; and encourage more favorable attitudes toward health profession. V. Welfare patients were poorer utilizers in a ratio of two to one.

Kegeles, S. S. Some motives for seeking preventive dental care. *Journal of the American Dental Association* 67 (July 1963): 90-98. I. Among the motives prompting persons to seek preventive dental care are the beliefs that one is susceptible to dental disease, that dental problems are serious, that dental treatment is beneficial; also a belief in natural causality, an esthetic concern for one's teeth, a lack of anxiety and fear about dental treatment and pain, and a positive appraisal of the dentist. II. Primary: interviews with 430 employees of a company that has a company-financed plan for dental care. III. Assess emotional impact of techniques and tools of dental practice to increase patient security.

Kegeles, S. S. A field experimental attempt to change beliefs and behavior of women in an urban ghetto. *Journal of Health and Social Behavior* 10 (June 1969): 115-24. I. Beliefs and attitudes incongruent with modern medical knowledge, particularly a skepticism in regard to vulnerability and effectiveness of treatment, lead to nonutilization. II. Primary: study of population in medium-sized metropolitan area. III. Black women in a heavily non-white area were given control and experimental educational material in an attempt to change beliefs about vulnerability to cervical cancer and the effectiveness of cytology, and to persuade them to visit a cytological clinic. IV. No significant difference in change of beliefs was noted between the control and experimental groups. The experimental group's utilization of clinic services was twice as great, however.

Kegeles, S. S., et al. Survey of beliefs about cancer prevention and taking Papanicolaou tests. *Public Health Reports* 80 (September 1965): 815-23. I. Factors: belief that self-diagnosis is as effective as professional diagnosis, early detection not viewed as important. II. Primary: studies from Alameda County and San Diego City, and a national probability sample of 1,493 noninstitutionalized adults, 20 years or older. III. Induce more private physicians to take cervical smears; explain to patients the benefits of periodic cervical examinations in doctors' offices; via a mass information program, alert women to the need of professional diagnosis and the benefits of early diagnosis of cervical cancer; solicit person-to-person those women who are not likely to be reached by mass communications; provide cervical cytology tests through a public health program to women who do not regularly visit physicians. V. Paper notes that women who were not motivated to take tests could develop a belief in preventive cancer care as a result of taking a test.

Keibuman, M. Poverty: A complex problem awaiting a thoughtful response. *Hospitals* 43 (July 1969): 29-33. I. The culture of poverty perpetuates itself, and too few individuals are committed to aiding the poor. III. Increase general consumer participation in health policy-making; make needed knowledge available and co-ordinate health services.

Kelly, C. Health care in the Mississippi delta. *American Journal of Nursing* 69 (April 1969): 759-63. I. Factors: no services available, extreme poverty, and transportation difficulties. II. Primary: OEO Health Center in Mississippi. III. Increase prenatal visits to decrease malnutrition. Improve overall environment as well as health care. Give *food* in addition to medicines (teach rural poor to grow food). Nurses need to follow up patients in their homes. IV. Both the general health and the economy of the community were greatly improved.

Kent, J. A., and C. H. Smith. Involving the urban poor in health services through accommodation—the employment of neighborhood representatives. *American Journal of Public Health* 57 (June 1967): 997-1003. I. Factor: "crisis orientation" of the poor toward health care. II. Primary: review of the Maternity and Infant Care Project, Denver Department of Health and Hospitals. III. Hire local poor to explain infant care clinic. Create programs that go beyond traditional public health practice. Create a new position of neighborhood representative to be filled by non-middle class, older females of long standing within the communities being served. IV. Innovations were successful.

Kessel, N., and M. Shephard. The health and attitudes of people who seldom consult a doctor. *Medical Care* 3 (January-March 1965): 6-10. I. No difference in social class was found among those who did not see a doctor regularly. The main reasons cited for non-attendance were "not ill enough," "too busy," and "couldn't afford to be ill." II. Secondary, and primary: from records of one physician in British National Health Service, 1949-1958. V. Non-attenders appeared to be as healthy as those who saw doctors regularly.

King, L., and L. Schwartz. Student activists see health in new ways. *Modern Hospital* 110 (May 1968): 118-20. I. Medical school graduates are less than fully capable of dealing with poor patients. III. Students in many medical schools have organized Student Health Organizations to offer seminars on human, social, and empathetic aspects of health care—topics conspicuously absent from formal curricula. OEO grant enabled students in California to work in poverty areas. IV. Students involved in California OEO program gained increased empathy and understanding for problems of the poor. V. Article describes "health team" of law students, economics students, ghetto area high school students, and community leaders.

Kissick, W. L. Effective utilization: The critical factor in health manpower. *American Journal of Public Health* 58 (January 1968): 23-29. II. Secondary: author's personal opinions and suggestions. III. Increase the efficiency of health manpower by: downward transfer of functions, education programs, career mobility, and better application of technology. V. This article details a general plan for the increased efficiency that will be required of the medical profession to deliver high-quality care to all people.

Kluger, J. M. The uninsulated caseload in a neighborhood mental health center. *American Journal of Psychiatry* 126 (April 1970): 1430-36. I. Most clinical services offered to the disadvantaged population involve covert barriers, physical and emotional. To assume that a prospective patient can wait for an appointment is to assume that he has the resources to sustain him over a period of crisis. This leads to a high rate of broken appointments and lower utilization. Staff frustration and feelings of powerlessness also lead to latent caseload insulation. II. Primary: the development of policies at a neighborhood mental health center in Denver neces-sitated by an administrative decree that there was to be no waiting list. III. A drop-in clinic was established; all patients were seen the first day they called. Open admission policy increased popularity with other agencies, and consultation services were provided so they might aid effectively with preventive services. IV. Same as above. V. Experiences of failure on the part of the staff gave them a sense of empathy with their clients; the staff became more cohesive and undertook honest evaluation of each person's abilities.

Knowlton, C. S. Cultural factors in the non-delivery of medical services to Southwestern Mexican Americans. In *Health Related Problems in Arid Lands*, ed. M. L. Reidesel, pp. 59-71. Tempe, Arizona: Arizona State University, April 1971. I. Conflict in values between Anglo-American health personnel and minorities. Anglo systems have been imposed on minorities who often reject them. High costs inhibit utilization. II. Secondary: author uses conclusions of research studies and his personal knowledge of cultures. III. Increase public subsidy of programs; drastically reorganize procedures; establish networks of clinics equipped for simple surgery and hospitalization; recruit Mexican-American students and motivate them to return to their own areas; and upgrade the economic and social conditions of Mexican-Americans in Southwest.

Koos, E. L. *The Health of Regionville*. New York: Columbia University Press, 1954. I. Social position in a community tends to carry with it values oriented to good or poor health practices. Doctors take narrow view of welfare patients. II. Primary: a sample of 514 families in upstate New York were surveyed over four years to determine health attitudes and practices. Doctors and the general conditions of health in the community were also reviewed. III. Health workers must overcome social class differences and learn to work with them. Doctors should be oriented to their responsibility as health educators and as participants in community. Greater emphasis needs to be placed on the desirability of having a hospital up to modern standards. V. The author describes varying health attitudes and behaviors of different social classes in a typical small town in upstate New York.

Koos, E. L. Metropolis: What city people think of their medical services. *American Journal of Public Health* 45 (December 1955): 1551-57. I. Lack of personalized service and the humaneness of old-time generalized practitioners were primary reasons for poor utilization. II. Primary: 1,000 personal interviews. V. Results: favorable response to G.P.s, not to specialists; 78 percent satisfied with Blue Cross, but only 49 percent satisfied with Blue Shield.

Kosa, J., et al. *Poverty and Health: A Sociological Analysis*. Cambridge: Harvard University Press, 1969. V. A valuable collection of articles on poverty and illness written especially for this volume. Authors include John Kosa, Monroe Lerner, Marc Fried, Irwin Rosenstock, David Mechanic, Julius Roth, Marvin Sussman, Arthur Shostak, John Stoeckle, Irving Zola, and Aaron Antonovsky. Extensive information on utilization of health services by the poor will be found in several of the chapters.

Kriesberg, L. The relationship between socio-economic rank and behavior. *Social Problems* 10 (Spring 1963): 334-53. I. Social rank and economic level are determinants of medical care utilization. II. Secondary: physician and hospital utilization has tended to equalize between socioeconomic groups, but there is still a strong relationship between socioeconomic rank and dental utilization. V. A good review of secondary sources.

Kriesberg, L., and B. R. Treiman. Socioeconomic status and the utilization of dentists' services. *Journal of the American College of Dentistry* 27 (September 1960): 147-65. I. Lack of money, childhood habits, and ideas about dental care affect utilization. II. Secondary: from household interviews with national sample of adults conducted by NORC in 1959; personal interviews with 1,862 adults. III. Stress early childhood training for dental care. V. Authors relate various sociocultural and socioeconomic variables to dental utilization.

Kriesberg, L., and B. R. Treiman. Preventive utilization of dentists' services among teenagers. *Journal of the American College of Dentistry* 29 (March 1962): 28-45. I. High-income teenagers receive more complete dental care, and their dentists are more apt to stress prevention. II. Secondary: from household interviews by NORC in 1959. III. Parental beliefs affect children. Create educational campaigns geared toward parents who will in turn teach their children. V. Underscores the striking relationship of financial resources to use: higher-income groups have greater dental utilization.

Lashoff, J. C. Medical care in the urban center. *Annals of Internal Medicine* 68 (January 1968): 242-45. I. Health care for poor is piecemeal, underfinanced, disorganized, and provided without concern for individual dignity. II. Secondary: editorial. III. Establish NHCs.

Laughton, K. B. Socioeconomic status and illness. *Milbank Memorial Fund Quarterly* 36 (January 1958): 366-85. I. Article reexamines hypothesis that low socioeconomic groups are ill more often than high socioeconomic groups and do not utilize medical services as often. II. Secondary: records of physicians' services in facilities where patients are enrolled in a comprehensive plan for prepaid medical care in Essex County, Ontario, 1948-1953. V. No appreciable trends were found in relationship to socioeconomic class, although lowest class was not included in study.

Lavenhar, M. A., et al. Social class and medical care: Indices of non-urgency in use of hospital emergency services. *Medical Care* 6 (September-October 1968): 368-80. I. Certain young and old segments of the patient population, particularly in the lower socioeconomic groups, utilize emergency room services routinely as an all-purpose clinic. II. Primary: sample of patient visits to Yale-New Haven Hospital Emergency Clinic during a two-week period. V. In addition to age distribution, other intervening factors such as marital status, family income, and usual medical care patterns are required to assist in discriminating between urgent and non-urgent use of emergency room services.

Lepper, M. H. Health planning for the urban community: The neighborhood health center. *Public Welfare* 25 (April 1967): 141-49. I. Initiation, availability, continuity and completeness of care affect utilization by poor. II. Secondary: authors conducted study. III. Suggestions for improving the four areas stated in I. Other proposals were: better community organization, an outreach program, more doctors, individualization of patient services, complete and continuous care, hiring of residents to work in neighborhood center, and coordination of all community facilities.

Lepper, M. H., et al. Approaches to meeting health needs of large poverty populations. *American Journal of Public Health* 57 (July 1967): 1153-57. I. Factor: there are 50 percent fewer M.D.s in poverty areas than elsewhere. II. Primary: statistical analysis by the Chicago Committee on Urban Opportunities, the State Department of Public Health, and the Chicago Board of Health. III. Develop three levels of care: public health nurses and aides, OEO NHCs, and teaching hospitals and medical schools.

Lepper, M.H., et al. An approach to reconciling the poor and the system. *Inquiry* 5 (March 1968): 37-42. I. Sociologic and economic developments bypass poverty groups. II. Secondary: statistics on use of services by poverty groups. III. Areas of social and psychological factors need most work. IV. OEO Clinic was established to meet needs of the poor.

Lerner, M., and O. W. Anderson. *Health Progress in the United States: 1900-1960.* Chicago: University of Chicago Press, 1963. II. Secondary. V. A classic examination of the major trends in health status and utilization in the first half of the century.

Lerner, R. C., et al. Social and economic characteristics of municipal hospital outpatients. *American Journal of Public Health* 59 (January 1969): 29-39. II. Primary: intensive interviews with

2,748 patients of New York City Free Clinics. V. Article concerns overutilization of city clinics, especially that segment (6.8%) classed as financially ineligible. For nearly half of these, their experience within the clinic system was of extremely short duration and seemed not to be based upon the desire to "cheat" the city by obtaining free care, but upon other circumstances.

Leveson, I. The demand for neighborhood medical care. *Inquiry* 7 (December 1970): 17-24. I. The high cost of services and the lost time and inconvenience involved in getting care are more than most poor people can cope with. II. Secondary: discussion of the economic and social costs of neighborhood health care. III. Provide health care at zero costs to the poor. If providing free health care will keep a man working and off the welfare rolls, it is public money saved.

Leveson, I. The challenge of health services for the poor. *Annals of the American Academy of Political and Social Science* 399 (January 1972): 22-29. I. The poor have less purchasing power, less knowledge, and less self-sufficiency than higher income groups. II. Secondary. III. Improve financing, physician-patient relations, and the coordination of health services with housing, welfare, and other agencies.

Leveson, I. Access to medical care: The Queensbridge experiment. *Inquiry* 9 (February 1972): 61-68. I. Substantial barriers to the receipt of ambulatory care exist for poor populations, even when it is provided without charge at a convenient location. Especially low utilization is noted for persons lacking alternative source of health care. II. Primary: utilization patterns of a Queensbridge Health Maintenance Service, offering free medical service to 1400 residents over age 60 at Queensbridge Housing Project on Long Island, New York. III. To make health services more accessible, it is not sufficient to remove financial and travel barriers. Health service programs for poor must be judged on how well they reach persons with health problems. IV. Generally low utilization was noted for population as a whole. Income appeared to be powerful determinant of health care patterns. Better educated and recently arrived residents were more likely to use services. Color was not significantly related to utilization.

Leverett, D. H., and A. Jong. Variations in the use of dental care facilities by low income white and black urban populations. *Journal of the American Dental Association* 80 (January 1970): 137-40. I. Factors: transportation costs and maldistribution of dental manpower. II. Primary: study of 457 families of children enrolled in Boston's Head Start Program, summer of 1968. V. Survey reported few social factors affecting dental care patterns, but blacks were higher utilizers of dental clinics than whites and traveled greater distances to receive treatment.

Light, H. L., and H. J. Brown. The Gouverneur Health Services Program: An historical view. *Milbank Memorial Fund Quarterly* 45 (October 1967): 375–90. II. Primary: NHC records of incoming patients. III. Tells of methods used and attitudes maintained by administrators and staff to achieve success in one of the earliest models for neighborhood health centers. IV. Community was involved   from   earliest   inception   of   the   facility.   A consumer–oriented attitude was maintained by all associated with the program. Local personnel were used to facilitate communication and integration with community. Experimentation and ingenuity in increasing efficiency and availability of health services was encouraged. Utilization and effectiveness were greatly increased.

Lowry, S. G., et al. Factors associated with the acceptance of health care practices among rural families. *Rural Sociology* 23 (June 1958):198–202. I. Rural persons of low socioeconomic status tend to not seek care as often as their more wealthy rural neighbors. Education had a positive correlation with seeking of services. II. Secondary: health agency records. V. Implications and suggestions for further social research are offered.

Ludwig, E. G., and G. Gibson. Self perception of sickness and the seeking of medical care. *Journal of Health and Social Behavior* 10 (June 1969):125–33. I. Subjects with low incomes, recent welfare contacts, and negative system orientations were most likely to fail in seeking medical attention. II. Primary: survey of applicants for social security disability benefits. V. Article suggests that negative orientations created by difficult situational factors can serve as rationalizations for failure to seek care.

Lurie, O. R. Parents' attitudes toward children's problems and toward the utilization of mental health services: Socioeconomic differences. *American Journal of Orthopsychiatry* 43 (March 1973): 251–52. I. Parents' attitudes and behavior reinforce deficiencies in availability of mental health services. Factors contributing to discrepancy are: the extent mother recognized behavior as deviant; kind of problems arousing mother's enxiety; whether parents felt satisfaction in life situation; mother's reactions to suggestions that child needed help; parents' conceptions about mental health professionals and appropriateness of mental health treatment for younger children; and preferences for alternative kinds of help. II. Primary: parents with income over $6500 were twice as likely to seek help as those with incomes under $6500. III. Mental health professionals should reexamine their roles and redefine their concepts of prevention and intervention in response to the needs of families of diverse social groups. It is suggested that parents would welcome new approaches that were applicable and relevant to their life problems.

McAtee, P. A. Poverty, relevance, and program failure. *Nursing Outlook* 17 (September 1969): 56–58. I. Factors: lack of understanding of illness and health and irrelevance of community nursing programs to life styles of minority groups. II. Secondary: opinions of author, in conjunction with a small local study of nurse-patient communications. III. Better attitudes of poor and public health nurses toward each other. Health care must include education. V. The expression "before every meal" implies a middle-class schedule of 8:00 a.m., noon, and 6:00 p.m.; it may not apply to the eating habits of the poor.

McBroom, W. H. Illness, illness behavior and socio-economic status. *Journal of Health and Social Behavior* 11 (December 1970): 319–26. I. Article concerns illness behavior; utilization behavior is only implied. II. Secondary: sample of 2,454 applicants for Social Security benefits from three regions of the United States. V. Study explores relationships between actual illness, illness reported, and responses to illness and social class membership. There were no indications that lower-class persons tend to overreact to illness or to overreport it; evidence suggests that upper-status persons do.

McKinlay, J. B.(a) The new latecomers for antenatal care. *British Journal of Preventive Social Medicine* 24 (February 1970): 52–57. I. Women from lower social classes feel inferior and thus underutilize antenatal services; they are more likely to become habituated to episodic and fragmented natal care. II. Primary: interviews with lower-class women in Scotland. III. Refocus attention on young primagravidae who are showing increasing tendencies to underutilize maternity care facilities. V. Article notes trends of primagravidae women to receive antenatal care later in pregnancy. Lower status groups remain the main contributors of underutilization.

McKinlay, J. B.(b) A brief description of a study on the utilization of maternity and child welfare services by a lower working class subculture. *Social Science and Medicine* 4 (December 1970): 551–56. I. Factors: values, norms, beliefs, definitions of women in a lower working-class subculture. II. Primary: interviews with 100 lower-class women in Aberdeen, Scotland. III. Underlying sociocultural characteristics should be determined and dealt with by reorganization of services. V. Article provides a theoretical model that can be used to examine subcultural characteristics.

McLaughlin, M. C. Issues and problems associated with the initiation of the large-scale ambulatory care program in New York City. *American Journal of Public Health* 58 (July 1968): 1181–87. II. Secondary: author's experiences. III. Neighborhood-based ambulatory care facilities are set up in New York City; eventual plans are for thirty such facilities, each serving ten to thirty thousand people in areas where needed. V. Article deals mostly with administrative, personnel, and financing problems of setting up ambulatory care facilities.

McNerny, W. J. Changing the health care system. *American Journal of Nursing* 69 (November 1969): 2428–35. I. The poor possess the same concern as others about health problems but are hampered by cost of care, lack of access to proper treatment, and lack of coping mechanisms for dealing with illness. II. Secondary. III. Reorganize health care system along nation- and area-wide lines; establish more group practice organizations; centralize major health services such as hospitals, doctors' office buildings, public health and health education agencies, into "health campuses"; establish neighborhood health centers in depressed areas and involve community in decision-making processes.

MacDonald, M. E., et al. Social factors in participation in follow-up care of rheumatic fever. *Journal of Pediatrics* 62 (April 1963): 503–513. I. Factors influencing participation are social circumstances, illness of others in the family, and the quality of interpersonal relations. II. Primary: study of 123 children admitted to a sanitarium. IV. The extent of illness among other persons in the family and problems in interpersonal relationship had a much greater effect on participation than social circumstances.

MacGregor, F. C. Uncooperative patients: Some cultural interpretations. *American Journal of Nursing* 67 (January 1967): 88–91. I. Uncooperative responses may often be explained by ethnic, social or religious background of patients. II. Primary: author cites three examples in which cultural interpretation and understanding achieved desired compliance. III. Educate professionals to cultural awareness; recognize differences in value orientations toward illness, hospitalization, and treatment. Be aware of overemphasizing psychologic determinants which may mask actual cultural problems.

Mahoney, M. E. Momentum for change. *American Journal of Nursing* 69 (November 1969): 2446–54. II. Subjective impressions of current trends in medical delivery. V. An outline of problems and possibilities in American health care philosophy. Major recommendations include increased use of paraprofessionals and medical assistants; extended educational opportunities for M.D.s; increased self-evaluation on the part of professional schools, medical centers, hospitals, and health agencies.

Maloney, W. F. The Tufts comprehensive community health action program. *Journal of the American Medical Association* 202 (October 1967): 411–14. I. Medical schools fail to work with people in the community and lack facilities to train doctors in community medicine. II. Secondary: a general description of the staffing and organization of two comprehensive, family-oriented NHCs. III. Change orientation of medical education from hospital medicine to community medicine. IV. Utilization and all aspects of health care delivery improved greatly in communities under study.

Martinez, C., and H. W. Martin. Folk diseases among urban Mexican-Americans. *Journal of American Medical Association* 196 (April 1966): 147–50. I. Social mechanisms within the ethnic population and society at large separate these people from the beliefs and actions of the large community. Folk beliefs and practices do not preclude the use of medical services for those health problems that are not defined by folk concepts. The lack of understanding of folk concepts by medical personnel inhibits treatment. II. Primary: interviews with 75 Mexican-American housewives living in public housing located in a large city; a high percentage knew of specific folk diseases and the therapeutic measures used in treating them. V. Paper deals with the extent of knowledge of folk concepts relating to health and disease, and a detailed account of etiology, symptomatology, and treatments.

Mechanic, D. The concept of illness behavior. *Journal of Chronic Diseases* 15 (February 1962): 189–94. I. Illness behavior refers to the various ways symptoms may be perceived, evaluated, and acted upon by different people. II. Secondary: author cites several other studies done on the subject of illness behavior. III. Learn more about the attitudes, values, and social definitions applied to symptoms and how these influence patient roles.

Mechanic, D. The influence of mothers on their children's health attitudes and behavior. *Pediatrics* 33 (March 1964): 444–53. II. Primary: data from 350 children and their mothers in Madison, Wisconsin. III. Consider the mother's attitude and its effect on a sick child. Mother may project illness onto her child. Educate both mother and child. V. Mothers who report more personal illness than average for themselves do the same for their children.

Mechanic, D. The sociology of medicine: Viewpoints and perspectives. *Journal of Health and Human Behavior* 7 (Winter 1966): 237–48. I. Factors: amount, visibility, and seriousness of aberrance; patient tolerance and understanding of abnormal state;

availability of resources; and certain social characteristics. II. Secondary: author cites many studies that contribute to placing medicine and health care in a larger social context. V. The article is primarily concerned with sociological research.

Mechanic, D. Response factors in illness: The study of illness behavior. In *Patients, Physicians and Illness*, 2nd ed., ed. E. Gartly Jaco, pp. 128–140. New York: The Free Press, 1972. I. Ethnic and cultural backgrounds influence patient perception. II. Secondary: author quotes many studies. V. There are many social factors that influence whether a patient seeks care for his illness, where he seeks care, etc.

Michal, M. L., et al. *Health of the American Indian: Report of a Regional Task Force*. Department of Health, Education, and Welfare Publication No. (HSM) 73-5118, April 1973. I. Factors: inadequate funds for IHS; limited staff; inadequate allotted monies for hospitalization of patients at off-reservation facilities; inappropriate recommendations from health providers due to social isolation and lack of cultural orientation; and jurisdictional disputes. II. Secondary: summary report using many statistical studies. III. Educate Indians to become involved in and to take responsibility for their own health care, including the reduction of accidents. Continue efforts to combat otitis media and to improve living conditions. Reorder priorities in IHS so that maternal and child-health activities make an increased impact on Indian morbidity and mortality. Expand and add nurse-midwife program to hospitals and field services.

Milone, C. L. The social sciences and dentistry: patterns of utilization of dental services in an urban neighborhood health center. *Journal of Public Health Dentistry* 33 (Summer 1973): 194–96. I. Spanish-speaking children were more likely than English-speaking children to use clinic. Black children completed treatment least often. Underutilization by whites may be caused by their having other sources of dental care, their feeling that the center is organized for minority groups, and their being unaware of their eligibility for certain dental services at the center. II. Secondary: utilization patterns at Hill Health Center, New Haven, Connecticut. III. Staff should attract more white children to center, attract and complete more treatment of the blacks, attract more patients age 15 years and over, and continue to attract and complete treatment for Spanish-speaking children.

Montiero, L. Expense is no object: Income and physician visits reconsidered. *Journal of Health and Social Behavior* 14 (June 1973): 99–115. II. Primary: data from the National Health Survey (1968) and a survey of Rhode Island residents (1971). V. Data show an inverse relationship between income and physician visits. Those who receive $3,000 per year or over $10,000 per year have equal rates of physician visits. Low-income persons have a higher need and are given publicly financed care; these conditions seem to stimulate more use of services.

Moody, P. M., and R. M. Gray. Social class, social integration and the use of preventive health services. In *Patients, Physicians, and Illness*, 2nd ed., ed. E. Gartly Jaco, pp. 250–261. New York: The Free Press, 1972. I. The poor are alienated from society in general and its organizations. The lower class participates less in preventive health services. II. Primary: a study of mothers with children under five years of age. III. Educate the poor and health personnel to a greater understanding of what each has to offer. Alter the perceptions and behavior of health personnel and the system rather than attempting to alter the life style of the poor.

Moore, F. J. Defining aggregations of the poor for community health center location. *Health Services Research* 4 (Fall 1969): 188–97. I. Factor: overcrowded health care facilities. II. Secondary: census data. III. Health centers should be located within one mile of the most distant point they serve. V. Study constructs socioeconomic indexes to identify poverty areas, then determines whether population density is adequate for efficient utilization of health centers.

Morris, N. M., et al. Deterrents to well-child supervision. *American Journal of Public Health* 56 (August 1966): 1232–41. I. Large family, low social-class status, and negative attitudes serve as deterrents to seeking well-baby health services. The greater the alienation, sense of powerlessness and social isolation, the fewer the number of inoculations. II. Primary: from household interviews with 246 black and white mothers in conjunction with the medical records of their 10-month-old babies enrolled in NC Memorial Hospital Well-Baby Clinic.

Muller, C. Income and receipt of medical care. *American Journal of Public Health* 55 (April 1965): 510–21. Low incomes make it difficult to afford proper medical care and to reach distant medical facilities. II. Secondary: a review of the literature and NCHs data. III. Public health workers have the responsibility to set a high priority on gaining a national financial commitment to providing medical services for the poor. V. Family spending on medical care rises sharply with income.

Muske, E. S. Health services at all levels of government: Desirable structure and relationship on the Federal level. *American Journal of Public Health* 58 (December 1968): 2198–2207. II. Secondary: data relates to the need to update health services because of popul-

ation statistics; statistics compare whites and non-whites. III. Coordinate state, local, and federal programs. Better planning and
design for agencies is needed.

Nall, F. C., and J. Speilberg. Social and cultural factors in the response of Mexican-Americans to medical treatment. *Journal of
Health and Social Behavior* 8 (December 1967): 299–308. I. The
environment of the Mexican-American subcommunity is unfavorable to the integrative and adaptive techniques involved in the
treatment of tuberculosis. II. Primary: sample of fifty-three Mexican-Americans in the lower Rio Grande Valley of Texas. III. More
research on the subject is needed. V. Study correlates attitudes of
households toward medical care and the medical profession. Integration into the ethnic subcommunity, especially into the family
unit, favors nonacceptance of tuberculosis treatment and vice
versa. Increased anomie correlated with increased acceptance of
treatment. No demonstrable impact of folk medicine beliefs and
practices on the acceptance of modern medical treatments was
found.

National Health Council, Inc. *Meeting the Crisis in Health Care Services in our Communities.* New York: National Health Council,
1970. I. Reasons for poor utilization from a consumer's and a
provider's point of view are enumerated in two chapters. II. Primary: a collection of reports from the 1970 National Health
Forum. III. Proposals for solutions are discussed in six chapters of
this volume.

Newman, H. N. Community leaders can help direct services to the
poor. *Hospitals* 43 (July 1969): 63–66. I. Hospitals are not responsive in dealing with the problems of the poor, thus the poor
will not utilize their services unless compelled to do so by an
emergency. II. Secondary: DHEW statistics. III. Hospitals should
"listen and learn" in dealing with poor and be flexible in policies
and procedures.

Nikias, M. K. Social class and the use of dental care under prepayment. *Medical Care* 6 (September-October 1968): 381–93. I. Behavior patterns with respect to dental care are the result of a
composite of interrelated causative factors, not just social class
differentials. II. Secondary: from administrative records of Group
Health Dental Insurance, Inc. III. Causative factors other than
social class must be considered in attempting to bring about uni-
form and optimum use of dentists' services. It is unlikely that
existing socioeconomic differentials in the use of dental care can
be eliminated by reducing financial barriers alone. IV. With financial barrier removed, lower social classes still have lower utilization. No comparison made with non-prepaid public behavior
patterns.

Nolan, R., et al. Social class differences in utilization of pediatric services in a prepaid direct service medical care program. *American Journal of Public Health* 57 (January 1967): 34–47. II. Primary: interviews with adults accompanying children enrolled at the Kaiser Foundation Health Plan facility in Oakland, California, over a four-day period in June 1964. III. Find out more about attitudes toward expectations of health care by ethnic minorities. Gear care to the life styles of the ethnic groups served. V. A thorough study with breakdowns of age, race, sex, social class, and number of visits. The elimination of financial barriers via prepayment did not result in equality of utilization of services among white and non-white population.

Norman, J. C. *Medicine in the Ghetto.* New York: Appleton-Century Crofts, 1969. I. The health problems of the poor are inextricably intertwined with problems of poverty, ignorance, and racial discrimination. II. Secondary: hard data are presented in some of the papers. III. Many suggestions are presented for improving black use patterns. IV. A series of papers presented at a conference on health in the ghetto at the National Center for Health Services Research. Excellent material on health care in ghetto areas; several of the presentations are highly emotional.

Notkin, H., et al. Knowledge and utilization of health resources by public assistance recipients. *American Journal of Public Health* 48 (March 1958): 319–27. I. Lack of knowledge of health resources available to public assistance recipients contributes to underutilization by this group. II. Primary: see *American Journal of Public Health* 48: 188–189 for information on survey population. V. An evaluation of health care delivery to welfare recipients.

Olendzki, M., et al. The significance of welfare status in the care of indigent patients. *American Journal of Public Health* 53 (October 1963): 1676–84. I. Irregular eligibility for welfare programs hinders support of the poor. II. Primary: study of 374 cases newly admitted to welfare program. V. Article concluded that the study population was highly unstable and that this had many implications for the continuity of care.

Olendzki, M. C., et al. The impact of medicaid on private care for the urban poor. *Medical Care* 10 (May-June 1972): 201–206. I. Clinics and emergency rooms in inner city, used as primary source of care by many indigent, are impersonal, fragmented, understaffed, bureaucratized, and demeaning to the poor. II. Primary: 729 former welfare clients in New York City were interviewed before and after the introduction of Medicaid. III. Medicaid attempts to give consumers a wider variety of choice in source of primary care. Study investigates extent to which study population switched from clinics to private practitioners after initiation of Medicaid.

IV. Proportion who considered private doctor their "main place" for medical care rose from 1 percent to 10 percent after Medicaid; a large majority continued to use and prefer clinics.

Osofsky, H. J.(a) After office hours: Some social-psychological issues in improving obstetric care for the poor. *Obstetrics and Gynecology* 31 (March 1968): 437–43. I. Factors: long waiting periods to see a different doctor every visit and perceived rejection by doctors. II. Secondary: other studies reviewed. III. Physicians should learn to approach the poor as human beings deserving respect. Professional-patient relationships should be based on need for professional help rather than social class. Physicians should be flexible in their roles and conform to individual needs. V. Doctors were found to base their relationships with patients on social class rather than medical needs. Patients of low income levels were found to lack value systems that allowed them to defer immediate gratification in the interest of long-term goals, a value especially important in prenatal and obstetric care.

Osofsky, H. J.(b) The walls are within: An examination of barriers between middle-class physicians and poor patients. In *Among the People*, ed. I. Deutscher and E. J. Thompson, pp. 239–257. London: Basic Books, 1968. I. Middle-class doctors have difficulties establishing meaningful doctor-patient relationships with lower-class patients; this affects overall medical care. II. Primary: sketches of five lower-class patients and two physicians.

O'Shea, R. M., and G. D. Bissell. Dental services under Medicaid: The experience of Erie County. *American Journal of Public Health* 59 (May 1969): 832–40. II. Primary: from fiscal records of recipients of Medicaid in Erie County, New York; cites results of Medicaid system of prepayment for dental services. III. Innovative new educational methods to alter dental attitudes drastically and to raise the low priority that dentistry has among welfare patients. IV. Those on welfare received less care than the "medically indigent" who were also eligible for Medicaid. Those in greatest financial need were less likely to visit the dentist than those enjoying a higher income.

Parsons, T. Definitions of health and illness in the light of American values and social structure. *Patients, Physicians, and Illness*, ed. E. Gartly Jaco, pp. 165–87. New York: The Free Press, 1958. I. The resistance of certain patients to dependence, the fear of losing status as an acceptable member of the group in some cultures, will prevent a person from going to the doctor. II. Secondary: author's observations of health behavior in American, British and Soviet societies. V. A classic article on the differences in health attitudes and behavior across culture.

Paul, B. D. *Health, Culture and Community.* New York: Russell Sage Foundation, 1955. I. In bringing modern medicine to various lesser developed cultures, one must learn to think like the people being served; one must start with people as they are. II. Primary: a book of studies, solving health problems in a wide variety of cultures. V. An interesting book dealing with various health problems around the world; but it offers no overall conclusions or suggestions for improvement.

Pearman, J. R. Survey of unmet medical needs of children in six counties in Florida. *Public Health Reports* 85 (March 1970): 180–96. I. Low family incomes and high dependency ratios severely limit family capacity to purchase medical services. II. Secondary: data from Headstart medical records, family interviews, county health departments, and school health records. III. Make medical services more available and less costly. V. Study undertaken to determine unmet medical needs of children under age 16. Results: 70 percent of Headstart children needed dental care; hypochronic anemia was common; over 50 percent of Headstart children were not immunized against smallpox and other diseases.

Penna, R. P. Pharmacy services in the health center. *Hospitals* 44 (July 1970): 70–72. II. Secondary: author's own opinions. III. Pharmacists can relieve the doctor of some of his duties in order to make health centers more effective, such as taking medication histories and counseling on nonprescription medication. V. A good article on the future of pharmacists in NHCs.

Perkins, R. A. *Health Care Patterns, Attitudes, and Resource Utilization of a Predominantly Indigent Population in Three Communities.* Ph.D. dissertation, Louisiana State University and Agricultural and Mechanical College. University of Michigan Microfilm File No. 72-28367:250, 1972. I. Gross morbidity was found to be related significantly to feelings of alienation at the personality system level; at the social system level, morbidity rates were found to be related significantly to incomplete family structure, position of a typical child, position of female head of household, and irregular church attendance and contribution. II. Primary: see title.

Peterson, M. L. What is needed is care as they see it, not as we do. *Modern Hospital* 113 (August 1969): 84–87. I. Factor: attitude of physicians that "they know best" without considering the wishes of those served; misunderstandings and distrust between consumers and medical practitioners. II. Secondary: personal experiences of the author with a community-sponsored clinic staffed by volunteer medical students and physicians. III. The poor must be allowed the opportunity to participate in decisions concerning the health policies of centers established for their use. IV. A growing empathy between professionals and consumers involved in clinic has resulted in increased utilization and cooperation.

Picken, B., and G. Ireland. Family patterns of medical care utilization; possible influences of family size, role and social class on illness behavior. *Journal of Chronic Diseases* 22 (August 1969): 181–91. I. High costs keep people away. II. Primary: study of 360 household records from a general practice in a village near Edinburgh. V. Authors test the hypothesis that patterns of illness behavior are influenced by psychosocial factors operating within the family. Results: No significant relationship was observed between social class or family size and the level of consultations of fathers and mothers.

Plaja, A. O., et al. Communication between physicians and patients in outpatient clinics: Social and cultural factors. *Milbank Memorial Fund Quarterly* 46 (April 1968): 161–212. I. Factors: lack of communication between physician and patient aided by factors such as social class, distance, and rural origin. II. Primary: fifty-nine interviews with outpatients. III. Develop an effective "social climate" in clinics to change rather than reinforce the patients' social conditions. V. The study analyzed the extent to which patients understood the doctor's vocabulary and instructions. Social scientists and M.D.s should work together for better communications in outpatient clinics. Study focuses on the relation of social class and vocabulary knowledge to patterns of doctor-patient communication.

Podell, L. *Studies in the Use of Health Services by Families on Welfare: Utilization of Preventive Health Services.* The Center for the Study of Urban Problems, Bernard H. Baruch College, City University of New York, Report No. PB 190:391, 1969. II. Secondary: survey drawn from New York welfare system rolls, mostly from Aid to Dependent Children categories. V. Major topics of this study were the mother's use of preventive services, prenatal care, and the health care of preschool children. Native-born whites were found to be the least receptive to preventive health care.

Podell, L., and R. Pomeroy. *Studies in the Use of Health Services by Families on Welfare. Special Population Comparisons — A) Between Husbands and Wives, B) With Other Low Income Families.* The Center for the Study of Urban Problems, Bernard M. Baruch College, City University of New York, Report No. PB 190:392, 1969. A) Between Husbands and Wives: II. Primary: sample of 161 black families; wives were surveyed in 1966 and husbands in 1968. V. Study shows health status perceptions and health services utilization of black husbands and wives. The wives were found to be more aware of existing services and tended to use them more frequently. B) With Other Low-Income Families. II. Primary: compares black families on welfare with other black low-income families; respondents were all mothers. V. The welfare mothers were more aware of health needs, had lower pain thresholds, utilized more medical care, and perceived their own health as being less sound.

Pomeroy, R., et al. *Studies in the Use of Health Services by Families on Welfare; Utilization by Publicly-Assisted Families.* The Center for the Study of Urban Problems, Bernard M. Baruch College, City University of New York, Report No. PB 190390, 1969. II. Primary: the first of a three-part study on the use of public facilities and services by New York City welfare recipients. V. Respondents, defined as White, Black, or Puerto Rican, were characterized by age, education, number of children, marital status, and place of birth. Stabilized welfare families coped well with the scattered health services and achieved as much care as lower-middle income families.

Pond, M. A. Interrelationship of poverty and disease. *Public Health Reports* 76 (November 1961): 967–74. I. Poverty conditions contribute to the spread of disease; the poor use medical care less frequently; illness is inversely related to income; and the lower the income, the less frequently dentists are seen. II. Secondary: author cites several studies. III. Removing the burden of poverty will contribute to the health of the poor and to their utilization of health services. IV. The poorer the family, the less healthy they are and the less tendency they have to use health services.

Pope, C. R., et al. Determinants of medical care utilization: The use of the telephone for reporting symptoms. *Journal of Health and Social Behavior* 12 (June 1969): 155–62. II. Primary: from medical records, interviews, and phone calls of 100 families in Kaiser Foundation Health Plan membership. V. Those with higher education, occupation, income and perceived social class were more likely to use telephone for reporting symptoms and less likely to use face-to-face contacts than those rated lower on the sociodemographic variables.

Pratt, L. The relationship of socioeconomic status to health. *American Journal of Public Health* 61 (February 1971): 281–91. I. Factors: low-income status, poor personal health practices. II. Primary: from detailed interviews with 401 currently married mothers in northern New Jersey city. III. Health programs should teach specific health practices, especially those regarding nutrition and exercise. V. Low-income women with good health practices were not found to be disadvantaged with regard to their level of health. They used fewer specialized and preventive medical services.

Rabin, D. L., et al. Use of health services by Baltimore Medicaid recipients. *Medical Care* 12 (July 1974): 561-70. I. Higher utilization of health services in Baltimore is explained by the fact that Medicaid recipients are sicker than the rest of the population. The higher rate of chronic illness accounts for higher hospital use for the working age population. II. Primary: survey of Medicaid recipients in Baltimore.

Rainwater, L. The lower class: Health, illness and medical institutions. In *Among the People: Encounters With the Poor*, ed. Irwin Deutscher and Elizabeth Thompson, pp. 259-79. New York: Basic Books, Inc.,1968. I. Health problems are less important than others, such as obtaining food and having rewarding social experiences. The lower class attach little worth to themselves or to their bodies. Illness is related to dysfunction in work, not symptoms. Team operations in health care programs do not meet the lower-class need for communication — psychosocial needs. II. Secondary: general discussions of lower-class attitudes. III. Create sub-professionals to take care of psychosocial needs of lower-class patients. Establish child-care programs next to (or near) schools.

Rayner, J. F. Socioeconomic status and factors influencing the dental health practices of mothers. *American Journal of Public Health* 60 (July 1970): 1250-57. I. Dental health behaviors are related to social class; dental values are a part of the family life style in the middle and upper classes. II. Primary: interviews with mothers of white school children, ages 11-14, in Buffalo, New York. III. Behavior precedes attitudes toward dental practices, so methods of adult education should be designed to influence children before attitudes are formulated.

Read, W. A. *Orientations to Health Services Among the Lower Class: Responses to Socio-Environmental Stress*. Ph.D. dissertation. Washington University. University of Michigan Microfilm File No. 71-19828, 391 pp., 1971. I. The survey showed that high-stress black families had a stronger orientation to public health care facilities than white families or low-stress black families. High-stress blacks had the lowest orientation to private physician care, this being mainly a low-stress white prerogative. Low-stress black families had the highest self-reliance in seeking health care and the highest skepticism about health care. II. Primary: a survey of 1,000 low-income households.

Rein, M. Social class and the utilization of medical care services. *Hospitals* 43 (July 1, 1969): 43-54. II. Secondary: data from

British National Health Survey. III. Offer free, on demand, comprehensive care, and use general practitioners for screenings and referrals. V. In England, the lowest social class makes the greatest use of the medical care services, and the care they receive appears to be as good as that received by other classes.

Reinhardt, U. E. Proposed changes in the organization of health care delivery: An overview and critique. *Milbank Memorial Fund Quarterly* 51 (Spring 1973): 169-222. I. The present health care system fails to deliver what is needed, where it is needed, and at the time it is needed. Available services are inefficient and costly. II. Secondary: various reform proposals and programs are examined in the light of pertinent empirical research. III. Author concludes that more empirical research needs to be done before the American health care system can be reorganized on a basis other than intuition or faith.

Richardson, W. C. Poverty, illness and use of health services in the United States. *Hospitals* 43 (July 1, 1969): 34-40. I. Author explores relationship of poverty to health status and utilization of services. The poor are sick more often than rest of the population, but make less use of services. II. Secondary: analysis of National Center for Health Statistics survey. The proportion of each income group that had a physician visit within the last year increased steadily as income increased.

Richardson, W. C. Measuring the urban poor's use of physicians' services in response to illness episodes. *Medical Care* 8 (March-April 1970): 132-42. II. Primary: data from three household surveys in three low-income neighborhood health centers. V. This article describes a new approach to the problem of measuring utilization of physician's services. Three factors were thought to influence response behavior: (1) severity of condition, (2) regular source of medical care, and (3) degree of poverty.

Richardson, W. C., and D. Neuhouser. First question in health planning: Does the public know what it wants, or not? *Modern Hospital* 110 (May 1968): 115-17. I. The public does not know what it needs and does not use what experts have provided; a disagreement between experts and the public. II. Secondary: general information. III. Public must be better educated to use health services. V. Authors debate who should decide what kinds of medical care should be provided, the provider or the consumer.

Riessman, F., et al. *Mental Health of the Poor.* New York: The Free Press, 1964. I. Factors: the poor face long waiting lists and private care costs beyond their means; bureaucratic requirements cause early withdrawals from health care programs; unskilled workers face noxious influences inherent in certain occupational tasks;

lower-class people have difficulty adjusting to middle-class culture, and they expect the therapist to assume a more active, medical role during interviews — which, when not forthcoming, often leads to discontinued therapy. II. Secondary: an anthology of readings. V. The authors question the Hollingshead-Redlich conclusion that "a distinct inverse relationship exists between social class and mental illness" (cf. *Social Class and Mental Illness*, 217). Analysis of the poor is best directed through appraisal of various subgroupings, rather than the disadvantaged as a whole. Treatment approaches for the poor should be based not only on more service, but on more appropriate service as well. Readings are grouped under four headings: Poverty, Mental Illness and Treatment; Low Income Behavior and Cognitive Style; Psychotherapeutic Approaches for Low Income People; and Rehabilitation of the Criminal, the Delinquent, and the Drug Addict.

Robertson, L. S., et al. Anticipated acceptance of neighborhood health clinics by the urban poor. *Journal of the American Medical Association* 205 (September 1968): 815-18. I. Health care of poor is fragmented, uncoordinated, etc. II. Primary: with respect to anticipated use of NHCs, families receiving comprehensive pediatric care were compared to similar families whose medical care was fragmented and uncoordinated in emergency clinics, well-baby clinics, etc. Families receiving comprehensive care continued in that program despite the greater convenience of the neighborhood clinics. The group receiving fragmented care said they would use the neighborhood clinic for health care, but only 58 percent expected to use it for illness care. III. Only to the extent that neighborhood clinics provide personalized, comprehensive care can we expect them to replace the present uncoordinated, fragmented pattern of health care prevalent in their target population.

Robinson, D. Obstetrical care and social patterns in metropolitan Boston. *Public Health Reports* 82 (February 1967): 117-26. I. Acute social problems experienced by unwed mothers lead to poor care and poor utilization. II. Secondary: from birth certificates filed in Boston in 1962. III. Better methods are needed to cope with high mobility of population; separation of childbearing women from community resources should be alleviated.

Robinson, D. Effectiveness of medical and social supervision in a multiproblem population. *American Journal of Public Health* 58 (February 1968): 252-62. I. Factors: lack of knowledge of how to treat complex social situations without turning to welfare agencies; patients unable to function in the private care system. II. Primary: report attempts to deal with social and medical problems of a 1,200-family housing project. IV. The effectiveness of the local center lay in providing some kind of ongoing supervision of medical cases after the crisis had been met and the family had failed to continue using outside medical agency care.

Roghmann, K. J., et al. *Child Health Services: Volume and Flow in a Metropolitan Community.* Rochester, New York: University of Rochester, 1967. I. Study assesses the motive for and pattern of child health services in a community. A larger proportion of low socioeconomic area residents had no doctor's visit within the last year. II. Primary: from interviews during 1967 Rochester Child Health surveys.

Roghmann, K. J., et al. Anticipated and actual effects of Medicaid on the medical-care pattern of children. *New England Journal of Medicine* 285 (November 1971): 1053-57. I. The study tested the theory that financial burden is the reason for nonutilization. II. Primary: interviews with 300 Medicaid-enrolled emergency room users. III. Marketing efforts are needed to bring consumer and services together. More manpower, improved transportation, outreach, culturally acceptable personnel and settings, and consumer participation in the program itself are required. Patients and staff must have a chance to develop personal relationships. V. The level of utilization remained the same with Medicaid as without it.

Rosenblatt, D., and E. A. Suchman. (a) Blue-Collar attitudes and information toward health and illness. In *Blue Collar World: Studies of the American Worker*, ed. Arthur B. Shostak and William Gomberg, pp. 324-33. Englewood Cliffs, New Jersey: Prentice-Hall, 1964. I. Organizational changes in medicine such as the replacement of the family physician by specialized professionals, have affected the blue collar world, which tended to receive care in the intimate confines of their own environment. II. Primary: major occupational groups were evaluated on their attitudes toward medical care. They were more dependent when ill and likely to have difficulty internalizing their sick role. III. More experimental demonstration projects are needed to determine the means of changing the organization of health care to deal with this population.

Rosenblatt, D., and E. A. Suchman. (b) The underutilization of medical-care services by blue-collarites. In *Blue Collar World: Studies of the American Worker*, ed. Arthur B. Shostak and William Gomberg, pp. 341-49. Englewood Cliffs, New Jersey: Prentice-Hall, 1964. I. Lower social classes tend to use lay referral network before turning to competent professional medical care. Other reasons for poor utilization are lack of preventive health orientation; the influence of nonrational thinking; prejudice on the part of health workers; and general "anomie" or normlessness.

II. Secondary: several studies cited. III. & IV. Relates success of demonstration projects experimenting with new methods of delivering and financing health care, including: Cornell Medical Welfare Demonstration Project; St. Vincent's Medical Care Project; Health Insurance Plan of Greater New York; Queensbridge Health Maintenance Service; and Cornell Navajo Project.

Rosenblatt, D., and E. A. Suchman. Awareness of physician's social status. *Milbank Memorial Fund Quarterly* 47 (January 1969): 94-102. I. Drab and low-status locations of public clinics are likely to hinder utilization by lower-class persons. II. Primary: a sample of 1,883 adults living in Washington Heights Health District (N.Y.), ranked according to SES. III. Communities should be willing to spend more money to see that clinics are properly "packaged"; the individuals most in need of outward symbols of success are most often the ones who attend public clinics. V. Folk-oriented and nonscientific groups tended to belong to the lower social class and tended to use outward symbols of success (office location, clothes worn, etc.) as the basis for judging a physician's competency.

Rosengren, W. R. Social class and becoming ill. In *Blue Collar World: Studies of the American Worker*, ed. Arthur B. Shostak and William Gomberg, pp. 338-40. Englewood Cliffs, New Jersey: Prentice-Hall, 1964. I. Low social class women more often defined pregnancy as being associated with sickness. Women with negative and escapist orientations were more often drawn into sick role. Women holding cultural values inconsistent with social class position were more prone to enact sick role. Women with low self-images regarded themselves as more ill. II. Primary: interviews with 115 obstetrical patients in a large lying-in hospital and 60 patients of obstetricians in private practice. V. A report of a study to examine the part social class position plays in motivating one to play the "ill" role.

Rosenkrantz, J. A. Community health centers offer high-quality care. *Hospitals* 43 (July 1, 1969): 67-69. I. Hospital outpatient departments are atrocious and ineffective. II. Secondary: general article. III. Full-time hospital-based health centers are needed. V. A general plea for hospitals to change their antiquated clinic systems.

Rosenstock, I. M. What research in motivation suggests for public health. *American Journal of Public Health* 50 (March 1960): 295-302. I. Health behavior is dependent upon a person's belief in the serious consequences of disease and the effectiveness of certain courses of action. Motives are frequently in conflict and the resolution depends on the individual's perception of the ultimate, greatest profit. Health-related behavior may give rise to nonhealth-related behavior, and vice versa. II. Secondary: author's opinions and suggestions. III. Successful public health programs must be based on adequate social research.

Rosenstock, I. M. Why people use health services. *Milbank Memorial Fund Quarterly* 44 (July 1966): 94-124. I. A decision to take health action is influenced by the individual's state of readiness to behave; by his socially and individually determined beliefs about the efficiency of alternative actions; by psychological barriers to action; by interpersonal influences, and by one or more cues on critical incidents which serve to trigger a response. II. Secondary: theoretical paper. III. Minimize barriers to action, increasing opportunities to act and providing cues to trigger responses. V. A review of literature on understanding and predicting health behavior. Paper presents a sophisticated model of medical decision-making based on present beliefs and perceptions of individuals.

Rosenstock, I. M., et al. Public knowledge, opinion, and action concerning three public health issues: Radioactive fallout, insect and plant sprays, and fatty foods. *Journal of Health and Human Behavior* 7 (Summer 1966): 91-98. I. A connection exists between income, education, and knowledge of health hazards. Nonwhite, poorly educated, and low-income groups tend to obtain health information primarily from face-to-face contact with neighbors. II. Primary: a stratified, multistage, probability sample survey of 1,493 adults 21 years of age and older living in private households in U. S. IV. While the mass media have been effective in reaching a majority of the public and in stimulating the learning of at least partially correct information, the nonwhite poorly educated, and low-income populace has been reached to a lesser degree.

Ross, J. A. Social class and medical care. *Journal of Health and Human Behavior* 3 (Spring 1962): 35-40. I. Education and income are directly related to the use of physician services. Reasons: purchasing power differentials; differing interpretations of illness; different orientation toward treatment; and knowledge and use of information differences. II. Secondary: analysis of National Center for Health Statistics Survey data, 1957-1959.

Salber, E. J., et al. Utilization of services at a neighborhood health center. *Pediatrics* 47 (February 1971): 415-23. II. Primary: from encounter forms for 1,989 children of 521 families registered over a five-month period at a neighborhood health center. III. Suggestions: easy accessibility, a reaching-out philosophy, and a more genuine staff concern. IV. After families were registered, variables such as race and education had little effect. Visits to physicians and dentists were higher than national norms for corresponding ethnic and socioeconomic groups.

Salber, E. J. et al. Health practices and attitudes of consumers at a neighborhood health center. *Inquiry* 9 (March 1972): 55-61. I. Eligibility requirements for participation in a neighborhood health center not known by residents. II. Primary: study of 200 households in a low-income housing project in Boston. III. Treat patients courteously, efficiently, and reduce waiting time; increase the quality of care. IV. The recorded responses taken from the study of the health center were favorable. V. A successful health center operation, with doctors patients like and trust.

Samora, J., et al. Medical vocabulary knowledge among hospital patients. *Journal of Health and Human Behavior* 2 (Summer 1961): 83-92. I. Doctors often use terms patients do not understand. Limited vocabulary, limited education, memberships in an ethnic group preserving a foreign language or having a low social class environment increased the probability of misunderstanding. II. Primary: 125 primarily low social class patients were asked to respond to terms commonly used by doctors.

Saunders, L. Healing ways in the Spanish Southwest. In *Patients, Physicians, and Illness*, ed. E. Gartly Jaco, pp. 189-206. New York: The Free Press, 1958. I. Factors: urbanization of Anglo medical services, high cost of services, lack of knowledge about services, and fear of them. Anglo medicine is impersonal and cold, while folk medicine provides familiar psychological rewards. II. Primary: author's own observations. III. Accept the vas cultural barriers separating Mexican and Spanish Americans from any aspect of Anglo society. Respect folk remedies and their importance to Mexican or Spanish patients. V. Author believes that despite hindrances, Anglo medicine will necessarily become a greater part of the care sought by the Spanish and Mexican Americans. For further reference see: Saunders, L. *Cultural Difference and Medical Care: The Case of the Spanish-Speaking People of the Southwest*. New York: Russell Sage Foundation, 1954.

Schneiderman, L. Social class, diagnosis, and treatment. *American Journal of Orthopsychiatry* 35 (January 1965): 99-105. I. Our health and welfare enterprise is bound by social class and culture; it is presently aimed toward a middle-class clientele. The current conceptual and knowledge base of how to work with the poor is inadequate. II. Secondary: author's own opinions. III. Move away from assuming the universality of our middle-class value systems; realize the implications of different life styles and value systems among various social class levels.

Schorr, D. *Don't Get Sick in America*. London: Aurora Publishers, Inc., 1970. I. The system fails to meet the medical needs of the poor. II. Primary: investigation by *Fortune* magazine of health care in America. III. Suggestions: increase National Health Insurance, HMOs, and neighborhood health centers. V. Chapter 8 is entitled, "Bringing the poor into the health system."

Schroeder, S. A. Lowering broken appointment rates at a medical clinic. *Medical Care* 11 (January-February 1973): 75-78. II. Primary: study of 503 patients at George Washington University Medical Clinic. V. Three methods of reducing broken appointments were evaluated: postcard to patient five days before appointment, phone call by nurse the day before appointment, and phone call by physician the day before appointment. Missed appointment rates: postcard, 13.9 percent; nurse calling, 19.5 percent; and physician call, 17.6 percent. The postcard notification system was instituted at the clinic.

Schulman, S. and A. M. Smith. The concept of health among Spanish-speaking villagers of New Mexico and Colorado. *Journal of Health and Human Behavior* 4 (Winter 1963): 226-34. I. The cultural definition of health is at odds with medical knowledge. So long as appropriately high energy level is maintained, and the person is well fleshed and free from pain, the villagers think of themselves as well and not in need of medical services. II. Primary: interviews were conducted with "insight-stimulating" informants both in and away from villages.

Schumaker, C. J. Change in health sponsorship: Cohesiveness, compactness, and family constellation of medical care patterns. *American Journal of Public Health* 62 (July 1972): 931-35. II. Primary: analyzes the changes in organization of health care in individuals and families before and after the introduction of a neighborhood health center. III. Patterns of organization of health care need to be understood in order to avoid costly, dysfunctional programs. IV. Operational change from a private practice to an ambulatory clinic of a large hospital resulted in a shift of medical care organization to less integrated, more diverse patterns.

Shannon, G. W., et al. The context of distance as a factor in accessibility and utilization of health care. *Medical Care Review* 26 (February 1969): 143-61. II. Secondary: an excellent review of the literature on this subject. V. Certainly physical distance alone is not the true variable nor is it all we are looking for; opportunity, cost—the price of foregoing alternatives—must also be considered.

Shapiro, S., and J. Brindle. Serving Medicaid eligibles. *American Journal of Public Health* 59 (April 1969): 635-41. II. Secondary: from analysis of Health Insurance Plan data in New York. III. Those responsible for financing, directing, and operating health programs must objectively assess the advantages, disadvantages, and results of their programs. V. A greatly increased enrollment of

Medicaid eligibles under the Health Insurance Plan of Greater New York caused many administrative and personnel problems.

Sheatsley, P. B. Public attitudes toward hospitals. *Hospitals* 31 (May 16, 1957): 47-49, 125-26. I. Financial inability, ignorance and lack of experience with hospitals, and resistance to hospitalization are noted, especially, among older people and those in low-income groups. II Primary: interviews with a cross section of American adults in 1955.

Sills, D. L., and R. E. Gill. Young adults' use of the Salk vaccine. *Social Problems* 6 (Winter, 1958): 246-53. I. Vaccination was clearly related to socioeconomic status; vaccination rate among those who said their friends were vaccinated was much higher than those who said their friends were not vaccinated. II. Secondary: interviews during a national survey in 1957. III. Make vaccination a topical subject; emphasize how attitudes against vaccination have changed. V. Living among people who have already been vaccinated is more important, as a motivating factor in having children vaccinated, than socioeconomic status.

Simmons, O. G. Implications of social class for public health. *Human Organization* 16 (Fall 1957): 7-10. I. Low-income groups relate well to health professionals of their own class — although they seldom have a chance to do so — whereas there is a natural conflict between middle-class health workers and lower-status patients that inhibits full use of services. II. Secondary: author's own opinions. V. Acceptance or rejection of health services to a great extent depends on how the services are offered to and perceived by low-income patients.

Simon, H. M. *Peer and Stranger Relationships between Public Health Nurses and Patients*, Ph.D. dissertation, Columbia University, University of Michigan Microfilm No. 67-15520, 377 pp., 1967. I. Verbal dominance affects communications between nurses and patients. When nurses were verbally dominant, discussion centered around matters requiring the advice and instruction of patients, leaving little time for patient complaints. Hence, nurse reassurance rates were low, and patient participation was confined to answering questions. When subject matter initiation and discussion were shared equally, patient complaints and nurse reassurance were higher. II. Primary: 176 taped conversations between nurses and patients. III. & IV. (See I.)

Solon, J., et al. Staff perceptions of patients' use of a hospital outpatient department. *Journal of Medical Education* 33 (January 1958): 10-21. I. Negative staff perceptions of patients act as a deterrent to utilizing facilities. Without a clear definition of the functions of the institution, each professional group interprets for itself what constitutes legitimate use of the clinic. II. Primary: from interview materials of physicians, nurses, and social workers involved in the outpatient program of a voluntary, medium-sized hospital. III. Hospitals should re-evaluate the purposes of the outpatient department in order to delineate policies in a rational manner.

Sparer, G., and L. M. Okada. Chronic conditions and physician use patterns in ten urban poverty areas. *Medical Care* 12 (July 1974): 549-60. II. Primary: household interviews, 1968-1971, in 10 urban areas. III. Provide health services tailored to specific poverty populations to increase utilization; provide broader medical care. V. National data understate illness levels in poverty areas. 85 percent are nonchronics, who are low utilizers of physician services.

Stein, B. The crisis in services to the poor: How we got into the mess and some suggestions for getting out of it. *American Journal of Orthopsychiatry* 42 (October 1972): 755-60. I. National economic conditions and governmental policies affect the economy of the nation and the overall ability of the nation to provide services to the poor. The unpopularity of welfare today (1972) is more extreme than at any time in recent history, a time when rising need collides with a tighter purse. When unemployment and inflation levy heavy taxes on many, the poor are the target of hatred and fear. II. Secondary, with documented statistics. III. Work for a climate of vigorous economic growth; raise the real income of the non-poor majority so as to make them better disposed toward helping the poor. Reduce unemployment so that there are fewer poor to serve. V. A good overview of the economic situation with particular emphasis on the forces that were at work in the early 60s and that led to the difficulties of the 70s. (Editor's note: the extreme inflation problem of the mid-70s further complicates the economic picture.)

Stephens, J. J. *Socio-economic Status and Related Variables that Influence the Initiation of Professional Medical Care among Montana Families.* Bulletin 631, Montana Agricultural Experiment Station, Montana State University, Bozeman, March 1970. I. Persons from low socioeconomic classes are less likely to seek preventive care or care for a serious condition because of high costs; poor are less likely to perceive illness symptoms as serious and requiring care. Misunderstanding exists between the poor and doctors; this has negative effect on any decision to seek care. Pessimism and feelings of powerlessness are prevalent among the poor. II. Primary: sample of 574 Montana low, middle, and upper-income persons. III. Provide funds for care and education of the poor; improve relationships between doctors and patients. V. Two variables discriminated most sharply in the utilization of care among different socioeconomic classes: (1) ability to pay (including health insurance), and (2) attitudes toward doctors.

Stockwell, E. G. Infant mortality and socio-economic status: A changing relationship. *Milbank Memorial Fund Quarterly* 40 (January 1962): 101-102. I. Infant children whose fathers have low earnings and low socioeconomic status tend to have a higher death rate. II. Secondary: based on well-documented statistics, one study done for the city of Providence, Rhode Island.

Stoeckle, J. D., et al. On going to see the doctor: The contributions of the patient to the decision to seek medical aid. *Journal of Chronic Diseases* 16 (September 1963): 975-89. I. In comparison with higher classes, the lower classes base expectations for medical care on interpersonal relations rather than on technical skills, and they are generally distrustful of medical personnel. II. Secondary: a good review of materials showing factors that influence the decision to see medical aid. III. Health programs should be directed toward the non-attending population; services should be geared to meet the concerns of lower-class patients.

Stoeckle, J. D., et al. The neighborhood health center: Reform ideas of yesterday and today. *New England Journal of Medicine* 280 (June 1969): 1385-91. I. NHCs are subject to conflicting pressures to bring services closer to the population and to efficiently organize the centers. V. Article details four ideas that have dominated the NHC movement since the early 1900s: district location, community participation, bureaucratic organization, and preventive care.

Strauss, A. L. Medical ghettos. *Transaction* 4 (May 1967): 7-15. I. Present medical organization and the planning for future development of medical delivery assume that hitherto medically disadvantaged groups can be reached without a radical transformation of the medical care system. Medical systems have never serviced lower-income groups in the past because they are not designed to do so. Professionals have not been trained in the special skills necessary to deliver quality care to poor. II. Secondary: a general article. III. Speed up initial visits for medical care; improve experiences with the medical system; improve communications about necessary regimens; increase the likelihood of compliance with regimens at home; increase likelihood of necessary visits to medical facilities; and decrease the time between necessary visits. Author suggests a number of recommendations aimed at reorganizing and increasing the effectiveness of the medical care system.

Stuart, B. C. National health insurance and the poor. *American*

Journal of Public Health 62 (September 1972): 1252-59. I. Most current proposals for national health insurance, and specifically the President's Family Health Insurance Plan, will actually reduce coverage now offered to the poor or continue discrimination against them. II. Secondary: analysis of Medicaid utilization and expenditure data. IV. Article details relative success of current Medicaid plan.

Suchman, E. A. Sociomedical variations among ethnic groups. *American Journal of Sociology* 70 (November 1964): 319-31. I. The more ethnocentric and socially cohesive a group, the more likely it is that the group is ignorant and skeptical toward the medical profession. II. Primary: personal interviews with 2,215 families in New York City. III. Break down resistance of groups to medical care in large cities, where groups of similar ethnic background band together. IV. Article stresses the perils of ethnocentricity.

Suchman, E. A. (a) Social patterns of illness and medical care. *Journal of Health and Human Behavior* 6 (Spring 1965): 3-16. I. Social structure was not found to be related to either health status or source of medical care. Social status and age affect a person's selection of health aid. II. Primary: interviews with a 1,883 sub-sample randomly selected from a probability sample of 5,340 adults in Washington Heights District in New York City. III. There needs to be more congruence between community and health services and new organizational methods that translate into accepta-ble forms for society. Social institutions should "reach out" to people needing services.

Suchman, E. A. (b) Social factors in medical deprivation. *American Journal of Public Health* 55 (November 1965): 1725-33. I. Lower socioeconomic groups are socially isolated and ethnocentric. Ethnocentricity is related to a lower level of knowledge about disease, unfavorable attitudes toward medical care, and depen-dency on lay support during illness. II. Primary: household health survey of representative cross section of 1,883 adults in low-in-come neighborhood compared with 1960 census. III. Gear medical services to low-income and minority groups. Increase communica-tion between the poor and health officials.

Suchman, E. A. (a) Ethnic and social factors in medical care orienta-tion. *Milbank Memorial Fund Quarterly* 47 (January 1969): 69-77. I. The less cosmopolitan and parochial the form of social organization of an ethnic group, the more likely it is to adhere to nonscientific health orientations. The more ethnocentric and cohe-sive the social group, the less likely it is to accept the objectives of the formal medical care system. II. Primary: a sample of 1,883 adults living in the Washington Heights Health District. III. It is doubtful that barriers interfering with medical care for minority groups in big cities can be removed, except as barriers to full participation in other aspects of American society are also removed.

Suchman, E. A. (b) Social factors in illness behavior. *Milbank Memorial Fund Quarterly* 47 (January 1969): 85-93. I. The more parochial the social structure in which an individual lives, and the more his health orientation tends to be popular (nonscientific) in character, the more difficulty he will have in accepting and adjusting to the modern medical care system. II. Primary: 137 cases from the Washington Heights Community Master Sample Survey. III. The strong group identification of individuals in parochial-popular groups provides a natural avenue for utilization of health services, if they can be organized in such a way as to receive the group's approval. To secure this approval, the medical care program must become part of the popular health culture of the group. V. Article analyzes the differences between parochial-popular and cosmopolitan-scientific groups in response to stages of symptom experience, assumption of the sick role, medical care contact, dependent-patient role, and recovery or rehabilitation.

Suchman, E. A. Stages of illness and medical care. In *Patients, Physicians, and Illness*, 2nd ed., ed. E. Gartly Jaco, pp. 155–171. New York: The Free Press, 1972. I. Selection of care is determined by knowledge, availability, convenience of services, and the influences of the social groups upon the individual. II. Primary: interviews with a 1,883 randomly selected sample of respondents in the Washington Heights District of New York City. V. Conclusion: a positive appraisal of the pathways and routines established by the medial system for care of the ill. Mechanics of current medical system work rather smoothly.

Tagliacozzo, D. L., and H. O. Mauksch. The patient's view of the patient's role. In *Patients, Physicians, and Illness,* ed. E. Gartly Jaco, pp. 172-85. New York: The Free Press, 1958. I. The ability of a patient to cooperate in his recovery is handicapped by inadequate communications, which fail to convey the proper expectations for his being a "good" patient. II. Primary: a study in a metropolitan voluntary hospital exploring the extent to which hospitalized patients understand their rights and the criteria for legitimate claims.

Tiven, M. B. *Older Americans: Special Handling Required.* Chapter III, Health, pp. 19-27. Washington, D. C.: National Council on Aging, 1971. I. Older people often think symptoms are a normal part of growing old and do not seek help. Limited mobility interferes with older people going to see the doctor. II. Secondary: a general discussion of the health needs and health care of older people. II. Encourage physicians and other health personnel to take a less negative attitude toward the elderly. Eliminate the gaps in Medicare coverage, such as nonpayment for preventive health services, extended care, and home care. Older people would use medical services more extensively if they could afford the cost and if they could get to the services with less difficulty.

Torrens, P. R., and D. G. Yedvab. Variations among emergency room populations: A comparison of four hospitals in New York City. *Medical Care* 8 (January-February 1970): 60-75. I. Emergency rooms often served as only source of medical care for the poor. II. Primary: 1,113 patients of four hospitals in New York City emergency rooms were interviewed as they waited to receive care. III. Reorganize facilities so that the poor do not have to use an emergency room as a "family physician."

Tranquada, R. E. A health center for Watts. *Hospitals* 41 (December 16, 1967): 43-47. I. Former health services were inaccessible, fragmented, unacceptable, discontinuous, and limited. II. Secondary: project director's description of program. III. Offer a group practice providing continuity from personal physicians and comprehensive care that is acceptable and accessible to the users.

Triplett, J. L. Failure avoiders—or success seekers? *Nursing Outlook* 17 (September 1969): 68-71. I. Poor users perceived high threat in past interactions, had little need for social experiences, and had little need for recognition as "good" mothers. In other words, they acted to avoid failure. High utilizers needed recognition as good mothers and social experiences, and these needs were stronger than any threat they perceived. II. Primary: study of 40 families connected with a midwest public health agency. III. Nurses should recognize the potential and actual threat in interactions, determine the needs of individuals, and provide successful experiences to those securing health services.

Tucker, M. A. Utilization and price analysis: Prospects for avoiding higher program costs in health care. *American Journal of Public Health* 59 (July 1969): 1226-42. I. Increased funding (Medicare) with neither control nor concern for the consequences (rise in prices) has resulted in lower utilization. II. Secondary: from the medical care components of Consumer Price Index: regression analysis techniques to determine health care price increase model. III. Policy makers should undertake detailed analysis of inflationary pressures of proposed programs.

Tucker, M. A. Effect of heavy medical expenditures on low income families. *Public Health Reports* 85 (May 1970): 419-25. I. Factors: lack of money; no health insurance. II. Secondary: 1963

National Opinion Research Center survey. III. Medical care at low cost should be made available to the poor. Paying for medical care now can be catastrophic to even middle and high-income families.

Tyroler, H. A., et al. Patterns of preventive health behavior in populations. *Journal of Health and Human Behavior* 6 (Fall 1965): 128-40. Part I of article: Acceptance of poliomyelitis vaccine within families. I. Lower acceptance of immunization by father in lower social class led to higher number of lower-class families with no members vaccinated. II. Primary: household interviews measuring response to oral immunization in Dade County, Texas. Part 2 of article: Levels of tooth salvage within families. I. Nonwhite and white lower class had lowest levels of tooth salvage because they had not seen dentists. II. Primary: from a statewide (Texas) survey of dental health.

United States Department of Health, Education, and Welfare. *Human Investment Program: Delivery of Health Services for the Poor.* Washington, D.C.: U. S. Government Printing Office, December 1968. I. Barriers to medical services for the poor include inability to pay, fragmentation of care, operational procedures of the services, attitudes toward health care, racial discrimination, and a lack of facilities and manpower. II. Primary: National Health Survey.

United States Department of Health, Education, and Welfare (a) Public Health Service. *Health Characteristics of Low-Income Persons.* Vital and Health Statistics. Washington, D. C.: U. S. Government Printing Office, July 1972. II. Primary—National Health Survey, 1972. V. Statistical report of number of physician visits, reasons for visit, and hospital use by age and family size among low-income persons.

United States Department of Health, Education, and Welfare. (b) *The Children and Youth Projects: Comprehensive Health Care in Low-Income Areas.* Washington, D. C.: U. S. Government Printing Office, July 1972. II. Factors: lack of doctors and dentists; crowded outpatient departments; long distances to source, particularly in rural areas; need for baby care at home while mother takes other children to get medical attention; language barriers; "crisis" attitude toward medical care; poor attitude toward medical care; poor attitude toward keeping appointments. II. Secondary: summary report of 59 Children and Youth projects in 28 states, the District of Columbia, the Virgin Islands, and Puerto Rico. III. Children require services that deal with basic physical needs, as well as social, emotional, and educational problems. Through parent education, the projects hope to instill the concept of preventive medicine. Cultural enrichment is offered through summer camps, arts and crafts, and recreational programs. Projects try to offer neighborhood locations, transportation and child care, convenient hours, and personalized care. Consumer participation is growing.

United States Department of Health, Education, and Welfare (c), National Center for Health Services Research and Development. *Health Service Use, National Trends—1953-1971.* (HSM) 73-3304, October 1972. II. Primary: data are based on four parallel studies of random samples of the nation's families conducted in 1953, 1958, 1964, and 1971. III. In order for health care to be equal for all classes, care for disadvantaged groups should be increased to compensate for a greater rate of illness and disability. V. This report highlights some of the major policy issues concerning the distribution of health services in the U. S. Findings from this report both support and contradict the view that the U. S. is attaining equalization of health care.

United States Department of Health, Education, and Welfare. *The Maternal and Child Health Service Reports on Research to Improve Health Services for Mothers and Children.* (HSM) 73-5116, May 1973. II. Primary: brief reports on ten studies, some of which are covered more fully in published reports. III. & IV. An infant mortality rate was reduced from 10.2 percent to 6.3 percent when a Care-by-Parent Unit was established at the University of Kentucky Medical Center High Risk Infancy Nursery. A study on "Adolescent Health in Harlem" suggests the need for comprehensive health services to deal with the variety and multiplicity of adolescent health problems. Another study showed the "Effectiveness of Counseling at the Time of Pregnancy Tests" by nurses.

Urvant, P. Health advocates. *Public Health Reports* 84 (September 1969): 761-66. I. The poor lack knowledge of the legal rights that would enable them to improve their unhealthy environment. II. Secondary: author's description of NHC in Bronx, New York City. III. Change the environment of the poor. Start health advocacy departments; give the poor knowledge of their legal rights regarding health and safety.

Vaughn, B. J. Maternal and infant care project: Results in Dade County, Florida. *Southern Medical Journal* 61 (June 1968): 641-45. II. Primary: personal interviews with 4,878 mothers. III. Increase comprehensive medical care. IV. Project resulted in reduced maternal morbidity, still birth rate, number of premature infants, neonatal morbidity, and infant mortality. Chief overall reduction was in the nonwhite group. V. The Dade County Maternal and Infant Care Project 515 has, in two and one-half years, given care to 4,878 medically indigent mothers. The result has been reduced maternal and infant mortality and morbidity.

Wallace, H. M., et al. Comprehensive health care of children. *American Journal of Public Health* 58 (October 1968): 1839-47. II. Secondary: authors' opinions. III. Article defines the objectives of a comprehensive health-care program for children which should include optional care, coordinated care, accessible care, and continuous care.

Wallach, R. C., and G. Blinick. Community prenatal care: An integrated approach. *American Journal of Obstetrics and Gynecology* 105 (November 1969): 808-12. I. Factors: lack of personal involvement with personnel because the patient comes to the clinic so late in pregnancy; physical setting of obstetrical clinics leaves much to be desired; prenatal care does not have high priority among the poor; transportation problems are severe; lack of continuity exists when patients are referred from gynecologist to obstretician. II. Secondary. III. Rehabilitate the physical setting of the clinic; increase the resident participation in clinic so continuity increases and more personal involvement results; integrate the clinic services (ob, gyn, and family planning) in the same location, and increase accessibility by providing night clinics. IV. After adopting the above measures, the clinic had a low rate of failed appointments, increased incidence of first trimester registration, and more clinic visits.

Walsh, J. L. Nurses, professional striving and the poor: A case of incompatibility. *Social Science and Medicine* 3 (August 1969): 217-27. I. PH nurses, who are members of a high-striving occupational group, approach poor patients less positively than they do middle-class patients. II. Primary: responses from 110 PH nurses in twa large urban PH departments in the East. III. Educational changes are needed to ensure adequate health care at all social levels; offer higher rewards to those who will work with the poor.

Walsh, J. L., and R. H. Elling. Professionalism and the poor—structural effect and professional behavior. *Journal of Health and Social Behavior* 9 (March 1968): 16-28. I. Members of high-striving occupational groups have negative orientation toward the poor. II. Primary: interviews with 207 health professionals, 16 M.D.s, 110 nurses, and 72 sanitarians. III. Occupational organizations may have to build into the system a greater form of reward for serving the impoverished and greater financial and professional rewards for those with the will and skill to serve the poor.

Wan, T. T. H., and S. J. Soifer. Determinants of physician utilization: A causal analysis. *Journal of Health and Social Behavior* 15 (June 1974): 100-108. I. Direct causal variables for predicting physician use are (1) the need for care, measured by the proportion of household members who have health disorders and respond to their illnesses; (2) the average cost per visit and health insurance coverage; and (3) the proportion of persons aged 65 and over and the percentage of females in each household. II. Primary: study of 2,168 households in a five-county area (New York and Pennsylvania). III. It is essential to develop and implement a public policy that will (1) pay in full for all physician visits, laboratory tests, hospitalization, etc.; (2) reduce the loss of income resulting from poor health and disability by increasing disability and rehabilitation coverage; and (3) provide counseling and referral programs to educate people more effectively to health problems and the importance of recognizing symptoms.

Watkins, E. L. Low-income Negro mothers—their decision to seek prenatal care. *American Journal of Public Health* 58 (April 1968): 655-67. I. Expectant mothers saw little value in prenatal care and lacked the money to choose preferred facilities. A higher proportion of early initiators described feeling sick in first four months of pregnancy. II. Primary: group of low-income, married, pregnant Negro women seeking prenatal care in first four months of pregnancy compared with group of women with similar characteristics who obtained care in last trimester. III. Health workers must find new ways of effectively promoting value of prenatal care and providing medical care in such a way as to convey concern for the individual. System for payment should give mothers choice of facilities.

Watts, D. D. Factors related to the acceptance of medicine. *American Journal of Public Health* 56 (August 1966): 1205-12. I. Factors: social problems, nonacceptance of middle-class values; difficulties in obtaining services from medical care facilities; long waiting periods for appointments; lack of financial aid for some who need it; and general "red tape." II. Primary: sample of 208 low-income and high social-problem families was studied to find social, psychological and cultural factors related to acceptance of modern medicine. III. Simplify procedures at medical facilities; assist persons with social problems; motivate them to seek care by informing them of their personal health status and future possibilities. IV. Article describes a demonstration project in which slum families were given full medical examination and were informed of health status and referred for further treatment. Eighty percent of the cases followed through on some or all of their medical referrals. Cases that received assistance with social problems were more likely to follow through on referrals.

Weinerman, E. R., et al. Yale studies in ambulatory medical care V. determinants of use of hospital emergency services. *American*

Journal of Public Health 56 (July 1966): 1037-60. II. Primary: two thousand patient visits to the emergency service of the Yale-New Haven Hospital during a two-week period were analyzed. III. Develop a community system of medical care which will provide personal, continuous, and comprehensive health care to all classes of the population. V. Lower-class persons tended to use the hospital emergency service more frequently than those of higher classes, and for a significant number of low-income cases the emergency service was their only source of medical care.

Weiss, J. E., and M. R. Greenlick. Determinants of medical care utilization: The effect of social class and distance on contacts with the medical care system. *Medical Care* 8 (November-December 1970): 456-62. I. The poor are less verbal and have a tendency to "walk in" rather than to use the telephone for appointments. II. Primary: from medical, administrative, and telephone-contact records of 3,106 members of the Kaiser Foundation Health Plan, Portland, Oregon, in 1967. III. Study suggests that more "walk in" clinics should be provided. V. Walk-in rates of the working class tend to decrease, although irregularly, with increased distances from a clinic, and the rates drop sharply at 15 miles. The use of emergency room increases sharply at 15 miles.

Weiss, J., et al. Use of mental health services by poverty and non-poverty members of a prepaid group practice plan. *Health Services Report* 88 (August-September 1973): 654-62. II. Primary: comparison in utilization rates between a poverty population of 7,000 in a prepaid health plan having access to a mental health clinic. V. Poverty and nonpoverty groups were compared in respect to utilization rate, referral patterns, and appointment keeping. The findings of this study suggest a need for further research and analysis of the social interaction processes influencing the mental health and subsequent referral system of poverty groups.

Welch, S., et al. Some social and attitudinal correlates of health care among Mexican Americans. *Journal of Health and Social Behavior* 14 (September 1973): 204-13. I. The article raised more questions than it answered. There was little evidence of Mexican-American folk culture; most respondents had a family doctor, went to a dentist and an eye doctor at least occasionally, and utilized other health services to a large extent. Questions raised included: "Why are medical pathologies among this group so high?" and "Why is the outcome of their utilization in terms of illness and mortality so different from other groups?" II. Primary: a sampling of four Nebraska communities with high Mexican-American population. Attitudinal characteristics made little difference in health-care seeking behaviors.

White, E. L. A graphic presentation of age and income differentials in selected aspects of morbidity, disability, and utilization of health services. *Inquiry* 5 (March 1968): 18-30. II. Secondary: analysis of National Center for Health Statistics survey, 1964-1967. V. Dental utilization was directly related to income, because this type of service is less affected by welfare and insurance programs. Low-income families tend to see physicians in outpatient clinics. Use of telephone consultations increased as family income rose.

White, K. L., et al. International comparisons of medical care utilization. *New England Journal of Medicine* 277 (September 1967): 516-22. II. Primary: data from household interviews conducted in small areas of England, Yugoslavia and the United States. V. There were some interesting conclusions drawn from this study besides the need for further research; people in the three vastly different communities appear to consult doctors in a similar fashion, but vary substantially in hospital utilization rates.

White, M. K., et al. Hard-to-reach families in a comprehensive care program. *Journal of the American Medical Association* 201 (September 1967): 801-806. I. High morbidity and family disorganization made continuous care almost impossible. II. Primary: families divided into easy-to-reach, hard-to-reach, and unwed-mother groups; personal interviews with female heads of household. III. Persistent calls and visits should be made to involve families. IV. 76 percent of hard-to-reach group came into program. V. Study measured amount of money per capita needed to bring different groups into program. Other social characteristics that affected the success rate of bringing people into program were examined. Special effort was made to contact unwed mothers.

Whitlock, R. P. Office of Economic Opportunity dental programs. *American Journal of Public Health* 59 (June 1969): 923-25. I. Dental care is the most universal health need of the poor. II. Secondary: dental programs in Head Start, Job Corps, Upward Bound, VISTA, and NHCs. (No sources listed.)

Williamson, J. W., and J. B. Tenney. *Health Services Research Bibliography*, United States Department of Health, Education and Welfare Publication No. (HSM) 72:3034, 1972-1973. II. Section IV of this bibliography is devoted to "Health Services Provision and Utilization" and lists 82 publications.

Willie, C. V. The social class of patients the public health nurses prefer to serve. *American Journal of Public Health* 50 (August 1960): 1126-36. II. Primary: Sixty four nurses were interviewed. V. Demonstrated attitudes of preference for patients by social class.

Wingert, W. A., et al. The demographical and ecological characteristics of a large urban pediatric outpatient population and implications for improving community pediatric care. *American Journal of Public Health* 58 (May 1968): 859-76. I. Factors: medical disorganization of low-income and uneducated group, lack of interest, residential instability, and cultural lag. II. Primary: 3,058 Los Angeles pediatric emergency room patients were interviewed. III. Improve public transportation; provide comprehensive and preventive medical services immediately in Emergency Room; give followup services in Emergency Room; use more auxiliary personnel; and design health literature for specific audiences.

Wingert, W. A., et al. Why Johnny's parents don't read: An analysis of indigent parents' comprehension of health education materials. *Clinical Pediatrics* 8 (November 1969): 655-60. I. Health pamphlets and other reading materials are written on a level beyond the comprehension of many mothers. II. Primary: mothers at a pediatric emergency room in Los Angeles were tested for reading comprehension. III. Health education materials must be written in a language comprehended by the reading clientele; a more simple approach is needed for the lower classes.

Winston, E. Health welfare partnership in programs for low-income groups. *American Journal of Public Health* 57 (July 1967): 1100-06. I. Poverty culture gives a low priority to health; there is a high acceptance of ailments, fatalism, and a distrust of doctors. III. Overcome fears by reaching out to the poor, and help deal with such practical obstacles as transportation and babysitting. V. Article describes teamwork between health and welfare officials.

Wise, H. B. Montefiore Hospital Neighborhood Medical Care Demonstration. *Milbank Memorial Fund Quarterly* 46 (July 1968): 297-307. I. Problems of communication between residents and health center. Health career professionals tend not to work in poverty areas, thereby creating a shortage of care. II. Secondary: evaluation of a health center in Southeast Bronx, New York City. III. Provide family medical care for all members at the same time and place; mobilize community interest to give medical care a higher priority; coordinate all health-related programs; use subprofessionals; and train people in low-socioeconomic communities to work directly in health program. IV. Article states specific problems dealing with training and implementation of health center objectives.

Wise, H. B., et al. (a) Community development and health education: I. Community organization as a health topic. *Milbank Memorial Fund Quarterly* 46 (July 1968): 329-39. II. Secondary: description of a successful health center by author. III. & IV. Article discusses successful operation of community health center and stresses the need to involve the community in health issues.

Wise, H. B., et al. (b) The family health worker. *American Journal of Public Health* 58 (October 1968): 1828-38. I. Many clinics utilized by the poor are organized for the convenience of the professional staff; health care lacks continuity and follow-up; and preventive medicine is often unknown. II. Primary: experiment in medical care delivery by Montefiore Hospital Neighborhood Medical Care Demonstration in the Bronx. III. Use a family health worker, trained in patient care and social-advocacy roles, to deal with populace instead of multiple case workers and counselors. IV. The lay worker, being a community member, was more accepted than the social case worker. V. Article emphasizes the consequences of simplifying health and social services.

Wolfe, S., and L. A. Falik. Effective health center (letter to the editor). *New England Journal of Medicine* 282 (March 1970): 643. III. Provide transportation and home visits for the poor. V. Failure to keep appointment does not mean disappointment. Ghetto residents are accustomed to receiving emergency care in an impersonal way, but they can learn to use the appointment system if assisted with transportation and home visits by neighborhood health workers.

Wolff, H. Disease and patterns of behavior. In *Patients, Physicians, and Illness*, ed. E. Gartly Jaco pp. 54-61. New York: The Free Press, 1958. III. Recognize the psychological components of illness as a causal factor; appreciate what actions and goals of an individual may cost in terms of disease, discomfort, and pain. V. Disease is related to attitudes, individual and group actions, goals, and conflict encountered.

Wood, E. C. Indigenous workers as health care expeditors. *Hospital Progress* 49 (September 1968): 64-68. I. A service gap exists between hospitals and the public, especially poverty groups. Hospitals make no effort to reach out to "consumers." II. Secondary: tells of health care expedition program at Mercy Hospital in Pittsburgh. III. Use of expeditors (trained residents in low-income groups) to follow up on patients who missed appointments and to reach out to the local community. V. An excellent article on the training of auxiliary personnel.

Yamamoto, J., et al. Racial factors in patient selection. *American Journal of Psychiatry* 124 (November 1967): 630-36. I. Ethnocentrism among therapists turns minority group patients away. II. Primary: study of 594 admissions to the Psychiatric Outpatient Clinic of Los Angeles County General Hospital; patients were followed for nine months. V. Object of the study was to determine if ethnicity led to differential treatment in a psychiatric clinic for the poor. The poor blacks, Chicanos, and Orientals dropped out of therapy more frequently than poor whites.

Yankauer, A., et al. An evaluation of prenatal care and its relationship to social class and social disorganization. *American Journal of Public Health* 43 (August 1953): 1001-10. I. Women of low socioeconomic groups tend to seek medical care late in pregnancy because of a greater degree of social disorganization and an outward manifestation of rejection of pregnancy. II. Primary: information collected from Rochester Community Hospitals, all maternity cases over a two-month period.

Yerby, A. S. The problem of medical care for indigent populations. *American Journal of Public Health* 55 (August 1965): 1212-16. I. Public health care is piecemeal, poorly supervised, and uncoordinated. It does not reach the needy poor who also need help in improving their environment, making it more conducive to good health. II. Secondary: a survey of infant mortality rates. III. Adequately finance services; competently supervise services; establish performance standards to govern use and payment of services; complement therapeutic care with social casework; and use preventive services.

Yerby, A. S. The disadvantaged and health care. *American Journal of Public Health* 56 (January 1966): 5-9. I. Care is inadequate, of poor quality, provided with little dignity or compassion, and rarely fulfills the total needs of the low-income family. It is basically inadequate, fragmented, underfinanced, and poorly organized. II. Secondary: author's own opinions and observations. III. Train, recruit, and retain more nurses and health personnel; build comprehensive neighborhood health centers; reorganize and refinance the whole system of medical care. V. This paper was given at the White House Conference on Health in November 1965.

Yerby, A. S., and W. L. Agress. Medical care for the indigent. *Public Health Reports* 81 (January 1966): 7-11. II. Secondary: editorial comments by the Director of Medical Care Services. III. Improve all types of care for welfare recipients; provide medical and dental care for prisoners as well as comprehensive mental care; improve medical services for the aged. IV. The results of the demonstration programs are not reported. V. A review of demonstrations and programs directed by the New York Department of Health aimed at improving welfare medical care.

Zola, I. K. Illness behavior of the working class: Implications and recommendations. In *Blue Collar World: Studies of the American Worker*, ed. Arthur B. Shostak and William Gomberg, pp. 350-61. Englewood Cliffs, New Jersey: Prentice Hall, 1964. I. People from different cultures tend to have different symptom response sets to the same illness; symptoms themselves tend to be relatively unimportant in the decision to seek medical aid; a decision to see a doctor is "triggered" by circumstances or conditions which vary from culture to culture. Triggers include interpersonal crises, social interference, presence of sanctioning, perceived threat to vocation or avocation, and the nature and quality of the symptoms. II. Primary: a list of references in which methodology is described is provided in this article. III. Acknowledge the motivational elements that lead an individual to see a doctor, and organize medical care and health education programs accordingly. Recognize qualitative differences between segments of population; make comparative studies of different sociocultural groupings.

Zola, I. K. Culture and symptoms: An analysis of patients presenting complaints. *American Sociological Review* 31 (October 1966): 615-30. I. The superficiality of medical care negatively influences the poor. Patterns of response to diseases vary with ethnic background. II. Primary: comparison of 63 Italians and 81 Irish patients admitted to a hospital in Massachusetts. III. Recognize ethnicity in patient response. V. A comparison of ethnic groups, not differing socioeconomically, in their response to respiratory disease.